Tissue Augmentation in Clinical Practice

BASIC AND CLINICAL DERMATOLOGY

Series Editors
ALAN R. SHALITA, M.D.
Distinguished Teaching Professor and Chairman
Department of Dermatology
SUNY Downstate Medical Center

Brooklyn, New York
DAVID A. NORRIS, M.D.
Director of Research
Professor of Dermatology
The University of Colorado
Health Sciences Center
Denver, Colorado

Tissue Augmentation in Clinical Practice

Second Edition

edited by

Arnold W. Klein

Department of Dermatology
David Geffen School of Medicine
University of California
Los Angeles, California, U.S.A.

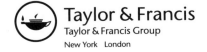

Taylor & Francis

Taylor & Francis Group

New York   London

Published in 2006 by
Taylor & Francis Group
270 Madison Avenue
New York, NY 10016

International Standard Book Number-10: 0-8247-5456-5 (Hardcover)
International Standard Book Number-13: 978-0-8247-5456-3 (Hardcover)
Library of Congress Card Number 2005052959

This book contains information obtained from authentic and highly regarded sources. Reprinted material is quoted with permission, and sources are indicated. A wide variety of references are listed. Reasonable efforts have been made to publish reliable data and information, but the author and the publisher cannot assume responsibility for the validity of all materials or for the consequences of their use.

Library of Congress Cataloging-in-Publication Data

Tissue augmentation in clinical practice / edited by Arnold Klein.-- 2nd ed.
    p. ; cm. -- (Basic and clinical dermatology ; 36)
  Includes bibliographical references and index.
  ISBN-13: 978-0-8247-5456-3 (alk. paper)
  ISBN-10: 0-8247-5456-5 (alk. paper)
  1. Tissue expansion. 2. Surgery, Plastic. 3. Biomedical materials. 4. Dermatology. I. Klein, Arnold William. II. Series.
  [DNLM: 1. Tissue Expansion. 2. Biocompatible Materials. 3. Dermatologic Agents. 4. Prostheses and Implants. 5. Surgery, Plastic--methods. WO 640 T616 2005]

RD119.5.T57T566 2005
617.9'5--dc22   2005052959

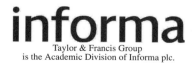
Taylor & Francis Group
is the Academic Division of Informa plc.

Visit the Taylor & Francis Web site at
http://www.taylorandfrancis.com

To Rabbi David Klein, my father, who taught me to be a scholar,

To Dr. Albert Kligman, who taught me to think, read, and be better than I could possibly be, and

To Dr. Joel Shulman, who showed me that you don't have to be famous to be a great doctor.

Series Introduction

During the past 25 years, there has been a vast explosion in new information relating to the art and science of dermatology as well as fundamental cutaneous biology. Furthermore, this information is no longer of interest only to the small but growing specialty of dermatology. Clinicians and scientists from a wide variety of disciplines have come to recognize both the importance of skin in fundamental biological processes and the broad implications of understanding the pathogenesis of skin disease. As a result, there is now a multidisciplinary and worldwide interest in the progress of dermatology.

With these factors in mind, we have undertaken this series of books specifically oriented to dermatology. The scope of the series is purposely broad, with books ranging from pure basic science to practical, applied clinical dermatology. Thus, while there is something for everyone, all volumes in the series will ultimately prove to be valuable additions to the dermatologist's library.

The latest addition to the series, volume 36, edited by Dr. Arnold W. Klein, is both timely and pertinent. The editor is a well-respected authority in cosmetic dermatology and tissue augmentation. We trust that this volume will be of broad interest to scientists and clinicians alike.

Alan R. Shalita
Distinguished Teaching Professor and Chairman
Department of Dermatology
SUNY Downstate Medical Center
Brooklyn, New York, U.S.A.

Foreword

It is with great pleasure that I write to introduce the second edition of *Tissue Augmentation in Clinical Practice* edited by my friend and colleague Dr. Arnold W. Klein. In the late 1970s, Dr. Klein and I, along with my late associates, Dr. Samuel J. Stegman and Theodore A. Tromovitch, were four of the original 14 investigators for Collagen Corporation to study a new medical injectable device, solubilized bovine collagen, developed originally at Stanford University by Rodney Perkins, M.D. (Otolaryngology), John Daniels, M.D. (Internal Medicine), Edward Luck (Medical Student), and Terrence Knapp, M.D. (Plastic Surgery). Because of the desire to limit the scope of the original trials, all investigators and patients in the original trials were within California.

My first introduction to Arnie was through Sam Stegman when Arnie came to our offices to film injection techniques with Sam. They were both at the right place at the right time. Sam was a master dermatologic surgeon who excelled at dermabrasion and deep chemical peeling and had incorporated Norman Orentreich's techniques of micro droplet silicone injection for acne scars into our practice. But the rumblings of discontent over the breast implants were already stirring, and both he and Arnie were uncomfortable with the injectable silicone and its lack of identifiable manufacturer and governmental approval. They both immediately embraced the new injectable filler substance as something that could fill a definite need. Sam pursued scar remediation and the nasolabial fold, as he had already identified and toyed with sleep lines and lines of repetitive expression in the face. Arnie rapidly taught himself the mastery of the wrinkle and became the undisputed master of lip augmentation, fulfilling the unspoken demand for what would eventually become known as "minimally invasive technique" in the land of unending demand for appearance enhancement, Los Angeles.

But the ascendancy of injectable collagen was aided by the eventual crash and burn of silicone until the FDA essentially banned breast implants in 1993 in a collision of quack science, the plaintiff's bar, and feminist politics. There was no turning back. For 25 years, from 1977 to 2003, Zyderm® and Zyplast® reigned as the only FDA-approved inject-ables for soft-tissue augmentation in the United States. They became the experiential gold standard for soft-tissue injectables, and some would say remain the standard against which all newcomers are measured.

With Sam's passing in 1990, no one is more readily identified with injectable fillers than Dr. Arnold W. Klein. With his obsessive (and I mean obsessive) devotion to the literature, Arnie has for years kept an unswerv-ing eye on the development of the field of soft-tissue augmentation. His predictions of the tidal wave of new agents coming into the United States from abroad have come true. With characteristic Hollywood verve, he can identify "The Good, the Bad, and the Ugly" in the field of soft tissue fillers. We have spent hours on the phone discussing such minutiae as the aesthetics of upper versus lower lip vermilion, the fibroblastic response to repeated injections of fillers, the flow characteristics of an injectable filler through 30- versus 32-gauge needles, etc.

In 1998 he gathered together his colleagues who are similarly obsessed, and with his guiding hand at the helm as editor, he put together the first edition of this book. In seven years much has changed. The num-ber of injectable agents in the worldwide market has tripled. But much has also remained the same. His credo has always been "The results should be natural. You should not be able to detect what was done." Sometimes easier said than done, but he has again gathered his friends together to provide the best advice they can on the use of these marvelous agents.

It is a new world of cosmetic surgery, totally dominated by mini-mally invasive techniques, built on a tripod of therapies with stunning synergies of aesthetic effect. We are utilizing injectable fillers for volume problems, botulinum toxin for problems related to repetitive muscular expression lines, and a variety of laser and light therapies aimed at cor-recting textural and color problems related to imprudent ultraviolet light exposure. But the first of the holy trinity of therapies was and remains volume correction with injectable fillers. So here is the current state of the art. I wonder what the third edition will bring.

Richard G. Glogau
Clinical Professor of Dermatology
University of California
San Francisco, California, U.S.A.

Preface

In her great one woman show "The Search for Signs of Intelligent Life in the Universe" Lily Tomlin appears as a homeless person with a shopping cart holding a can of Campbell's soup asking the audience "is this soup or is this art—soup or art?"

As a freshman at Penn I remember the arrival of Andy Warhol, together with Edith Sedgwick, on campus. They had come to introduce his Pop Art. Joan Kron (now one of the editors of *Allure*) had staged the show and to me it was revolutionary. With his philosophy "Everything is beautiful, Pop is everything," Warhol took elements of everyday life and created art.

Later, during my undergraduate years, I would study in a tower that overlooked the Alfred Newton Richard's Medical Building designed by Louie Kahn. It was not a traditional structure but perched on cement columns hung like an alien spacecraft over the campus. Later I would get to know this mighty wizard of design. As I entered the great rotunda of Penn's School of Medicine the mighty image of the Agnew Clinic by Thomas Eakens cast its powerful gaze on me. Although medical school was not the best of times for me (I lost my Father and brother), I went to England after my third year to study drug abuse, but more importantly to see if there was a form of it where doctors were more interested in people than the disease. The singular ability of a gifted English dermatologist to diagnose a barbiturate overdose from patterns on the skin amazed me and changed my life forever. Dermatology and not psychiatry became my career goal. Yet as far apart as they seemed in those days, I now realize they are so very close together.

After an internship in Los Angeles I returned to Penn for residency. Walter B. Shelly and Albert Kligman both amazed me. It would be Kligman, the greatest mind in dermatology, who taught me to think and to read everything. Furthermore, he encouraged me not to be the best I can be, but better.

As the West beckoned, the intellectual freedom as well as the California light I had once experienced, lured me back to Los Angeles and I transferred residences to UCLA. Suddenly I found myself in a surgical subspeciality wherein they did everything but appendectomies. After I graduated as Chief Resident I opened a small 800 square foot office in Beverly Hills. Then came injectable collagen and my love affair with the syringe.

It was while making a film on collagen in the offices of the late great Stegman and Tromovitch where I met the quiet yet brilliant Richard Glogau. To this day Rick and I produce a nightly "mind meld" on the phone. Also into my life came Frank Gehry, Ed Moses, Bob Graham, Ed Rusha, Ellsworth Kelly, and John Baldesarri who revolutionized my vision of art and architecture.

We are now in 2005. I finally realize that art and medicine are profoundly similar. My passion for both is in fact a singular emotion. It is now obvious that the best of each arises from human creativity. Medicine at its best is raised to an art form and aesthetic medicine is not just ok, but as Al Capone would say, "It is the 'cherries.'" Minimally invasive aesthetic enhancement defines my existence and I am honored to be part of this revolution. Life is not simple; I have survived the BOTOX® lawsuit, my nurse's marriage, and all those who imitate me. Just remember that integrity and passion are the critical aspects of a physician, and never believe something simply because it has been written down by others.

Arnold W. Klein

Contents

Contributors

Leslie S. Baumann Division of Cosmetic Dermatology, Department of Dermatology and Cutaneous Surgery, University of Miami School of Medicine, Miami, Florida, U.S.A.

Frederick C. Beddingfield, III Division of Dermatology, Department of Medicine, David Geffen School of Medicine, University of California, Los Angeles, California, and Dermatology Research and Development, Allergan, Inc., Irvine, California, U.S.A.

Andres Boker Department of Dermatology, University of Miami School of Medicine, Miami, Florida, U.S.A.

Fredric S. Brandt Department of Dermatology, University of Miami School of Medicine, Miami, Florida, U.S.A.

Alastair Carruthers Division of Dermatology, University of British Columbia, Vancouver, British Columbia, Canada

Jean Carruthers Department of Ophthalmology, University of British Columbia, Vancouver, British Columbia, Canada

David M. Duffy Department of Dermatology, University of Southern California, Los Angeles, California, and Department of Dermatology, University of California, Los Angeles, California, U.S.A.

Melvin L. Elson Cosmeceutical Concepts International, Inc., Nashville, Tennessee, U.S.A.

Ellen Gendler Ronald O. Perelman Department of Dermatology, New York University Medical Center, New York, New York, U.S.A.

Richard G. Glogau University of California, San Francisco, California, U.S.A.

Carolyn I. Jacob   Chicago Cosmetic Surgery and Dermatology, and Department of Dermatology, Northwestern Medical School, Chicago, Illinois, U.S.A.

Derek H. Jones   Department of Dermatology/Medicine, University of California, Los Angeles, California, U.S.A.

Michael S. Kaminer   SkinCare Physicians of Chestnut Hill, Chestnut Hill, Massachusetts; Department of Medicine, Dartmouth Medical School, Dartmouth College, Hanover, New Hampshire; and Department of Dermatology, Yale School of Medicine, Yale University, New Haven, Connecticut, U.S.A.

Arnold W. Klein   Department of Dermatology, David Geffen School of Medicine, University of California, Los Angeles, California, U.S.A.

Gary P. Lask   David Geffen School of Medicine, Dermatologic Surgery and Laser Center, University of California, Los Angeles, California, U.S.A.

Gottfried Lemperle   Division of Plastic Surgery, University of California, San Diego, California, U.S.A.

Anna-Sophia Leone   Orentreich Medical Group, LLP, New York, New York, U.S.A.

Corey S. Maas   Division of Facial Plastic Surgery, Department of Otolaryngology–Head and Neck Surgery, University of California, San Francisco, California, U.S.A.

Rhoda S. Narins   Department of Dermatology, New York University Medical Center, New York, New York, and Dermatology Surgery and Laser Center, New York, New York, U.S.A.

David S. Orentreich   Orentreich Medical Group, LLP, New York, New York, U.S.A.

David Charles Rish   Los Angeles Medical Center, University of California, Los Angeles, California, U.S.A.

Teresa T. Soriano   David Geffen School of Medicine, Dermatologic Surgery and Laser Center, University of California, Los Angeles, California, U.S.A.

Howard D. Stupak   Division of Facial Plastic Surgery, Department of Otolaryngology–Head and Neck Surgery, University of California, San Francisco, California, U.S.A.

James M. Swinehart   Colorado Dermatology Center, Denver, Colorado, U.S.A.

Joshua A. Tournas   Irvine Department of Dermatology, University of California, Los Angeles, California, U.S.A.

Justin J. Vujevich   Department of Dermatology and Cutaneous Surgery, University of Miami School of Medicine, Miami, Florida, U.S.A.

1

Fat Transfer with Fresh and Frozen Fat, Microlipoinjection, and Lipocytic Dermal Augmentation

Rhoda S. Narins
Department of Dermatology, New York University Medical Center,
New York, New York, and Dermatology and Laser Center,
New York, New York, U.S.A.

Fat transfer or microlipoinjection of autologous fat is a safe, effective method for correcting contour defects that result from aging, trauma, surgery, and various atrophic diseases. Most people have an unlimited source of fat from tissues available for transfer to other areas. The technique for harvesting fat from the donor site and reinjecting it into recipient sites is easily done and easily taught. There is no significant morbidity, and there are no significant complications.

HISTORY

Injectable fat is the oldest material used for tissue augmentation (1–7, 9,14,15,30). More than 100 years ago, Nueber, in Germany, reported on results of small adipose grafts transplanted from the arm for reconstruction of a soft tissue defect on the face (1). In the twentieth century, free fat grafts were used for tissue augmentation until the technique was replaced by the use of pedicle flaps and then the subsequent use of paraffin or silicone as filling agents. In 1911, Brunnin was the first to inject autologous fat into subcutaneous tissue. His grafts showed absorption and this technique did not catch on. Peer, in the late 1950s, utilized free fat grafts and reported that 50% of their volume dissipated after transplantation and, therefore, many individuals questioned their efficacy.

With the advent of liposuction surgery, the technique of microlipoinjection took on new life (8,11,13,16,17,24,34,40). Dr. Yves-Gerard Illouz first reported reinjecting viable fat that had been obtained during liposuction surgery (8,9) to correct body-contour defects some patients had had after having liposuction performed by other surgeons. He published his findings in 1985 in France and in 1986 in the United States (8).

1

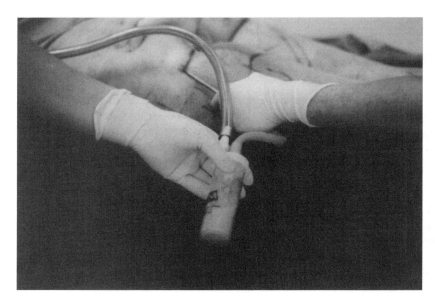

Figure 1
Fat collected during liposuction.

In 1986, at the annual meeting of the American Society for Dermatologic Surgery, Dr. Pierre Fournier presented his technique of syringe extraction of fat and reinjection (37,39).

Today, fat is usually harvested by hand using the syringe technique or, rarely, with a collecting system during liposuction surgery (Fig. 1). I always harvest by hand and the technique I use is adapted from that described by Coleman (49), who stressed the use of small aliquots of fat injected with a blunt cannula at multiple levels in the subcutaneous tissue, muscle, etc. However, I do not overcorrect my patients and I freeze fat for later use. After harvesting and preparing the fat, some of the material is injected into the recipient site and the rest is kept in a freezer dedicated to fat storage for up to two years when subsequent injections are necessary. This makes it easier for patients because they do not need to have the material harvested each time they have fat injected. Fat can be used to correct folds, wrinkles, depressions, and scars and can even be used to achieve a mini–face-lift, especially when combined with liposuction of the face, neck, and jowls.

CONSULTATION: PATIENT SELECTION

When performing any cosmetic procedure, it is important that the patient understands the parameters of what can be achieved. Thus, selecting a patient who is realistic and likely to be happy with the results of the procedure is one of the main goals of consultation. Sometimes, the use of autologous fat for tissue augmentation is used as an adjunct to other procedures to get the best result. These procedures include face-lifts, resurfacing with chemical peels, dermabrasion, nonablative lasers or the CO_2 laser, injections of BOTOX®, liposuction of the face, neck, jowls, etc. At the initial consultation, the procedure itself, as well as any possible complications, should be discussed with the patient. Autologous fat transfer is not a totally predictable technique, but this problem has largely disappeared because of our ability to freeze additional fat for future use. There are also those patients who would benefit from the use of autologous fat injections but who do not have enough fat on their bodies for this procedure. Usually, these patients have thin faces and submalar atrophy, and need large quantities of fat to correct these defects. They are best helped by the use of other filling substances. Sometimes fat can be harvested from multiple sites even in these patients but there may not be enough fat to freeze. If this is possible, the results from filling up the hollows in cheeks are remarkable and usually permanent. Fat may be the best answer for some patients who are allergic to collagen and the only answer for those patients who need a large amount of filling substance for correction, those who want a mini–face-lift with fat, or those who would like more permanent results than that possible with collagen.

INDICATIONS

Transplanted fat tissue seems to last longest in those areas with the least movement (Table 1). Most surgeons see longer and often permanent improvement in the buccal fat hollows as opposed to the nasolabial lines (38). When fat is used to enhance the zygoma and the lateral mandible, as well as the submalar cheek hollows, the cheek flap is pulled up, making the nasolabial and puppet lines less deep.

Table 1
Indications For Autologous Fat

Face	Nonfacial areas
Nasolabial folds	Rejuvenation of hands
Commissures of the mouth	Body contour defects
"Puppet lines"	Depressions caused by liposuction
Under eye hollow and tear trough	or trauma
Submalar depressions	Breast enlargement
Lip augmentation	
Chin augmentation	
Malar augmentation	
Congenital or traumatic defects	
Surgical defects	
Wide based acne scarring	
Idiopathic lipodystrophy	
Facial hemiatrophy	

Face

There are many areas on the face where autologous fat can be used. These include the nasolabial folds (Figs. 2 and 3), the commissures of the mouth and "puppet lines," submalar depressions (Figs. 4 and 5), lip augmentation, chin augmentation, malar augmentation, zygoma enhancement, ear lobe augmentation, congenital or traumatic defects, surgical defects (Figs. 6 and 7), wide-based acne scarring, idiopathic lipodystrophy, under eye hollow and tear trough, and facial hemiatrophy (31,32,43,44).

Autologous fat has also been used in nonfacial areas for rejuvenation of the hands (Figs. 8 and 9) (45) for body-contour defects, as well as for depressions caused by liposuction or trauma. Less commonly, it has been used for breast enlargement (35).

Nonfacial Areas

Fat has a soft consistency and is easily injected into areas of the face, resulting in a completely natural look (16,26,28).

Fat is the obvious tissue to correct small or large defects after liposuction surgery and to correct body-contour defects such as trochanteric depressions; this can be done at the time of surgery (27). If there is scarring, sometimes subcision must be done before the fat transfer to lift the skin off the underlying muscle to which it has adhered.

Fat can also be used for breast augmentation but further studies are necessary to standardize the procedure and to understand long-term results. Calcifications, similar to those that occur with other types of breast surgery, are caused. Although radiologists say that these are not to be confused with malignant calcifications, more studies need to be done. Microlipoinjection of autologous fat is also used to camouflage the skeleton-like appearance of the hands that occurs with sun damage and aging. Even though the overlying skin does not change after the procedure, the hand itself is given a more youthful plumper appearance. Intense pulsed light treatments, chemical peels, and lasers can be combined with fat transfer to enhance the appearance of the skin.

PREOPERATIVE CONSIDERATIONS

Preoperative Instructions

The patient is advised to wear comfortable clothing to the office. Patients take a wide-spectrum antibiotic for a period of five days, beginning the morning of surgery. They are advised to avoid aspirin, aspirin-containing compounds, vitamin E more than 200 units, and nonsteroidal anti-inflammatory agents for two weeks prior to surgery, even if only reinjection is being done.

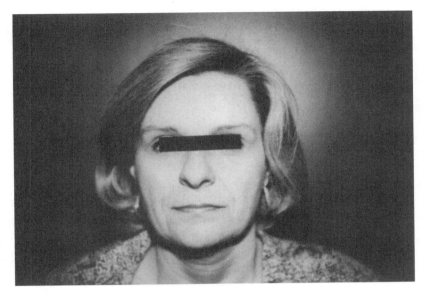

Figure 2
Preoperative nasolabial lines.

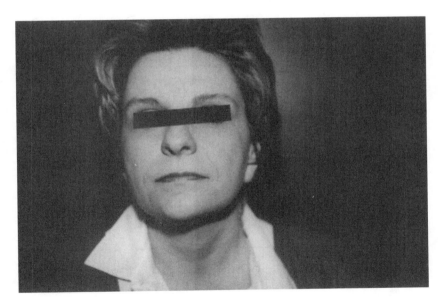

Figure 3
Four-week postoperative nasolabial lines.

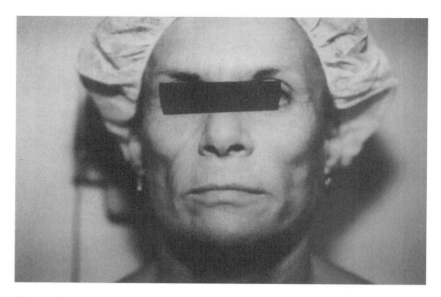

Figure 4
Preoperative cheek submalar depression under eye hollows.

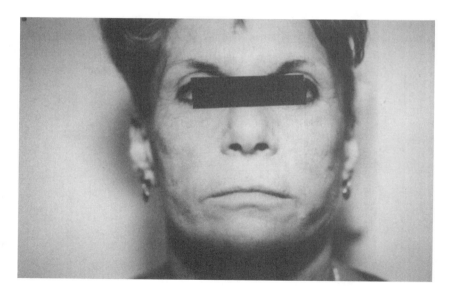

Figure 5
Postoperative submalar depression under eye hollows.

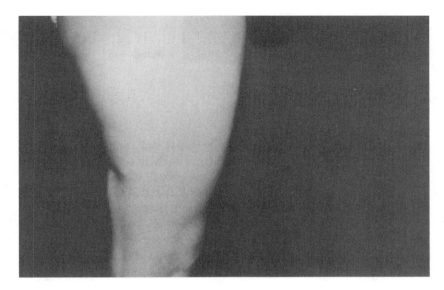

Figure 6
Preoperative photo showing trauma from previous surgery.

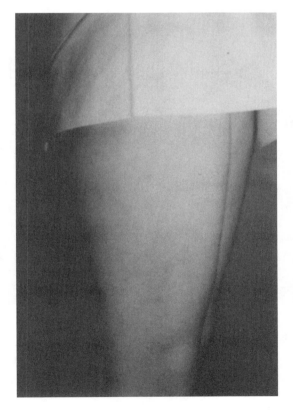

Figure 7
Postoperative photo showing results of postsurgery trauma correction.

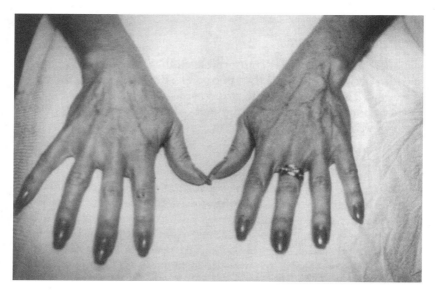

Figure 8
Preoperative hands.

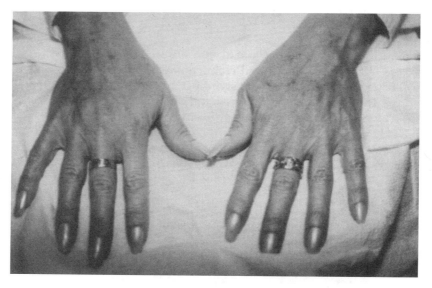

Figure 9
Hands two months postoperative.

Donor Sites

Sometimes the surgeon has no choice but to take fat from whatever donor site is available. Some patients have no donor site. Sometimes, to get enough, fat must be harvested from multiple sites. These problems occur in thin patients with little body fat. In most people, the abdomen, buttocks, hips, lateral thighs, inner thighs, knees, or flanks can be used for harvesting. Pinski and Roenigk reported that adipose tissue from the thigh lasted longer than that from the buttock or abdomen (46). Katz prefers the buttock for donor fat, while Scarborough and colleagues prefer the fat from the medial knee. Most physicians feel that harvesting fat by syringe is preferable to harvesting via liposuction procedures because of damage to fat from high negative suction pressure.

Day of Surgery

Care is taken to make sure that the patient has complied with all preoperative instructions. Photographs are taken of the donor and recipient areas, and the donor and recipient areas are marked while the patient is standing. Circles should not be drawn around the entire donor area because these marks last longer than any possible problem with the donor area and are cosmetically unacceptable to the patient. A dot is sufficient marking in the donor area. All questions should be answered, and the risks, benefits, and options reviewed again with the patient. The consent form is then signed and witnessed.

TECHNIQUE

Equipment

Very little equipment is necessary for this surgery. A sterile tray with several 10-cc syringes, a female-to-female Luer-lock adapter (Fig. 10), a test tube rack for the syringes to stand in, various needles including 30-gauge 0.5 inch

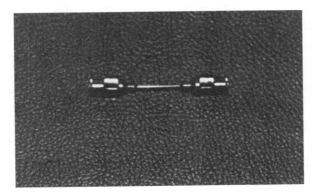

Figure 10
Female-to-female adapter.

Table 2
Tumescent Solution (TS) for Smaller Areas

	250 cc	Normal saline	0.09%
	25 cc	Lidocaine	1%
	1/4 cc	Epinephrine	1/1000
	4 cc	Bicarbonate	8.4%
Total	250 mg	Lidocaine = 1/1 million epinephrine	0.1%

and 16, 18, 22-gauge spinal needles, Coleman® extraction and injection cannulas, red syringe caps, and gauze pads. Some setup for administration of local anesthesia is necessary, which should include tumescent solution, spinal needles, and a pressure pump with IV tubing or 10-cc syringes.

Preoperative Preparation and Anesthesia

The recipient and donor sites are prepped with Betadine®, and the patient is placed on the surgical table (Table 2). A small amount of tumescent anesthetic is injected with a 30-gauge 0.5-inch needle using a 3-cc syringe in the "incision" area of the donor site (Fig. 11). Tumescent anesthesia is injected radially through this incision site using either 10-cc syringes (Fig. 12) and a spinal needle, or the Klein® pump (very low setting) and IV tubing with an 18- or 20-gauge spinal needle.

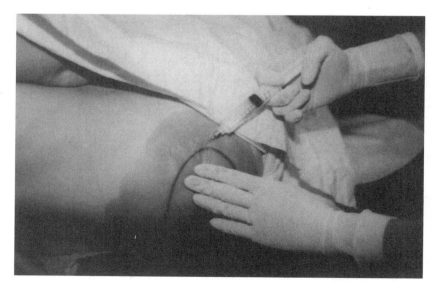

Figure 11
Donor area.

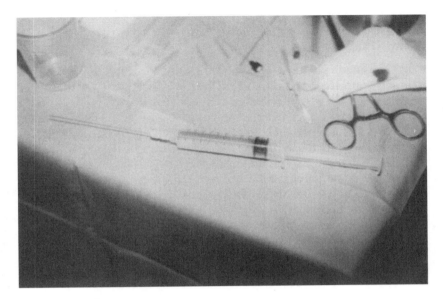

Figure 12
Syringe with anesthetic solution.

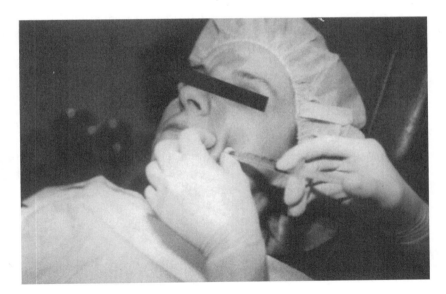

Figure 13
Preoperative injection of anesthetic along nasolabial lines.

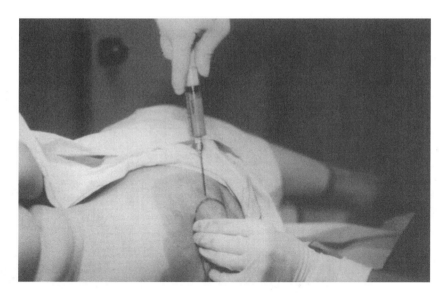

Figure 14
Harvesting fat.

Recipient Site

The incision sites of the recipient areas are injected using a 30-gauge 0.5-inch needle and a 3-cc syringe (Fig. 13). A tiny amount of tumescent anesthetic is delivered radially into the reinjection area using a 30-gauge 1-inch needle or, if the area is large, a 22-gauge spinal needle. In this area, very little anesthesia is needed and should be delivered under barely any pressure using a syringe so that there is no distortion of the tissue. This slight anesthesia of the recipient area makes reinjection much more comfortable for the patient. Tiny needles are necessary to minimize the risk of bleeding, especially in fat that is very vascular. When augmenting the nasolabial fold and the commissures of the mouth, lips, puppet lines, and cheeks, one reinjection site can be used on each side just lateral to the lips. If the chin or area anterior to the jowls is being enhanced, two incision sites are used and the fat is injected at multiple levels from both incision sites.

HARVESTING THE FAT

Syringe Harvesting

An incision is made with a 16-gauge needle used as an awl or a 16-gauge NoK® or needle currently in frequent use. No mark is left from this incision and no suture is necessary. Through this opening, a Coleman extractor attached to a 10-cc syringe can be inserted and used to harvest the fat (Fig. 14). Negative pressure is obtained in the syringe by pulling out the plunger and holding it in that position while the syringe is moved

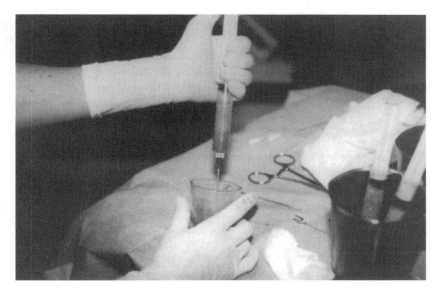

Figure 15
Syringe with fat and some blood. The infranate can easily be expelled by a push of the plunger.

back and forth in the subcutaneous tissue. Fat and fluid fill the syringe, which is then placed in the container with the plunger up; the fluid can then settle to the bottom and the fat can rise to the top. This procedure can be repeated with as many syringes and donor sites as are necessary. The negative pressure on the plunger should be small; when it is pulled back 0.5 to 1 cc, the fat comes out easily.

The fluid infranate collects at the bottom of the syringe (Fig. 15) and is easily expelled by a push of the plunger. A cap is put on the tip of the syringe and the plunger is removed before centrifuging for one to two minutes. The lock on the tip is removed and any remaining infranate drained; the oily supranate is then poured off and any remaining supranate removed with sterile gauze. The plunger is replaced and the fat can then be used for transplantation (Fig. 16). The fat appears yellow and clean. The fat that will be used at the time of harvesting is transferred into 1-cc Luer-lock syringes through a female-to-female adaptor. The rest of the fat is frozen in the 10-cc syringes with the syringes capped. The patient's name, social security number, and the date are carefully placed on each syringe to be saved and all placed in the same container, which is also labeled with the patient's name and the date. This container is then put in the freezer in alphabetical order.

Liposuction Harvesting

Fat is harvested by hand as described above and then the liposuction is done. Fat for harvesting is not obtained using the liposuction aspirator because of the high pressure involved.

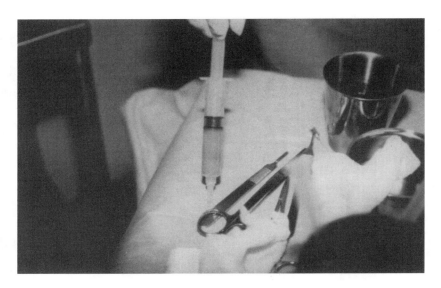

Figure 16
Syringe of fat.

REINJECTING FAT

Fresh Fat

The fat is reinjected through an incision with an 18-gauge NoKor needle using a 1-cc Luer-lock syringe attached to a Coleman injection cannula using one or two reinjection sites per area. This is to prevent extrusion of the fat through multiple openings. The cannula is inserted to the farthest point, and a tiny aliquot of fat is injected as the syringe is pulled out. This is done at multiple levels of the skin and subcutaneous tissue.

After reinjection, the surgeon should massage the injected fat so that it fills the area smoothly (Fig. 17). When injecting, the surgeon should keep a hand on the outside of the area so that the fat remains in the desired area. Some surgeons overcorrect because some of the fat may disappear within the first few days after the procedure. I find that I do not need to overcorrect and my patients prefer this approach, as they want to go back to their normal lives as soon as possible.

When injections are done to the hands, I use one injection site on the back of each hand at the wrist and inject 5 cc of fat per hand. I then have the patient make a fist and massage the injected area to make the fat spread easily over the entire hand.

Frozen Fat

After checking with the patient the day before to confirm the scheduled treatment, the amount of fat necessary for reinjection is removed from the freezer a few hours prior to the appointment. The syringes are placed upright in a container and the tray is set up as for fresh fat. The fluid, if there

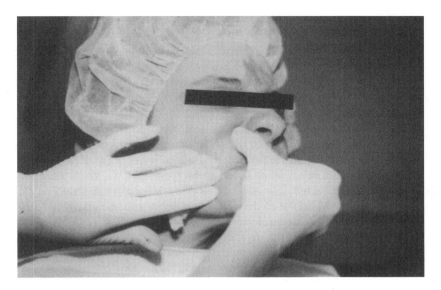

Figure 17
Massaging the injected fat.

is any, is allowed to drain off and the top 0.5 to 1 cc is not used as it is usually just triglyceride and other fatty acids. It is then pushed through a female-to-female adaptor into 1-cc Luer-lock syringes that are then attached to a Coleman injector, a blunt-tipped instrument. Local anesthesia is the same as for fresh fat. Some physicians use a sharp 18-gauge needles to reinject fat monthly, with no local anesthetic. With a blunt-tipped instrument like the Coleman injector, find that I need reinject less often; also my patients prefer local anesthesia. I also think that there is more undermining or sub-cision with the blunt-tipped instrument that adds to the results.

POSTOPERATIVE CARE AND DIRECTIONS

Recipient Site. An antibiotic ointment is placed over the injection site, and the area is iced.

Donor Site. An antibiotic ointment is placed over the harvesting site, and a piece of French tape is placed over the gauze as a pressure dressing to be kept on for 24 hours.

Two cubic centimeters of IM Celestone® is given. The patient is told to finish the antibiotic and to avoid aspirin, aspirin-containing compounds, and nonsteroidal anti-inflammatory agents for two to three days. Patients are encouraged to contact my staff or me if any untoward reactions occur, such as ecchymosis, swelling, or pain. They are advised against eating chewy foods or talking excessively on the first postoperative day. Patients are also counseled that occasional ice packs can help in minimizing any swelling.

COMPLICATIONS

Postoperative problems are very rare but include infection, hematomas, and swelling. There are known cases of blindness resulting after fat transplantation in the glabella (13); similar case was reported with collagen in that area. I prefer to use BOTOX, sometimes with Zyderm, in this area. No other problems with fat embolism have been reported. Although infections are possible, none have been reported. This is a very safe procedure. With the techniques currently in place, complications are extremely rare.

CONTROVERSIES

Campbell et al. (41) have shown that there is adipocyte viability after extraction during liposuction and reinjection. Skouge et al. followed the results in patients with syringe-extracted fat and, again, there was viable adipose tissue nine months after transplantation (12). Glogau reported a great deal of individual variation (29). Moscatello et al. (50) showed that frozen fat was not viable although most practitioners know that it works. Narins (51) has shown that frozen fat is sterile for up to two years.

Many other influencing factors are currently unknown: Is there a best donor site? Is there a difference in the recipient site based on its vascularity? Is there a way to treat the fat that can make it last longer (33)? Work still has to be done in all of these areas. Certainly we know that the more active recipient sites do not have as good a long-term result as locations of the body that do not have a lot of movement (36). Multiple treatments may result in long-term results.

Amar (42) feels that fat should be injected into muscle; his Fat autograft muscle injection (FAMI) procedure has become very popular.

LIPOCYTIC DERMAL AUGMENTATION

Lipocytic dermal augmentation is the breakdown of fat that is then processed into a less viscous form for injection into the dermis. First proposed by Pierre Fournier in Paris in the early 1980s as "autologous collagen," lipocytes are ruptured and the triglyceride contents are removed, and the remaining cell walls are used as a fibrous tissue filler for correction of dermal abnormalities (37,39). When combined with fat transfer, lipocytic dermal augmentation provides a two-layered approach to improve wrinkles and scars (47).

Coleman et al. (48) theorized in *The Journal of Dermatologic Surgery* in 1993 that the improvement from lipocytic dermal augmentation was due to an initial inflammatory response that led to the formation of fibrous tissue and collagen at the injection site. They interpreted that there was more stimulation of collagen, than injection of collagen, so they changed the name from "autologous collagen" to "lipocytic dermal augmentation."

The technique consists of harvesting the fat in the usual manner. After the infranate is discarded, 2 cc of fat is transferred into a 3-cc syringe with 1 cc of sterile water, which is a hypotonic solution. These syringes are capped and flash frozen in liquid nitrogen and immediately thawed in warm tap water. After standing upright for a few minutes, the infranate is again discarded. The syringes are then centrifuged for one minute at 1000 RPM to further separate the ruptured cell walls from the free triglyceride. The material can be injected after transfer to 1-cc Luer-lock syringes. A 23- to 25-gauge needle is necessary to get the fat through. Some physicians dilute the fat with saline to get it through a 30-gauge needle. Small amounts of anesthetic may be needed as a block, so the physician must carefully plan how much fat will be used prior to injecting the anesthetic.

Fat for lipocytic dermal augmentation can be frozen for later use after the initial freeze in liquid nitrogen and the same steps followed after defrosting. This procedure is often combined with fat transfer for a two-layered approach.

SUMMARY

Autologous fat transplantation provides cosmetically significant correction for many filling defects. It is relatively easy to perform and results in very few complications (13). It is a safe and effective procedure. Small amounts of fat can be injected to obtain a mini–face-lift. Autologous fat transplantation is a tool that should be in the armamentarium of every dermatologic surgeon.

REFERENCES

1. Neuber F. Fat transplantation. Chir Kongr Verhandl Dsch Gesellsch Chir 1893; 22:66.
2. Neuhof H. The Transplantation of Tissues. New York: Appleton & Company, 1923.
3. Barnes HO. Augmentation mammoplasty by Iipotransplant. Plast Reconstr Surg 1953; 11:404.
4. Peer LA. Loss of weight and volume in human fat grafts with postulation of "cell survival theory." Plast Reconstr Surg 1950; 5:217.
5. Boering G, Huffstadt AJ. The use of derma-fat grafts in the face. Br J Plast Surg 1968; 20(2):172.
6. Roy JN. War surgery: plastic operations on the face by means of fat grafts. Laryngoscope 1921; 31:65.
7. Stevenson TW. Fat grafts to the face. Plast Reconstr Surg 1949; 4:58.
8. Illouz YG. The fat cell "graft": a new technique to fill depressions. Plast Reconstr Surg 1986; 78:122.
9. Peer LA. The neglected "free fat graft," its behavior and clinical use. Am J Surg 1956; 92:40.
10. Peer LA, Paddock R. Histologic studies on the fate of deeply implanted dermal grafts. Observations on sections of implant buried from one week to one year. Arch Surg 1037; 34:268.
11. Wetmore SJ. Injection of fat for soft tissue augmentation. Laryngoscope 1980; 90:50.
12. Skouge JW, Canning DA, Jefs RD. Long term survival of perivesical fat harvested and injected by microlipo injection techniques in a rabbit model. 16th Annual American Society for Dermatologic Surgery Meeting, Fort Lauderdale, FL, March 1989.
13. TeimourinB. Blindness following fat injections (Letter to the editor). Plast Reconstr Surg 1988; 82(2):361.
14. Katocs AS, Largis EE, Allen DO. Perfused fat cells: effects of lipolytic agents. J Biol Chem 1973; 248(14):5089–5094.
15. Sidman RL. The direct effect of insulin on organ cultures of brown fat. Anat Rec 1956; 124:723.
16. Illouz YG. Present results of fat injection. Aesth Plast Surg 1988; 12:175.
17. Gormley DE, Eremia S. Quantitive assesment of augmentation therapy. J Dermatol Surg Oncol 1990; 16:1147.
18. Horl HW, Feller AM, Biemer E. Technique for liposuction fat reimplantation and long-term volume evaluation by magnetic resonance imaging. Ann Plast Surg 1991; 26:248.
19. Billings E Jr, May JW Jr. Historical review and present status of free graft autotransplantation in plastic and reconstructive surgery. Plast Reconstr Surg 1989; 83:368.
20. Chajchir A, Benzaquen I. Liposuction fat grafts in face wrinkles and hemifacial atrophy. Aesthetic Plast Surg 1986; l0:115.
21. Roenigk HH, Rubenstein R. Combined scalp reduction and autologous fat implant treatment of localized soft tissue defects. J Dermatol Surg Oncol 1988; 14:67.
22. Gurney CE. Experimental study of the behavior of free transplants. Surgery (St. Louis) 1938; 3:680.
23. Johnson G. Body contouring by macroinjection of autogenous fat. Am J Cosmet Surg 1987; 4:103.
24. Agris J. Autologous fat transplantation: a 3-year study. Am J Cosmet Surg 1987; 4:111.
25. Saunders MC, Keller JT, Dunsker SB, et al. Survival of autologous fat grafts in humans and in mice. Connect Tis Res 1981; 8:81.
26. Asken S. Autologous fat transplantation: Micro and macro techniques. Am J Cosmet Surg 1987; 4:111.

27. Hudson DA, Lambert EV, Bloch CE. Site selection for autotransplantation: Some observations. Aesth Plast Surg 1990; 14:195.
28. Matsudo PKR, Toledo LS. Experience of injected fat grafting. Aesth Plast Surg 1988; 12:35.
29. Glogau RG. Microlipoinjection. Arch Dermatol 1988; 124:1340.
30. Gurney CE. Studies on the fate of free transplants of fat. Proc Staff Meet Mayo Clin 1937; 12:317.
31. Lisman RD, Smith BC, Nassid J. Current concepts in dermis-fat graftins. Int Ophthalmol Surg Oncol 1990; 16:12.
32. Roenigk H Jr, Rubenstein R. Combined scalp reduction and autologous fat implant treatment of localized soft tissue defects. J Dermatol Surg Oncol 1988; 14:1.
33. Nguyen A, Pasyk KA, Bouvier TN, Hassett CA, Argenta LC. Comparative study of survival of autologous adipose tissue taken and transplanted by different techniques. Plast Reconst Surg 1986; 78:122.
34. Smahel J. Adipose tissue in plastic surgery. Ann Plast Aurg 1986; 16:444–453.
35. Barnes HO. Augmentation mammoplasty by lipotransplant. Plast Reconstr Surg 1953; 11:404.
36. Hiragun A, Sato M, Mitsui H. Preadipocyte differentiation in vitro: Identification of a highly active adipogenic agent. J Cell Physiol 1988; 1345:124–130.
37. Fournier PF. Facial recontouring with fat grafting. Dermatol Clin 1990; 8:523.
38. Chajchin A, Benzaques I. Fat grafting injection for soft tissue augmentation. Plast Reconstr Surg 1989; 84:921–934.
39. Fournier PF. In: Collagen Autologue: Liposculpture Ma Technique. Paris: Arnette, 1989:277–279.
40. Zocchi M. Methode de production de collagene autologue par traitement du tissue grasseaux. J Med Esthet Chirur Dermatol 1990; 17, 66:105.
41. Campbell GL, Laudslager N, Newman J. The effect of mechanical stress on adipocyte morphology and metabolism. Am J Cosmet Surg 1987; 4:89–94.
42. Amar RE. Microinfiltration adipocytaire (MIA) au niveau de la face, ou restructuration tissulaire par greffe de tissu adipeux. Ann Chir Plast Esthet 1999; 44(6):593–608.
43. Afifi AK, Bergman RA, Zaynoun ST, Bahuth NB, Kraydieh M. Partial (localized) lipodystrophy. J Am Acad Dermatol 1985; 12:199.
44. Moscona R, Ullman Y, Har-Shai Y, Hirshowitz B. Fat free injections for the correction of hemifacial atrophy. Plast Reconstr Surg 1989; 84:501–507.
45. Lauber JS, Abrams H, Coleman III WP. Application of the tumescent technique to hand augmentation. J Dermatol Surg Oncol 1990; 16:369–373.
46. Pinski KS, Roenigk HH. Autologous fat transplantation: long term follow-up. J Dermatol Surg Oncol 1992; 18:179–184.
47. Coleman WP III. Lipocytic dermal augmentation. In: Klein WA, ed. Tissue Augmentation in Clinical Practice. New York: Marcel Dekker, 1998:49–62.
48. Coleman WP III, Lawrence N, Sherman RN, Reed RJ, Pinski KS. Autologous collagen. Lipocytic dermal augmentation: a histopathologic study. J Dermatol Surg Oncol 1993; 19:1032–1040.
49. Coleman SR. Facial recontouring with lipostructure. Clin Plast Surg 1997; 24(2):347–367.
50. Moscatello DK, Dougherty M, Narins R, Lawrence N. Cryopreservation of human fat for soft tissue augmentation: viability requires use of cryoprotectant and controlled freezing and storage. Dermatolog Surg (Fall 2005). In Press.
51. Narins RS. Long term sterility of fat frozen for up to 24 months. Drugs Dermatol 2003; 2(5):505–507.

2
Dermal Grafting

James M. Swinehart
Colorado Dermatology Center, Denver, Colorado, U.S.A.

Is it possible to identify a soft tissue augmentation substance that is autologous, readily accessible, available in solid graft form, easily inserted in an accurate manner, offers permanent correction of contour defects, with a minimum of side effects and without risk of allergy or rejection? Dermal grafting, properly performed, can offer all of these advantages (Table 1). This minor surgical procedure, although employed by various specialties for more than six decades, is surprisingly underutilized by cosmetic surgeons. It is hoped that this chapter will stimulate the practicing surgeon to revisit and to perfect this versatile technique.

BACKGROUND AND RATIONALE

"Dermal grafting" may be defined as the insertion and implantation of appropriately sized, dissected, and contoured solid segments of deep dermis and attached fibrous fat into correspondingly sized recipient sites under depressed scars, facial lines, or other soft tissue contour defects, in order to provide long-term elevation and correction of these defects.

Dermal grafts or derma-fat grafts have been in use for at least 60 years (1). In earlier years, surgeons focused on their use in ophthalmology. For example, large dermal grafts, taken from the abdomen, have been utilized to fill the postenucleation orbital defect prior to the fitting of a (flat) glass eye. Ophthalmic surgeons have inserted dermal grafts into the orbital region following "blow out fractures" and other contour defects (2–4). Fat grafting has been described for therapy of vocal cord paralysis (5). Maxillofacial surgeons, utilizing buccal fat pad grafts, have been able to correct intraoral defects (6). Neurosurgeons have implanted dermis–fat grafts following lumbar spinal decompression (7). Similarly, cosmetic surgeons have, for many years, sought to correct facial contour defects with grafts of fat, dermis, or both (8,9,12–14). Fournier has expertly utilized postblepharoplasty fat pads and dermal grafts

Table 1
Properties of an Ideal Filler Substance

Ready availability
Lack of rejection (autologous substance)
Nonallergenic and nonirritating
Permanent correction in unaltered state
Low cost
Accurate placement
Implanted by a single, simple maneuver
Office procedure

remaining after face-lift surgery, for simultaneous implantation into other facial areas (10). In earlier years, previous problems noted included epidermal inclusion cyst formation following implantation of attached epithelium, inflammation, and unpredictable "take" or behavior (8,9). These, and other potential problems, may be largely prevented by new methods of donor and recipient site preparation, graft harvesting and dissection, and proper patient selection. These methods are fully described in this chapter.

With all the other methods and materials available for soft tissue augmentation, why do we need dermal grafting? An examination of these methods will not only answer this question but also provide the rationale for design of the ideal dermal graft.

Punch grafting, scar excision, or punch elevation can be successful in the correction of deep acne "ice pick" scars or "large pores"—but generally cannot correct scars greater than 3 to 4 mm in diameter due to the resultant scar from the excision or graft.

Depressed facial scars or lines are similar to the tufting on a sofa; the surface is held down by fibrous bands attached to deeper structures, including fascia or facial musculature. Subcision (simple scar undermining) has been shown to improve facial acne scars (11) by interruption of these fibrous bands. However, in the absence of a filler substance or "spacer," these bands may reattach, or regenerate, resulting in reappearance of the defect.

Dermabrasion, chemical peeling, and laser resurfacing can often beautifully correct finer facial lines, small- to moderate-sized rhytides, and smaller, soft acne scars. However, with broad, deep, facial defects, the dermabrasion wheel is like a "row boat in the ocean"; it floats over the larger elevations and dells, but is unable to be taken deeply enough into the peripheral elevations around the central defect without the risk of scarring. In other words, in order to correct deeper problem areas, one must not only "sand down the mountains" but also must "fill up the valleys."

With respect to other filling substances, injectable bovine collagen implant (Zyderm®, Zyplast®, Collagen Corp., Palo Alto, California, U.S.) may not be practical for the correction of larger, deeper cutaneous

Table 2
Indications for Dermal Grafting
Broad, soft, depressed, or linear acne scars
Glabellar lines or folds
Nasolabial folds
Perioral lines
Other soft, wide, distensible facial defects
–Lip augmentation
–Cellulite correction
Post-traumatic or postsurgical scars

defects because of the need for repeated injections of larger volumes, with resultant cost outlay. Silicone, banned years ago, has recently been reapproved in the United States by the Food and Drug Administration. At the time of writing, nearly three dozen substances are available, either in the United States or abroad, for soft tissue augmentation.

"Autologous collagen," described elsewhere in this text, may be utilized for soft tissue augmentation. However, because of the fact that the fat from which it is derived contains only approximately two percent of actual collagen, its actual mode of action may be to attempt to stimulate the synthesis of autologous neocollagen in the dermis. Similarly, autologous fat implantation, in liquid form, may be difficult to exactly localize into small or linear defects. Instead, it seems to stimulate the production of autologous tissue and scar formation via "lipocytic dermal augmentation"; and, because the injected fat cells may lose the race with time with respect to nourishment from existing tissues, its use often yields unpredictable correction (16–18).

Using solid fat grafts quite often results in successful augmentation of larger soft tissue defects (19–21). However, many physicians feel that a graft simultaneously containing both dermis and fat will take better and more predictably. It is theorized that this superior rate of success is due to the process of inosculation, whereby existing capillaries in the graft immediately reattach to capillaries in the adjacent recipient sites, resulting in rapid reestablishment of local circulation, and hence, graft nourishment and success (22,23).

INDICATIONS AND PATIENT SELECTION

Dermal grafting is presently indicated for the correction of relatively deep, broad, flexible, distensible soft tissue defects (Table 2). It is not as effective for finer lines or wrinkles or small, fibrotic, pitted acne scars. Acne scars that seem to respond best are those at least 4 to 5 mm in diameter. Recipient rhytides should be at least 2 to 3 mm wide, prominent, and able to accept undermining. Because of the fact that the recipient incision sites, though small, may leave a tiny scar, and because concomitant scars, lines,

| **Table 3** |
Dermal Grafting Test Areas
Perform on one to three small, but representative lesions
Insert 3-mm dermal grafts
Compare with/without prior undermining (subcision)
May combine with dermabrasion, chemical peel, or laser test spots
Evaluate for degree of correction, surface changes, and possible side effects

or other entities are usually present, the patient often must accept the need for, and consent to, a subsequent resurfacing procedure(s).

During the initial consultation, prospective patients should be educated about the possible benefits, risks, and side effects of the procedure. Before and after photographs of previous patients with similar indications may be shown. In addition, the surgeon should discuss alternative surgical techniques, filler materials, and resurfacing methods with each patient. Patient motivation, expectations, and sincerity should be evaluated as thoroughly as possible. The postoperative course (including bruising, need for repeat dermal grafting sessions, and possible need for subsequent resurfacing, with its respective healing time) must be emphasized.

In the event that the patient or physician is unsure about the successful outcome or risks of the operation, one or more test areas may be performed (Table 3) (24). One may select one or several acne scars or facial lines to evaluate the efficacy of dermal grafting alone, dermal grafting in combination with dermabrasion or resurfacing, or dermabrasion, resurfacing, or chemical peel alone. Of course, the results of one test area may not always predict the outcome of a full facial procedure, and test areas are certainly not indicated in all patients. However, the patient and physician may be able to assess healing time, pigmentary match, degree of correction, and postoperative appearance; in addition, patient anxiety, with respect to larger procedures, may be diminished. In other words, it is often helpful to have the additional knowledge gained rather than to not receive it.

Once the patient has requested dermal grafting, a preoperative visit is usually scheduled at least two weeks in advance. At this time, a detailed plan and timetable for facial rejuvenation can be discussed and solidified. This plan should include a schedule for test spots, facial undermining, dermal grafting, and dermabrasion for subsequent resurfacing. Appropriate consent and/or arbitration forms are read, explained, understood, and signed. Reproducible preoperative photographs are taken without makeup and with consistent lighting. A physical examination is usually performed. Preoperatively, the author obtained the following tests: a complete blood count, biochemical panel, urinalysis, serum pregnancy test in females, prothrombin time, partial thromboplastin time, serum HIV, and serum hepatitis B and C surface antigens. Whenever there is a question about the patient's health, a letter or release from the patient's personal physician might be obtained. Detailed pre- and postoperative instructions are provided and explained. Preoperative medications may include a cephalosporin started one day preoperatively and continued for five days, as well as Hibiclens® scrub (with eyes avoided) started two days preoperatively. Postoperative medications can include a triamcinolone or medrol dosepak for swelling, Dalmane® for sleep, and a pain reliever of choice (most postoperative discomfort is seen in the postauricular donor sites).

SURGICAL TECHNIQUES

Upon arrival at the private office procedure room, the patient is greeted by the surgical staff. The patient is then carefully photographed again in the sitting position from a variety of angles and distances, depending on the areas that will receive treatment. Utilizing a tangential light source, the scars or facial contours are delineated with a permanent marker. Different colors may be used to identify areas or defects scheduled to receive other therapy (such as punch grafting or lipoinjection). The patient is provided with a hand mirror during this extremely important marking process. The light is moved in several directions, providing the patient and physician with the opportunity to evaluate and mark all areas of concern; the patient should be in complete agreement with the procedure to follow. Photographs may again be taken of the markings.

ANESTHESIA AND ANALGESIA

If desired, preoperative sedation may be obtained with oral or sublingual diazepam, intramuscular Versed®, or oral narcotics such as Percocet®, or oral Dramamine®. In the event that preoperative sedation is used, the author maintains an intravenous line and monitors the patient with blood pressure monitor, cardiac monitor, and pulse oximetry.

The use of the ice–saline–xylocaine technique may facilitate local anesthesia (25).

For larger procedures, one can first perform supraorbital, supratrochlear, lateral zygomaticotemporal, mental, and nasal nerve blocks, as well as anesthetize the tumescent entry sites and the postauricular donor sites. Cryogel ice "pillows" are first applied to the skin to provide surface analgesia. Normal saline containing benzyl alcohol (a weak local anesthetic) is then injected over the sites to be blocked. The actual blocks can be performed with a solution containing 1% xylocaine with epinephrine 1:1,000,000 mixed 50/50 with 0.5% Marcaine®. Generally, a mixture of 10 cc of the above solutions will be necessary for facial sites, and another 5 cc for both postauricular areas should suffice. All previously marked recipient areas may also be infiltrated with tumescent solution containing xylocaine 0.1% (1 g/L), epinephrine 1:1,000,000 (1 mg/L), and sodium bicarbonate 10 to 12.6 MEq/L in normal saline. Infiltration may be expedited via a 22- to 25-gauge spinal

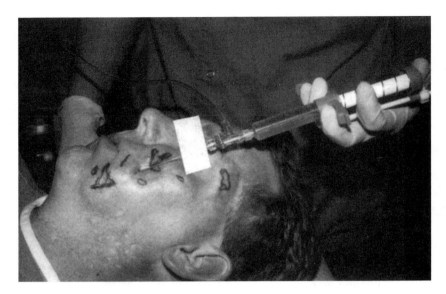

Figure 1
Infiltration of recipient areas with tumescent solution via McGhan® tissue expander fill kit.

needle on a McGhan® tissue expander fill kit attached to the solution utilized above (Fig. 1).

UNDERMINING OF FACIAL DEFECTS

Simple undermining of acne scars, without subsequent soft tissue augmentation, has been employed for many years by dermatologic surgeons for improvement of these defects. Orentreich (11) has recently described the use of this technique, called "subcision," and has achieved good results. The rationale for this maneuver is based on the concept that undermining with a small blade or large, flat needle will lead to fibrin production, stimulate the formation of new collagen, and create granulation tissue, all of which serve to augment the soft tissue defect.

However, in a number of instances, the undermined scars or rhytides will eventually reattach to the underlying fibrous bands that have been sectioned.

Therefore, it is advantageous to insert a "spacer" (i.e., a dermal graft) during the grafting operation that follows. Although a paired comparison study of undermining alone versus a pretunneling operation prior to subsequent dermal grafting has not been completed, the author feels that such an initial procedure is beneficial. Preliminary undermining can promote initial soft tissue augmentation of the scars or lines, and can generate a vascular bed of granulation tissue that is receptive to a graft inserted subsequently into the same area. Indeed, one may discover that a number of smaller scars or finer lines undermined in this way may improve to the point that dermal grafting may not be necessary. Therefore, at the initial phase, undermining of all identifiable defects is undertaken with an 18-gauge NoKor® needle (Becton, Dickinson, Cockeysville, Maryland, U.S.), with an attempt made to remain in a mid-dermal plane. One can often feel a considerable "gritty" resistance as the fibrotic bands are sectioned by the sharp end of the needle.

However, as discussed in this chapter, larger defects, including those defects remaining after subcision, generally require a dermal graft session or sessions. This grafting procedure may be performed two to six weeks after the initial undermining (Fig. 2). For this operation, similar preoperative sedation, local anesthesia, monitoring, and sterile techniques are employed.

THE DONOR AREA

One or both postauricular regions serve as excellent sources for dermal grafts. These areas are free of hair follicles and relatively free of other appendages, contain compressed fibrous fat attached to the dermis, are relatively avascular, and yield a scar hidden in the postauricular crease (similar to a face-lift scar) after closure and healing. The resultant collagen bundle formation in this scar, incidentally, can serve as an excellent source of material for subsequent dermal grafting sessions should this become necessary.

Under local anesthesia, this area is dermabraded to the level of the deeper dermis, visualizing ragged collagen bundles, with a coarse diamond fraise (Figs. 3 and 4). This level is much deeper than what one would reach with facial dermabrasion, but serves to prevent the accidental implantation of epithelium. The epidermis could be removed with a scalpel, a CO_2 or erbium laser, dermasanding, or other means, but dermabrasion offers the advantage of speed, precise depth control, and generation of a broad donor surface.

DERMAL GRAFT HARVESTING

Smaller dermal grafts (primarily for acne scars or touch-up procedures) may be harvested from one or both postauricular donor sites with circular punches (with or without subsequent harvesting of the remaining "serrated island") (Figs. 5 and 6). If larger numbers or sizes of grafts are desired, a more convenient and effective en bloc excision with a No. 15 scalpel blade is performed (Fig. 7). The latter method serves to remove all of the available, exposed donor tissue, down to the level of the retroauricular fascia if necessary, but with avoidance of the postauricular muscles (Fig. 8). This donor tissue is placed immediately into chilled

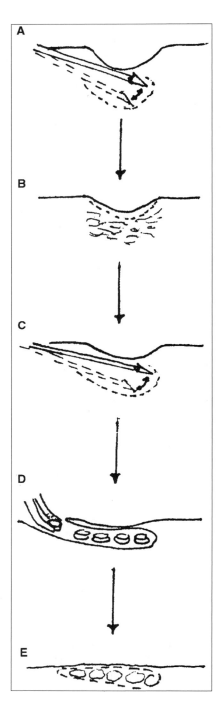

Figure 2
Pocket grafting with dermal grafts.

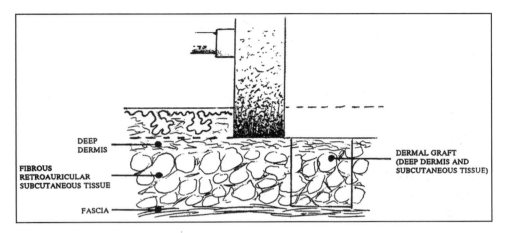

Figure 3
Dermabrasion to the level of deep dermis, removing epidermis and appendages prior to harvest of dermal grafts.

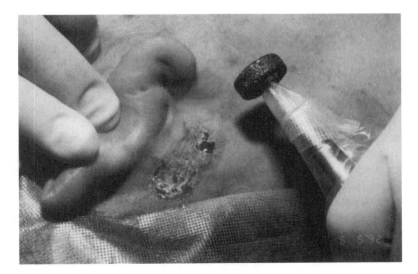

Figure 4
Postauricular dermabrasion with a coarse diamond fraise on a Bell hand engine to the level of deep dermis.

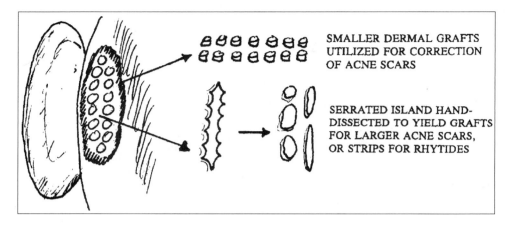

Figure 5
Dermal grafts harvested from non-hair–bearing postauricular region.

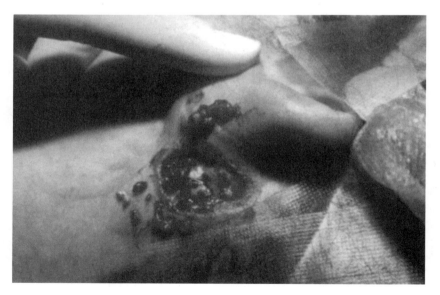

Figure 6
Excision of dermal and derma-fat grafts from the postauricular donor area.

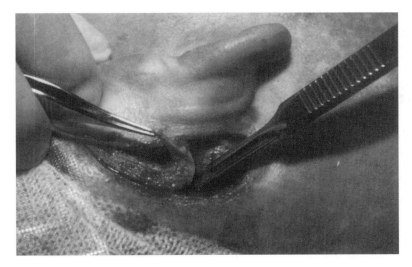

Figure 7
Excision on en bloc dermal grafts with a No. 15 blade.

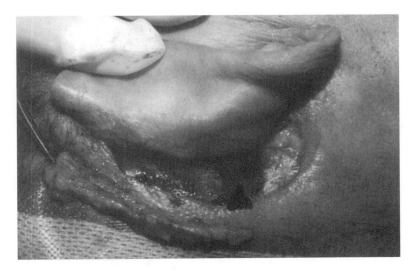

Figure 8
Excised dermal graft. Note the underlying postauricular muscle.

sterile saline. Closure of donor sites with running horizontal mattress 4/0 PDS, vicryl, or other degradable sutures everts the wound edges and obviates suture removal (Fig. 9).

DERMAL GRAFT DISSECTION

Surgical attention is then directed toward graft dissection. One of the prime advantages of the elliptical method of donor harvesting is the opportunity afforded by this large strip for precise dissection of grafts customized to fit each and every recipient site. Small 3- to 6-mm grafts work well for smaller acne scars, whereas large blocks of linear tissue can be inserted under larger scars; smaller "julienne" strips serve to correct smaller lines or glabellar folds, and long, relatively wide strips can be dissected for nasolabial folds augmentation (Fig. 10). The dissection is performed with good lighting under magnification with a sterile tongue blade and No. 10 Personna® (teflon-coated) blade in a manner similar to that used during hair transplant microdissection. The surgeon can trim away excess fat if necessary, but some should be left attached to the dermis. The dissected grafts are graded, sorted, and reinserted into chilled sterile saline while they await their ultimate fate (Fig. 11).

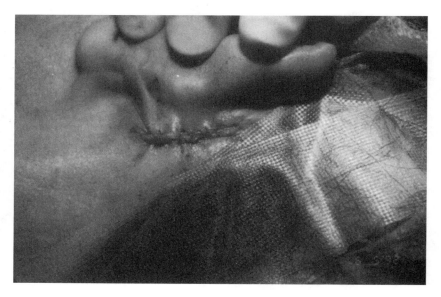

Figure 9
Closure with running 4/0 horizontal mattress degradable sutures.

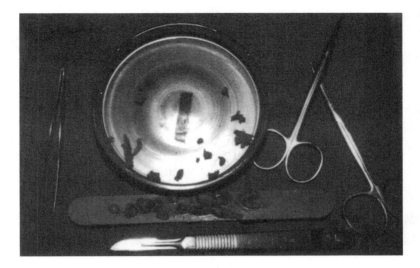

Figure 10
Dissection of the dermal graft block into grafts customized for the patient's defects.

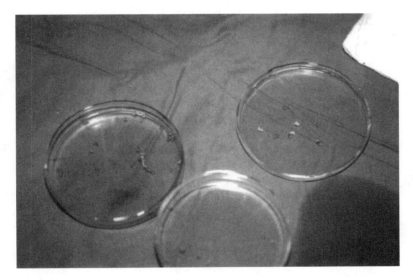

Figure 11
Dermal grafts are sorted and stored in iced saline in petri dishes.

INTRAOPERATIVE RECIPIENT SITE CREATION

Acne scars, glabellar folds, mental creases, and smaller lines or defects are then undermined in the mid-dermis with an 18- or 16-gauge NoKor needle or similar device possessing a sharp terminal blade (Fig. 12). A to-and-fro "windshield wiper" method is helpful for creating a pocket under larger scars or defects (Figs. 13 and 14). A Rhytisector® (Byron Instruments, Tucson, Arizona, U.S.) is utilized for undermining nasolabial folds in the dermal–subcutaneous plane between two small stab wounds placed lateral to the nasal ala and lateral to the corner of the mouth. Hemostasis is generally rapid following this undermining.

DERMAL GRAFT INSERTION

Implantation of smaller or short linear dermal grafts is then undertaken with a pair of curved jeweler's forceps in the dominant hand, and a pair of straight jeweler's forceps (to prevent extrusion) in the nondominant hand. One grasps the dermal portion of the end of a graft and meticulously maneuvers it, one step at a time, through the needle hole and into the defect (Fig. 15). With patience it is possible to insert a fairly large graft through the seemingly small needle hole due to the elasticity of facial skin. The graft is then positioned precisely with jeweler's forceps (Fig. 16). More than one graft may be inserted into larger defects (Fig. 17). An even correction, or slight overcorrection, should be attempted and perceived.

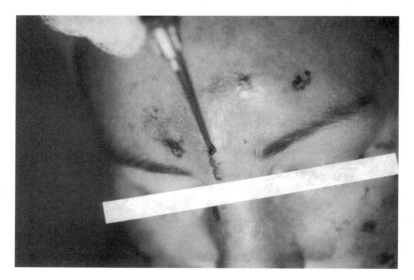

Figure 12
Undermining of the glabellar crease with 18-gauge NoKor® (Becton, Dickinson) needle, immediately prior to dermal grafting.

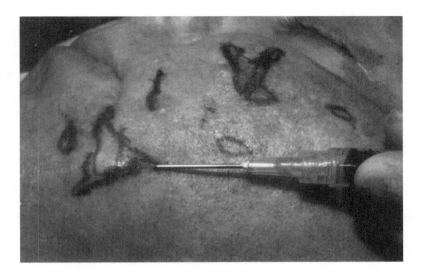

Figure 13
Undermining of a large depressed lipotrophic acne scar with 18-gauge NoKor®
(Becton, Dickinson) needle.

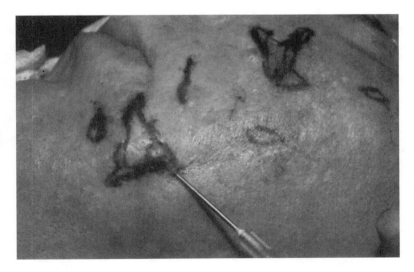

Figure 14
The same needle is rotated superiorly to cut under the fibrotic bands and create
a "recipient pocket."

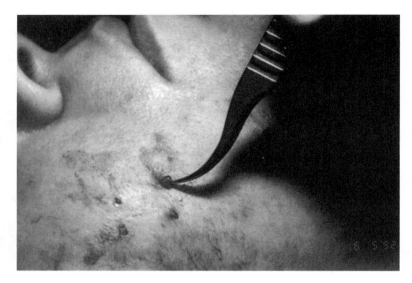

Figure 15
Insertion of dermal graft into a tiny hole made with 18-gauge NoKor® needle.

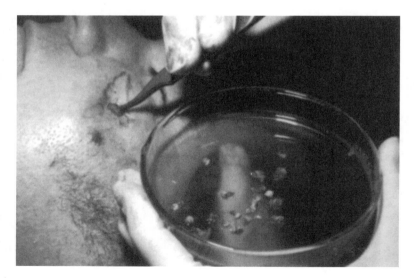

Figure 16
Larger scars may need more than one graft. Note that various sizes of grafts
have been prepared, corresponding to the different sizes of acne scars.

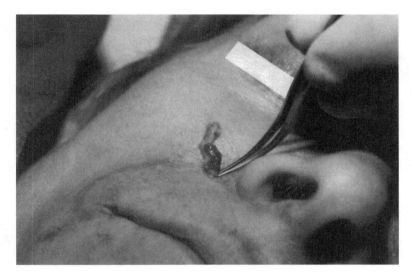

Figure 17
Insertion of linear dermal grafts into the superior aspect of the nasolabial fold.

For correction of larger, longer contour defects, such as those of nasolabial folds or for lip augmentation, long thin dermal grafts (the length of the donor incision) should be used (Figs. 18–20). The linear dermal grafts should be 5 to 10 mm longer than the distance between the upper and lower incision sites.

One technique employs a 3/0 Prolene® suture on a Keith® (straight) needle tied to one end of the graft. This needle, containing the graft, is then pulled through the nasolabial tunnel until the graft is visualized at the top and bottom (Fig. 21). The 3/0 Prolene is snipped and removed, taking care not to allow the graft to disappear.

A second method, now in use by the author, utilizes a thin snare to grasp and pull the graft through the recipient area (Figs. 25 and 26).

A 4/0 or 5/0 degradable suture is then placed at both the superior and inferior ends of the tunnel, catching (in sequence) skin, dermal graft, and opposing skin, and back, with a horizontal mattress suture (Fig. 22). Thus, as the interrupted suture is tied, the skin edges will be opposed yet the graft will be secured in place preventing further slippage (Fig. 23). All areas are then cleansed with hydrogen peroxide and dried. In general, all 18-gauge NoKor needle sites may be closed with steri-strips, although occasionally a degradable suture may be necessary (Fig. 24). Mastisol can aid in steri-strip permanency, with care taken to avoid the wounds themselves.

DRESSINGS AND POSTOPERATIVE CARE

Following the procedure, a nonadherent dressing should be applied to all surgical fields. Vigilon® or Second Skin® represent excellent choices, as

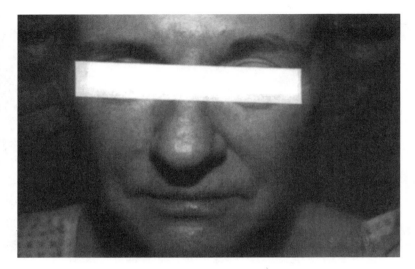

Figure 18
Preoperative view of a female patient with prominent nasolabial folds.

do Omiderm® or an antibiotic ointment plus a telfa or release pad. This dressing can be secured with Hypafix®, which conforms well to facial contours. Following the surgical recovery period, the patient is discharged from the office operatory.

The initial dressing may be removed in one to two days, with steri-strips removed in three to four days. Generally, the face may be

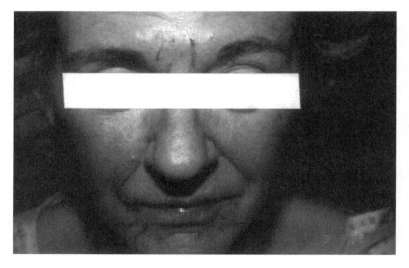

Figure 19
Areas to receive dermal grafts are delineated with violet marker.

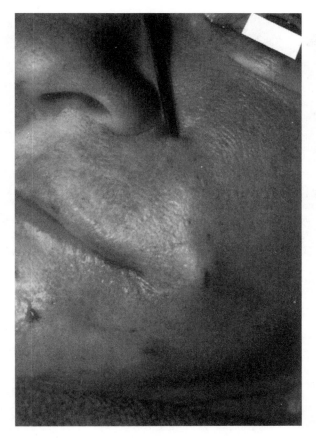

Figure 20
The nasolabial fold is undermined with Rhytisector® (Byron, Tucson, Arizona, U.S.).

washed on the third postoperative day. Postoperative care of the donor sites generally consists of application of hydrogen peroxide and antibiotic ointment. It is often helpful and supportive to see the patient on the third or fourth postoperative day. In addition to examination of the donor and recipient sites, instructions can be provided for coverage of bruising or discolored areas. The use of colored concealers (green for red areas, violet for yellow areas, and yellow for purple areas) followed by beige makeup can help to camouflage any problem areas and assist the patient in appearing in public or returning to work.

Follow-up can then be arranged in two to four weeks to assess the results of the dermal grafting. At that time, planning for subsequent dermal grafting sessions or resurfacing can be undertaken. Long-term follow-up at three months, six months, 12 months, and beyond should be advised as well.

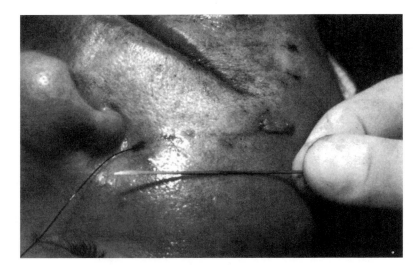

Figure 21
A linear dermal graft is pulled through the nasolabial fold via 3/0 Prolene tied to
one end.

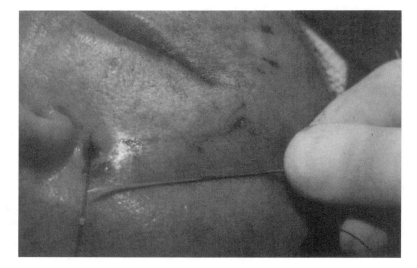

Figure 22
A dermal graft has been anchored at the inferior aspect with a 5/0 degradable
suture. A top knot of 3/0 Prolene will be removed as the superior aspect of the
graft is anchored in a similar fashion.

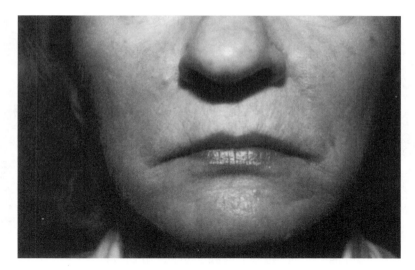

Figure 23
Approximately one year following dermal grafting. Note the absence of nasolabial folds with permanent correction.

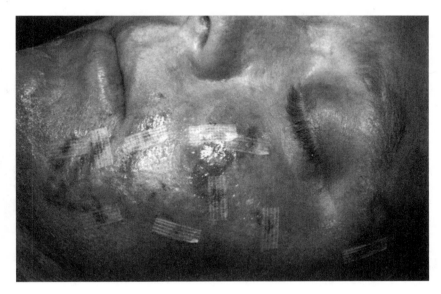

Figure 24
Postoperative closure of recipient sites with steri-strips alone.

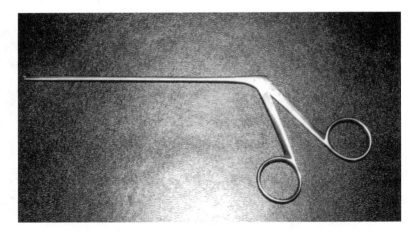

Figure 25
Snare used to pull long graft through nasolabial fold.

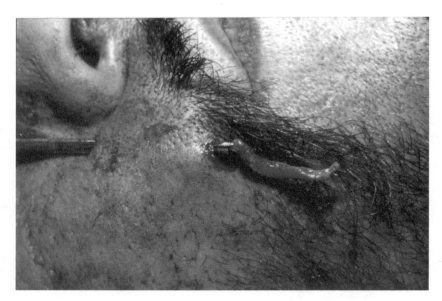

Figure 26
Dermal graft pulled through with the snare.

SIDE EFFECTS AND COMPLICATIONS

Untoward results, although infrequent, must be anticipated with any surgical procedure, no matter what the initial expectations on the part of the surgeon or the patient may have been. Short-term difficulties that are to be expected include bruising, hematoma formation, discoloration, crusting, and edema. Secondary infection has not been seen with the use of perioperative antibiotics, but it is possible. Pain or discomfort is to be expected but should be controlled with analgesics. The author has encountered two acute cystic lesions while inserting over a thousand dermal grafts; these resolved promptly with incision and drainage. Long-term epidermal inclusion cysts are rare when using a proper technique. Overcorrection of one scar required intralesional triamcinolone for treatment. Undercorrection, necessitating a subsequent dermal grafting procedure, is certainly possible and is to be expected; one operation treating up to 50 facial defects should never be expected to be 100% successful. On one occasion, a graft extruded during steri-strip removal. On another occasion, a nasolabial fold graft migrated inferiorly, necessitating the insertion of another dermal graft at the superior end. The number of dermal grafts inserted in a second operation is nearly always lower than that during the initial operation. Scarring from the 18-gauge NoKor needle holes or Byron rhytisector incision sites is uncommon, but is occasionally seen. These scars can be removed during the planned dermabrasion that follows. One or two dermal grafts could also be inserted at the time of this resurfacing.

ANTICIPATED RESULTS

Long-term follow-up with patients who have received dermal grafts has revealed an approximate correction of 40% to 70% on average after one session, and 50% to 100% after two sessions. Grafts that persist longer than six months appeared to maintain a permanent degree of correction. Any settling seems to occur between one and six months. Patients have maintained their correction for up to five years on long-term follow-up (Figs. 27–39).

Soft acne scars and smaller folds seem to respond best to dermal grafting. Nasolabial folds have also maintained their permanent augmentation. Dermal implants into glabellar creases have been somewhat less effective, probably because of the intact corrugator muscles. Further long-term follow-up is desirable.

DISCUSSION

Dermal grafts, therefore, possess many of the advantages seen in an ideal filler substance (Table 4).

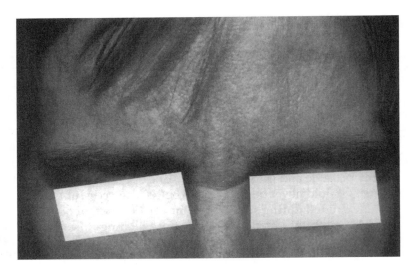

Figure 27
Prominent glabellar folds in a 33-year-old white female.

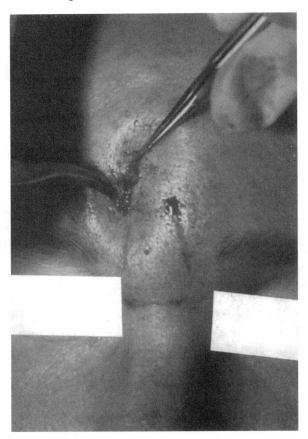

Figure 28
Dermal grafts are inserted superiorly into the undermined tunnel.

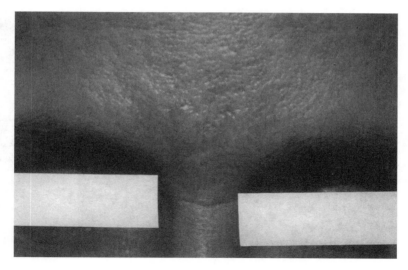

Figure 29
Three-month postoperative appearance showing correction of defects. Tiny "pores" represent entry sites.

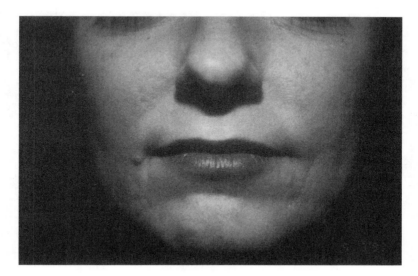

Figure 30
A 35-year-old white female with acne scars on the chin.

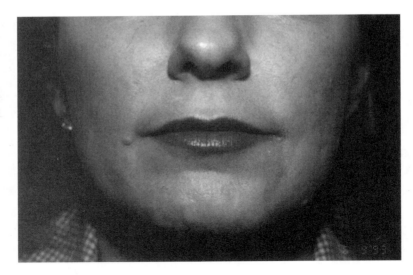

Figure 31
Same patient five weeks after dermal grafting, showing an approximate 50% to 70% improvement.

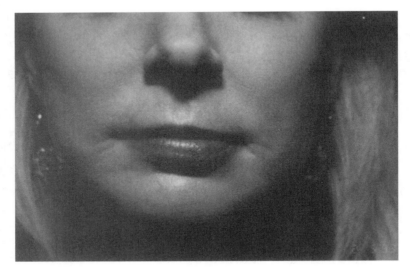

Figure 32
A 29-year-old white female with horizontal perioral lines that developed secondary to aggressive undermining during a face-lift.

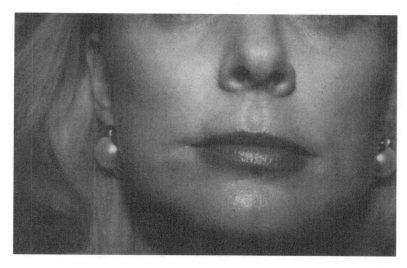

Figure 33
Correction of defects following placement of dermal grafts via an intraoral approach.

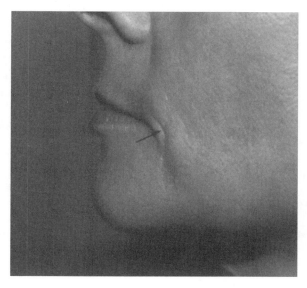

Figure 34
Female patient with prominent vertical perioral folds.

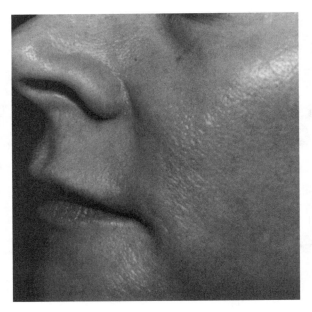

Figure 35
Correction of approximately 50% following one dermal grafting session.

As with any operation, several disadvantages can be identified (Table 5). Some of these concerns can be met by other means described later in this text.

Dermal grafting may be combined with other operations. The prior deployment of subcision has been discussed. Punch grafting or elevation can be performed simultaneously on adjacent scars. The use of botulinum toxin injections leads to successful treatment of the paralysis of underlying corrugator or procerus muscles, whereas dermal grafting works better to treat the overlying skin folds. The author has combined fat injections for elevation of deeper subcutaneous planes with dermal grafting placed more superficially on the same patient in the same operation. Resurfacing procedures, including chemical peeling, dermabrasion, or laser planing, can be utilized to "sand down the mountains." Since dermal grafts are inserted much more deeply than the level reached by the above modalities, it should be theoretically possible to perform these procedures simultaneously. Careful trials with these combinations should hence be performed.

CONCLUSIONS

The future for dermal grafting appears bright, but many areas remain to be explored. Does prior undermining enhance the results? Would dermal grafts from other sources (such as the upper back, hard palate, surgical

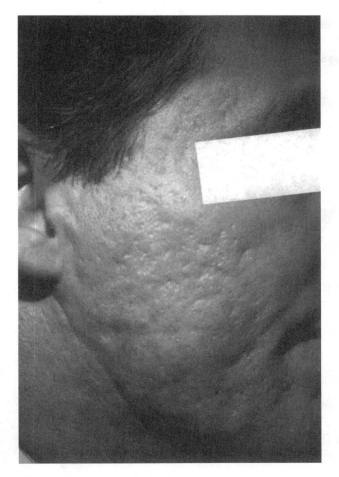

Figure 36
Male patient in mid-thirties with deep, severe, fibrotic acne scarring.

scars, or fibrous capsules from tissue expanders) prove to be even more efficacious? Can dermal grafts or derma-fat grafts correct cellulite "dimples" not improved by liposuction? Is the lip augmentation obtained via dermal grafting superior to that seen when fat, collagen, or Gortex® is used? And, finally, how long do the grafts really last? It is difficult to perform postoperative biopsies from the face in cosmetic surgical patients. However, the use of appropriate histologic markers identifiable in sequential biopsies, combined with repeated optical profilometry, might shed light on these questions.

When one considers the obvious advantages with relatively few drawbacks, it is evident that dermal grafting is an underutilized procedure (26,27). The author, in this chapter, has introduced several new concepts, including the harvesting of elliptical solid donor grafts, use of dermal graft test areas combined with other modalities, customized

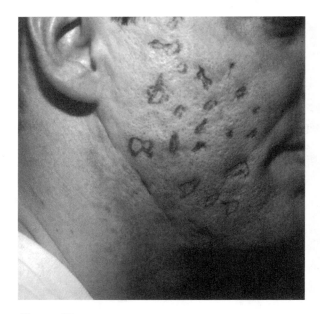

Figure 37
Areas to receive dermal grafts have been delineated with aid of tangential light source.

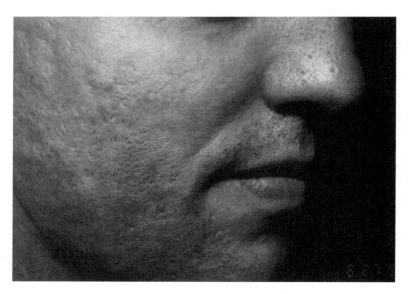

Figure 38
Result after two dermal grafting sessions.

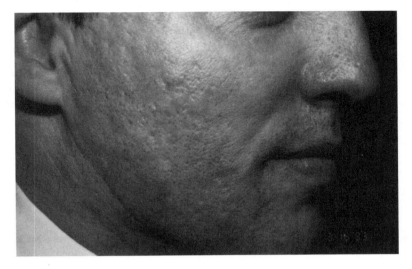

Figure 39
Final results one year later after subsequent full face dermabrasion showing permanent correction of approximately 90% of the scars.

| **Table 4** | |
Dermal Graft Advantages	
Autologous material	Dermis attached to fat allows inosculation to occur
Readily available	Grafts can be contoured to fit defect
Easily inserted with precision	Office procedure, easily repeated
Firm structure gives good correction	No allergic reactions or extrusions

| **Table 5** |
Dermal Graft Disadvantages
Separate harvesting step
Donor scar
Surgical skill needed for insertion
Length and cost of procedure
Risk of cyst formation
May need repeat procedure and/or subsequent resurfacing

dissections to fit a variety of soft tissue defects, and the "pull through" technique for nasolabial fold and lip augmentation. It is hoped that the reader will be stimulated not only to consider this operation in clinical practice, but also to develop the science of dermal grafting even further into the twenty-first century.

REFERENCES

1. Peer LA, Paddock R. Histologic studies on the fate of deeply implanted dermal grafts: Observations on sections of implants buried from one week to one year. Arch Surg 1937; 34:268.
2. Migliori ME, Putterman AM. The domed dermis–fat graft orbital implant. Ophth Recon Surg 1991; 7(l):23–30.
3. Meyer DR, Wobig JL. Diamond shaped incision for obtaining dermis–fat grafts. Am J Ophth 1990; 109(6):746–748.
4. Rose GE, Collin R. Dermofat grafts to the extraconal orbital space. Br J Plast Surg 1992; 76(7):408–411.
5. Mikaelian DO, Lowry LD, Sataloff RT. Lipoinjection for unilateral vocal cord paralysis. Laryngoscope 1991; 101(5):465–468.
6. Loh FC, Loh HS. Use of the buccal fat pad for correction of intraoral defects. J Oral Maxillofac Surg 1991; 49(4):413–416.
7. Stromqvist B, Jonsson B, Annertz M, Holtas S. Cauda equina syndrome caused by migrating fat graft after lumbar spinal decompression. A case report demonstrated with magnetic resonance imaging. Spine 1991; 16(1):100–101.
8. Sawhney CP, Banerjee TN, Chakravarti RN. Behavior of dermal fat transplants. Br J Plast Surg 1969; 22:169.
9. Boering G, Huffstadt AJ. The use of derma-fat grafts in the face. BR J Plast Surg 1968; 20(2):172.
10. Fournier PF. Facial recontouring with fat grafting. Dermatol Clin 1990; 8(3):523–537.
11. Orentreich DS. Soft Tissue Augmentation Seminar, AAD. San Francisco, CA, December 1992.
12. Loeb R. Nasolabial fold undermining and fat grafting based on histological study. Aesth Plast Surg 1991; 15:61–66.
13. Asaadi M, Haramis HT. Successful autologous fat injection at 5-year follow up. Plast Reconstr Surg 1991; 91(4):755.
14. Ersek RA. Transplantation of purified autologous fat; a 3-year follow up is disappointing. Plast Reconstr Surg 1991; 87(2):219–227.
15. Coleman W, Hanke CW, Alt TH, Asken S. eds. Cosmetic Surgery of the Skin. Philadelphia: B.C. Decker, 1991.
16. Naomi L. Soft Tissue Augmentation Seminar, ASDS, Charleston, SC, March 1993.
17. Coleman W. 4th Annual Cosmetic & Reconstructive Seminar, Colorado Society of Dermatologic Surgery, Snowmass, CO, April 1992.
18. Skouge JW. Soft Tissue Augmentation Seminar, ASDS, Charleston, SC, March 1993.
19. Liposuction Seminar, AACS, New Orleans, LA, May 1987.
20. Horl HW, Feller AM, Biemer E. Technique for liposuction fat reimplantation and long-term volume evaluation by magnetic resonance imaging. Ann Plast Surg 1991; 25(3):248–258.
21. Ellenbogen R. Free autogenous pearl fat grafts in the face—A preliminary report of a rediscovered technique. Ann Plast Surg 1986; 16(3):179–194.
22. Hynes W. The early circulation in skin grafts with a consideration of methods to encourage their survival. Brit J Plast Surg 1954; 6:257.
23. Mordick TG, Larossa D, Whitaker L. Soft tissue reconstruction of the face: a comparison of dermal-fat grafting and vascularized tissue transfer. Ann Plast Surg 1992; 29(5):390–396.
24. Swinehart JM. Test spots in dermabrasion and chemical peeling. J Dermatol Surg Oncol 1990; 16(6):557–563.
25. Swinehart JM. The ice–saline–xylocaine technique: a simple method for minimizing pain in obtaining local anesthesia. J Dermatol Surg Oncol 1990; 18:28–30.

26. Swinehart JM. Pocket grafting with dermal grafts: autologous collagen implants for permanent correction of cutaneous depressions. Am J Cosmet Surg 1995; 12(4):321–331.
27. Swinehart JM. Dermal pocket grafting: Implants of dermis, fat, and 'autologous collagen' for permanent correction of cutaneous depressions. Int J Aesth Restor Surg 1994; 2(l):43–52.

3

Soft Tissue Augmentation Using Human Allografts and Autografts

Carolyn I. Jacob
*Chicago Cosmetic Surgery and Dermatology, and Department of Dermatology,
Northwestern Medical School, Chicago, Illinois, U.S.A.*

Michael S. Kaminer
*SkinCare Physicians of Chestnut Hill, Chestnut Hill, Massachusetts; Department of Medicine,
Dartmouth Medical School, Dartmouth College, Hanover, New Hampshire; and Department
of Dermatology, Yale School of Medicine, Yale University, New Haven, Connecticut, U.S.A.*

INTRODUCTION

Soft tissue augmentation has been popular for restoring the loss of volume and elasticity of the face for over 20 years. Bovine collagen and autologous fat transplantation remain two of the most widely used filler substances. Both have their advantages and drawbacks. Because the general consensus among physicians is that an ideal filler substance is yet to be developed, both human- and nonhuman-derived products continue to be developed and evaluated.

Bovine collagen injections are a nonsurgical approach for patients desiring temporary correction of rhytids. Two skin tests are recommended to exclude over 97% of allergic reactions, which manifest as erythema and edema of the treated site (1,2). Rare reactions to gluteraldehyde cross-linking (used in the thicker form of collagen, known as Zyplast®) have also been known to occur. Over the past five years, the concern of contamination of bovine substances with transmissible spongiform encephalopathies has raised public concern and caused a reduction of cosmetic bovine collagen injections in Europe (3). Fortunately, injectable bovine collagen in the United States is derived from an Angus/Hereford secluded donor herd in California, which has never been fed bovine protein. In addition, the injectable collagen, made from the hides of these cows, is prepared under sterile conditions with virus inactivation procedures (4). Despite these safety precautions, some patients remain wary of using bovine collagen.

Autologous fat transplantation provides long-term correction, with treatment requiring a mini-liposuction procedure for fat harvesting.

In addition, two to three touch-up procedures performed approximately every two to four months are usually required to achieve the desired filling. Unfortunately, there are many patients for whom autologous fat transplantation is not possible owing to lack of adequate donor fat supply (e.g., HIV wasting syndrome, extremely thin body types).

The search for nonsurgical, nonallergenic, longer-lasting filler substances has led to the development of allografts, or material harvested from a different individual of the same species, for implantation or injection.

HUMAN-DERIVED HOMOLOGOUS FILLER SUBSTANCES (ALLOGRAFTS)

There are several human tissues, that have been investigated, and some are currently used to create filler substances for human soft tissue augmentation. These include dermis, fascia lata, human cell cultures derived from neonatal foreskin, human placental collagen, recombinant human collagen, and dura mater (Collagenesis, Inc., Beverly, Massachusetts, U.S.; Lifecell Corporation, Branchburg, New Jersey, U.S.; Fascian Biosystems, LLC., Beverly Hills, California, U.S.; Inamed Corporation, Santa Barbara, California; Cohesion Technologies, Palo Alto, California, U.S.) (Table 1).

Human Dermis

Cosmetic injectables derived from human tissue banks are currently available for human implantation. These tissues are viewed as devices by the U.S. Food and Drug Administration (FDA), and manufacturing companies are required to screen their tissue bank donor pool. These human tissue banks were not regulated by the FDA until April 3, 2001, with the implementation of Current Good Tissue Practice of Manufacturers of Human Cellular and Tissue-Based Products. The FDA currently inspects human tissue banks every two years (5).

Dermaplant®

Dermaplant (Collagenesis Inc. Beverly, Massachusetts, U.S.) is a solid sheet of dermis with the split below the basement membrane. It therefore does not contain lamina densa collagen (type IV). It can be stored at room temperature, has a sterile inner pack, and appears to be more flexible and stronger than AlloDerm® (6).

AlloDerm® and Cymetra®

AlloDerm and Cymetra (LifeCell Corp., Branchburg, New Jersey, U.S.) are acellular dermal materials harvested from the American Association

Table 1
Human Derived Filler Substances

Material	Anesthesia	Placement site	Needle gauge	Over-correction	Skin test	Duration
AlloDerm®	Regional/ local	Subdermal	N/A	N	N	Up to 20 months
Amnion®	Unknown	Unknown	Unknown	Unknown	N	Unknown
Autologen®	Local	Upper dermis	30	Y	N	Unknown
CosmoDerm/ Cosmo-Plast®	Topical	Upper/lower dermis	30	N	To be determined	Unknown
Cymetra®	Regional/ local	Dermal/ Subcutaneous junction	21–25	N	N	Partial up to 1 year
Dermalogen®	Topical/ local	Mid-upper dermis	30	N	N	2–3 months
Dermaplant®	Regional/ local	Subdermal	N/A	N	N	Unknown
Dura mater	Unknown	Unknown	Unknown	Unknown	N	Unknown
Fascian®	Regional/ local	Dermis	16–25	Y	N	3–4 months
Isolagen®	Regional/ local	Upper dermis	30	N	N	Unknown
Recombinant human collagen	Unknown	Unknown	Unknown	Unknown	N	Unknown

of Tissue Bank (AATB) screened cadavers. The tissue is freeze-dried and processed, and major histocompatibility complex (MHC) antigens are removed to prevent immunological rejection. Electron microscopic analysis has shown that collagen types IV and VII, laminin, and elastin reside in the resulting matrix.

Available in sheets, AlloDerm has been used in scar revision, lip augmentation, nasolabial and glabellar frown line correction, and revision rhinoplasty, to name a few (7). One side of the graft contains reticular dermis and the other side is composed of the basement membrane complex of the dermal–epidermal junction. The sheets are reconstituted with saline, and rolled or cut to create the desired shape for implantation. For scars or nasolabial folds, lidocaine with epinephrine is used to anesthetize the prepared recipient site surgically and tunneling is performed to create a pocket for the material. Some authors advocate subcutaneous suturing to secure the graft placement. Closure of the skin incisions is performed with 6/0 polypropylene. For lip augmentation, infraorbital and mental nerve blocks as well as local anesthesia may be desired. Insertion sites are created with a No. 11 blade on the vermillion commissures (without crossing the white roll), and a tunnel gently created with the smooth end of a Freer periosteum elevator. Care must be taken to avoid the labial artery, which courses deep to the lip mucosa. Alligator forceps are then placed within the tunnel, and at the distal opening of the tunnel, the rolled AlloDerm can be grasped and gently pulled back through the lip. Closure of the incision sites is performed using 6-0 silk sutures.

Integration of AlloDerm into surrounding tissue has been demonstrated both histologically and immunologically (8). Achauer et al. (9) retrospectively reviewed 11 patients with facial soft tissue defects treated with AlloDerm, and determined the stability of the product up to 20 months after implantation. They speculate that AlloDerm provides a template, that the fibroblastic and endothelial cells repopulate, resulting in a permanent, integrated graft. Castor et al. (10) showed lip augmentation with AlloDerm along with fat autograft to be superior to autologous fat injection alone. They demonstrated the clinical persistence of the graft at three months.

Cymetra is made from processing the same AlloDerm collagen matrix in liquid nitrogen into small particles. The particulate nature of this processed dermal matrix allows for easy delivery of liquid concentrations up to 330 mg/mL, which exceeds that of other currently used products (11). Available in a powdered form prepackaged in syringes, Cymetra requires reconstitution with lidocaine or saline for injection. A 21- to 25-gauge needle is also recommended due to the particulate size, thereby requiring local anesthesia for patient comfort. Cymetra may be used for shallow boxcar and rolling acne scars, nasolabial folds, HIV-related facial lipodystrophy, and lip augmentation. Longevity has been shown to exceed that of intradermal collagen at one month in a study performed with implantations postauricularly (12). Patients who receive three treatments may have partial correction for over a year (13).

Dermalogen®

No longer available for purchase, Dermalogen® (Collagenesis, Inc., Beverly, Massachusetts, U.S.) is composed of intact collagen fibrils extracted from cadaver tissue. Extensive screening of donors for HIV, hepatitis B and C, HTLV-1, syphilis, and bacterial contamination is conducted by the AATB-accredited Musculoskeletal Transplant Foundation. This injectable human tissue matrix is also treated with antiviral agents. Skin testing may be indicated for patients with multiple sensitivites such as allergy to bovine collagen. Available in prefilled 1-cc syringes, Dermalogen is injected with a 30-gauge needle. As Dermalogen does not contain lidocaine, topical or local anesthesia may be used for patient comfort. Current treatment techniques include intradermal placement, without overcorrection, and a second injection two weeks later for best results. Patients have been followed up for up to six months and a greater increase of longevity has been reported with Dermalogen than with bovine collagen. At 12 months they were equal (6).

Human Fascia Lata

Fascian® (Fascian Biosystems, LLC, Beverly Hills, California, U.S.) is preserved particulate fascia available in preloaded syringes. It is screened according to the AATB standards. It is freeze dried and preirradiated with gamma radiation. It does not require refrigeration and, because of low allergenicity, test implantation is not indicated. It is available in multiple particle sizes such as <0.25 mm, <0.5 mm, and <2.0 mm. Larger gauge needles, such as 16- to 27-gauge, are required for the larger particle sizes. The freeze-dried particles are reconstituted and agitated with lidocaine. The larger particles require 20 minutes or more to optimally hydrate the particles. Injections are performed with regional blocks or local anesthesia.

Injections are placed subdermally or, in the case of lip augmentation, in the layer of the submucosal glands. Clogging of the material in the syringe hub may occur if the needle is too small to permit an even flow of the particles. If this occurs, an additional 0.5 cc of saline may be aspirated in the syringe, or the needle may be changed. Clogging is more common with the <2.0 mm preparation. Application of firm pressure and ice after treatment may help in reducing edema. In one study, no incidents of local or systemic hypersensitivity reactions occurred. Minimum local tenderness and ecchymoses may occur postoperatively. In this same study, graft persistence was clinically evident at three to four months follow-up (14).

Human-Cultured Skin Derived from Neonatal Foreskin

CosmoPlast® and CosmoDerm® I and II (INAMED Corp., Santa Barbara, California, U.S. and Advanced Tissue Sciences, La Jolla, California, U.S.) are tissues synthesized from prescreened human neonatal foreskin culture. It is packaged with lidocaine in prefilled syringes, similar to Zyplast® and Zyderm® I and II. CosmoPlast is cross-linked with gluteraldehyde, which may cause rare allergic reactions in gluteraldehyde-sensitive patients, yet pretreatment tests are not required. The substance is directly injected into the dermis using 30-gauge needles, as performed with bovine collagen. Clinical studies of longevity have not been performed.

Human Placental Collagen

Gamma-irradiated amnion collagen from human placentae has been suggested for soft tissue augmentation and tested in animal studies (15,16). Placentae are readily available and living donors could be followed up for evolving HIV or hepatitis infection. Placentae also have the potential to provide autologous collagen akin to Autologen from harvested skin. No human testing has begun at this time.

Recombinant Human Collagen

Research in recombinant human collagen (Cohesion Technologies, Palo Alto, California, U.S.) is underway to produce material for reinjection. It would eliminate the necessity for donor tissue, eradicate the need for proteolytic cleavage of animal collagen with its attendant degradation, and have no potential for allergy. Human collagen is grown in the cow and separated from the cow's milk. Concern for potential bovine allergy cross-contamination is evident; as of the date of publication, no real product has come to the U.S. market (6).

Dura Mater

Dura mater has been studied as an allograft, but the risk of Creutzfeldt–Jakob disease transmission remains a valid concern (17). Disease transmission can occur through inadvertent use of transmissible spongiform encephalopathy–contaminated dura or instruments contaminated with prions (5). As there is no current method of sterilization for prions, dura mater will not likely become a cosmetic implant in the near future (18).

HUMAN AUTOLOGOUS FILLER SUBSTANCES (AUTOGRAFTS)

Autologen®

Autologen (no longer available) is a suspension of intact collagen fibrils, elastic tissue, and proteoglycans aseptically prepared from the patient's own tissue. Host skin from an earlier procedure is forwarded to Collagenesis, Inc. (Beverly, Massachusetts, U.S.) for processing. Three square inches of skin produces 1 cc of Autologen at a 3.5% concentration, and is returned to the physician in prefilled syringes. It is used for superficial placement in fine lines and lip augmentation (6).

Isolagen®

Isolagen (Isolagen Technologies, Paramus, New Jersey, U.S.) consists of cultured autologous fibroblasts. Processed from a 3-mm punch biopsy, a test dose is first performed, then treatments are begun two weeks afterwards. There is a temporary halt in production as their use of growth factors in processing classifies Isolagen as a medical device. FDA approval will likely be necessary for the use of the product (6).

DISCUSSION

The quest for the perfect substance for soft tissue augmentation continues, and there is a growing array of choices for patients and physicians. To this end, development of human allografts and autografts is an exciting area in the reconstructive and cosmetic surgery arena. It has become clear over the past decade (or longer) that patients desire cosmetic treatments, that require minimal time lost from their daily activities, as well as a favorable risk/benefit profile. For these and other reasons, including the trend toward minimally invasive surgery, the role of soft tissue augmentation is likely to expand over the coming years.

Therefore, the development and refinement of the agents used for soft tissue augmentation are paramount to the future success and utility of this form of cosmetic treatment. The use of human-derived substances for soft tissue augmentation is a concept that has met with some success in recent years. Although the relative utility of some of the available agents yet to be proven, the concept has merit. Yet, the limiting factor in the overall success of human tissue as a soft tissue augmentation agent is not only the ability of the scientific community to create new and better products, but the continued acceptance of this concept by our patients. Safety ranks one, two, and three on the list of important items in product development. One case of disease transmission from donor to recipient by a human-derived agent can literally doom the concept. It is for this reason that the scientific community must make a commitment to safety over profit.

All too often the cosmetic industry has hailed a new device or substance as the latest, greatest breakthrough, only to have those claims later proven to be less than accurate. The prudent practitioner must be careful to fully evaluate potentially risky treatments before bringing them to his or her patients. But in this case, it appears to be the industry's responsibility to carry the burden of proof regarding safety. The industry cannot sacrifice safety in the name of profits.

Efficacy is certainly an important issue and one that will likely continue to drive the search for new and better means of using human-derived tissue for soft tissue augmentation. The products currently available should certainly be considered by physicians skilled in the art of soft tissue augmentation. When carefully matched to patient expectations, they can be superb complements to a well-planned skin care and cosmetic treatment plan.

REFERENCES

1. Stegman SJ, Chu S, Armstrong R. Adverse reactions to bovine collagen implant: Clinical and histologic features. J Dermatol Surg Oncol 1998; 14(suppl):39–48.
2. Elson ML. The role of skin testing in the use of collagen injectable materials. J Dermatol Surg Oncol 1989; 15:301–303.
3. Stephens B. Mad Cow Disease 101. Wall Street Journal. December 21, 2000.
4. McGhan Medical Corporation. What you should know about collagen replacement therapy. Santa Barbara, CA, McGhan Medical Corp, 2001.
5. Carruthers J, Carruthers A. Mad cows, prions, and wrinkles. Arch Dermatol 2002; 138:667–670.
6. Klein AW, Elson ML. The history of substances for soft tissue augmentation. Dermatol Surg 2000; 26(12):1096–1105.
7. Jones FR, Schwartz BM, Silverstein P. Use of a nonimmunogenic acellular dermal allograft for soft tissue augmentation: A preliminary report. Aesth Surg Quart 1996; 16:196–210.
8. Livesey SL, Horndon, DN, Holloak MA, et al. Transplanted acellular allograft dermal matrix. Potential as a template for the reconstruction of viable dermis. Transplantation 1995; 60:1.
9. Achauer BM, VanderKam VM, Celikoz B, Jacobson DG. Augmentation of facial soft-tissue defects with AlloDerm dermal graft. Annals Plas Surg 1998; 41(5):503–507.
10. Castor SA, To WC, Papay FA. Lipo augmentation with AlloDerm acellular allogenic dermal graft and fat autograft: A comparison with autologous fat injection alone. Aesth Plast Surg 1999; 23:218–223.
11. Griffey S, Schwade ND, Wright CG. Particulate dermal matrix as an injectable soft tissue replacement material. J Biomed Mater Res 2000; 58(1):10–15.
12. Sclafani AP, Romo T III, Jacono AA, McCormick S, Cocker R, Parker A. Evaluation of acellular dermal graft in sheet (AlloDerm) and injectable (micronized AlloDerm) forms for soft tissue augmentation. Clinical observations and histological analysis. Arch Facial Plast Surg 2000; 2(2):130–136.
13. Alam M, Omura N, Kaminer MS. Longevity of result after facial injection of human collagen (Cymetra). Poster Presentation, Society for Investigative Dermatology, 63rd Annual Meeting, Los Angeles, CA, May 15–18, 2002.
14. Burres S. Preserved particulate fascia lata for injection: A new alternative. Dermatol Surg 1999; 25:790–794.
15. Liu B, Harrell R, Davis RH, et al. The effect of gamma irradiation on injectable human amnion collagen. J Biomed Mat Res 1989; 23:833–844.
16. Spira M, Liu B, Xu Z, et al. Human amnion collagen for soft tissue augmentation–Biochemical characterizations and animal observations. J Biomed Mat Res 1994; 28:91–96.
17. Nordstrom MR, Wang TD, Neel HB. Dura mater for soft-tissue augmentation. Evaluation in a rabbit model. Arch Otolaryngol Head Neck Surg 1993; 119:208–214.
18. Shimizu S, Hoshi K, Muramoto T, et al. Cruetzfeld-Jakob disease with florid type plaques after cadaveric human dura mater grafting. Arch Neurol 1999; 56:357–362.

4

Injectable Collagen

Arnold W. Klein
*Department of Dermatology, David Geffen School of Medicine,
University of California, Los Angeles, California, U.S.A.*

Richard G. Glogau
University of California, San Francisco, California, U.S.A.

Injectable bovine collagen, Zyderm® collagen implant, has been in use in the United States since 1977 (1). Originally developed by the Collagen Corporation (Palo Alto, California, U.S.) in 1979, the product became widely available to interested physicians in the United States under a phase III protocol. Ultimately, in July of 1981, the Zyderm collagen implant received the approval of the Food and Drug Administration (FDA), representing the first time an FDA-approved injectable device was available for soft tissue augmentation. This approval sparked interest in the entire field of filling substances and, to date, more than 1,300,000 individuals have received injectable collagen treatments. Following the approval of the first injectable form, Zyderm I® collagen implant, the FDA cleared two additional formulations, Zyderm II® collagen implant and Zyplast® implant. Subsequently, a special packaging of Zyderm I collagen, which contains a 32-gauge needle, was made available. The barrel of the syringe for this product—Zyderm I with Fine-Gauge Needle—is specifically suited for use with the supplied metal-hub needle.

FORMULATIONS

Zyderm collagen (ZC) is a sterile-purified fibrillar suspension of dermal collagen derived from cowhide (Fig. 1). The substance is taken from the skin of a closed American herd, which has been sequestered since production began in the 1970s. The herd has never been exposed to animal proteins in their feed, nor have the animals been permitted contact with other ungulates, negating the possibility of contamination with the bovine spongiform encephalopathy virus, the pathologic agent in "mad cow disease" (2). The cowhide undergoes purification, pepsin digestion,

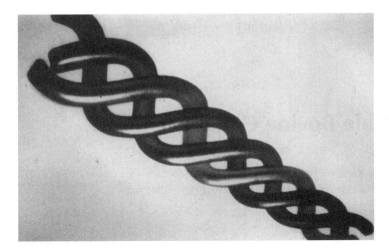

Figure 1
Bovine collagen with the telopeptides removed, with preservation of the helical structure.

and sterilization during the fabrication process. The pepsin hydrolysis is critical because it removes the more antigenic telopeptide regions without disturbing the helical structure. It is the helical structure that is thought to contribute substantively to the product's characteristics upon implantation. Furthermore, the removal of the telopeptides makes the product more immunologically compatible with humans. ZC contains 95% to 98% type I collagen; the remainder is type III collagen (3). The collagen is suspended in phosphate-buffered physiologic saline with 0.3% lidocaine. It is provided in prefilled syringes, which are stored at a low temperature (4°C), so that the dispersed fibrils remain fluid and small. This allows passage of the product through a 30- or 32-gauge needle. Once implanted, the human body temperature (37°C) causes the product to undergo consolidation into a solid gel, as intermolecular cross-linking occurs in the suspension with the generation of a high proportion of larger fibrils.

ZC is currently available in three forms (Fig. 2). Two of these differ only in the concentration of suspended material. These are Zyderm I collagen (ZI), the original material, which is 3.5% by weight bovine collagen (35 mg/mL), and Zyderm II (ZII), introduced in 1983, which is 6.5% by weight bovine collagen (6.5 mg/mL). The third agent, Zyplast implant (ZP), was approved in 1985. This product is unique in that the bovine dermal collagen is lightly cross-linked by the addition of 0.0075% glutaraldehyde. Glutaraldehyde produces covalently-bonded cross-linked bridges between approximately 10% of the available lysine sites on the bovine collagen molecules. These bridges are produced intramolecularly, intermolecularly, and between fibrils. This more substantive product is in actuality an injectable lattice work of bovine collagen (4). In addition to being more resistant to proteolytic degradation, ZP is less immunogenic than ZI or ZII (4–6). Furthermore, the more robust nature of ZP compared to other

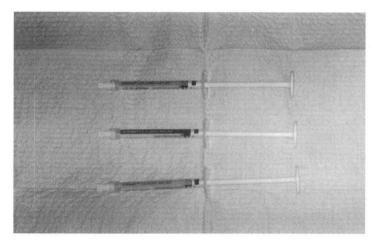

Figure 2
Top to bottom: Zyderm I®, Zyderm II®, and Zyplast®.

forms of ZC makes it applicable for deeper contour defects previously not amenable to correction with injectable bovine collagen (7,8).

In addition to the various forms of ZC, a special packaging of ZI collagen is available, which contains a syringe specially suited for use with a 32-gauge needle. This product—Zyderm I with Fine-Gauge Needle (Z-FGN)—contains a syringe barrel specifically designed for use with the supplied metal-hub needle. Nevertheless, since 32-gauge metal-hub needles are easily affixed to the other ZI syringes, some individuals have not found this packaging particularly necessary (Fig. 3).

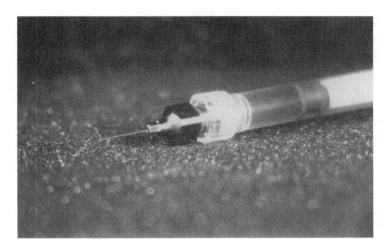

Figure 3
32-gauge metal-hub needle.

PATIENT SELECTION AND SKIN TESTING

Proper patient selection and skin testing are of paramount importance in the application of bovine collagen therapy. Individuals who have lidocaine sensivity, a history of anaphylaxis for any reason, or previous sensitivity to bovine collagen are excluded from testing and treatment. Potential hypersensitivity to injectable collagen therapy is reliably determined by intradermal skin testing. Skin-test syringes, that contain 0.3 cc ZI collagen are utilized to screen for allergy to all forms of injectable collagen (ZI, ZII, or ZP). A tuberculin-like test is performed in the volar forearm, using only 0.1 cc of the material contained in the test syringe. The test site is evaluated at 48 to 72 hours and again at four weeks. A positive-skin test response will be seen in 3.0% to 3.5% of individuals even in the absence of prior treatment with injectable collagen. Seventy percent of these reactions will manifest in 48 to 72 hours, indicating a pre-existing allergy to bovine collagen (9–12). Thus, it is mandatory to observe the test site at 48 to 72 hours, as well as the standard four-week interval.

A positive skin test is defined as any swelling, palpable induration, persistent tenderness or evanescent, and intermittent or persistent erythema and including any redness that persists or occurs six hours or longer after the test implantation. Most authorities recommend a second test as an additional precaution (13–16). This can be placed in the contralateral forearm or the periphery of the face. It is administered either two weeks after the initial test with treatment commencing at four weeks after initial testing, or four weeks after the initial test with treatment commencing six weeks after first testing. The volume utilized for the second test is the same as that used for the first test; again, skin test syringes are employed.

As the majority of treatment-associated hypersensitivity reactions occur shortly after the first treatment, double testing greatly reduces the frequency of this most undesirable sequela by changing the first-treatment exposure to a second-test exposure. Additionally, treatment-associated hypersensitive reactions that do occur after two negative-skin tests tend to be, in general, milder, indicating that the physician has selected out the most severely allergic individuals. Single retesting of individuals who have not been treated for more than one year, or who were successfully tested or treated elsewhere, is strongly recommended. An interval of two weeks is recommended for test-site evaluation after retesting before commencing treatment, although 48 hours is the minimum interval after retesting that is necessary to capture the vast majority of sensitized patients.

TECHNIQUES OF INJECTION

Injection technique is the most important factor in the successful application of bovine collagen implants. It is an evolutionary process for the

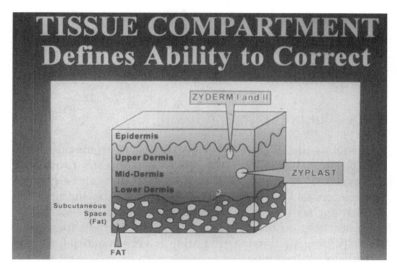

Figure 4
Zyderm® is placed superficially in the upper dermis to fill defects while
Zyplast® is placed at the mid-dermal plane.

treating physician, yet there are basic principles that can be gleaned
from others' experiences. First, the value of good positioning, lighting,
and magnification cannot be overstated. The patient must be in the
seated position because many contour defects all but disappear in the
supine position. Additionally, tangential halogen lighting is very beneficial because many subtle defects are best revealed in this type of light.
Finally, magnification will enable the treating physician to implant
more precisely and control many technique variables associated with
injection, such as position of the needle bevel, angle of needle entry
into the skin, avoidance of small superficial veins, telangiectasia, etc.

ZI TECHNIQUE

ZI is the most versatile of all forms of injectable collagen. It is also
the most technique sensitive and the most forgiving. Since it has
good flow characteristics, meaning it tends to disperse evenly and
without resistance when placed correctly into the papillary or upper
dermis, it will smoothly fill superficial defects (Fig. 4). This is best
done with a 32-gauge metal-hub needle regardless of the syringe
type chosen (0.5 cc, 1.0 cc, or Z-FGN). One holds the treatment site
taut with the thumb and forefinger of the opposing hand. Next, the
needle tip is guided horizontally with the bevel down along the skin
surface until it barely penetrates the skin. The hub of the needle is
then gently rocked over the thumb of the opposing hand, tenting
up the skin with the needle tip, and a flow of material is created in

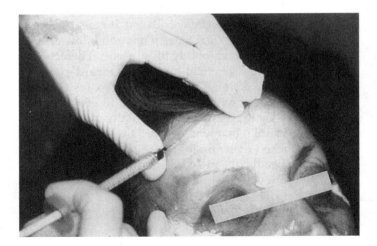

Figure 5
Zyderm I® in a 1-cc syringe with 32-gauge needle. Note the wide and flat flow of material. Collagen appears more yellow and not overly white after injection.

the upper dermis as a smooth, yellowish mass that is both wide and flat (Figs. 5 and 6).

A technique originally advocated by the manufacturers–to place the material "as superficial as possible"– is to be avoided because residual whiteness at the treatment sites can be experienced as a result. This is particularly true where the skin is very thin, e.g., around the eyes and areas of crows feet.

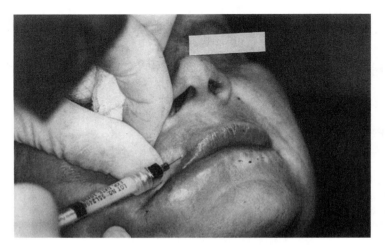

Figure 6
Zyderm I®. Note the smooth flow of material along the skin above the upper lip.

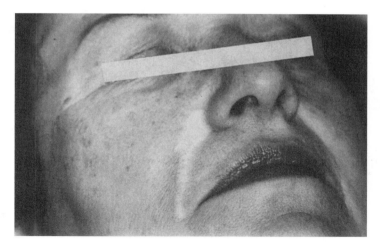

Figure 7
Zyderm I®. Smooth flow of material in the nasolabial fold.

With ZI, an upper dermal flow is created by applying each subsequent injection at the edge of the previously injected volume. This continuous, wide, and flat flow in the upper dermis smoothly fills superficial soft tissue defects, providing the most satisfying cosmetic results.

Initially, deliberate overcorrection was promoted as a desirable injection technique with ZI based on the theory that, after condensation and resorption of the saline and lidocaine, only 30% of the implant remained. Nevertheless, as one becomes more proficient with ZI implantation technique, deliberate overcorrection should be avoided because it often results in persistent overcorrection (17).

Lesions most amenable to correction with ZI are soft, distensible, superficial defects, and lines. Shallow acne scars, horizontal forehead lines, crow's feet, glabellar lines/furrows, nasolabial lines, accessory nasolabial lines, perioral lines, drool grooves, and the like also respond well (Figs. 7–9).

ZII TECHNIQUE

ZII is a more concentrated form of ZI. It requires greater mechanical force to inject than ZI does and it undergoes less condensation, leaving approximately 60% of the material at the implantation site. It is useful for deep scars and deep glabellar furrows. Additionally, when certain defects expected to respond to ZI do not, ZII can be employed successfully. Owing to its viscous nature, it can be injected only with a 30-gauge needle. Otherwise, techniques for injection with ZII are almost identical to those outlined for ZI.

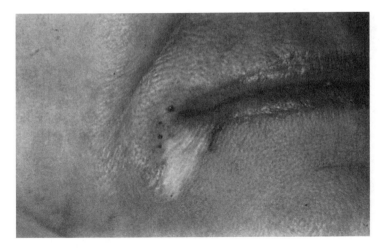

Figure 8
Zyderm I®. Angle of mouth immediately after proper augmentation.

ZP TECHNIQUE

ZP is a robust form of injectable bovine material. Two critical factors—the rigid cross-linked lattice network and the absence of microfibrils—greatly reduce the ability to flow this material if it is placed too superficially (7). Furthermore, the material undergoes little syneresis or condensation upon implantation, so overcorrection with ZP should be avoided. Nevertheless, if ZP is placed too deeply, unnecessarily large amounts of the material will be utilized and the resultant correction will be very short lived. ZP works best

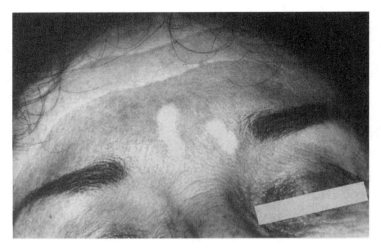

Figure 9
Zyderm I®. Glabellar frown immediately after augmentation.

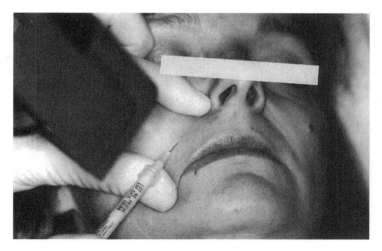

Figure 10
Zyplast® collagen. Note that the material is placed in the mid-dermis going up the nasolabial line. The material is injected medially to the line/fold at a 30° angle.

when placed at a mid-dermal level by means of a 30-gauge needle at a 10° to 20° angle from the skin's surface (Figs. 4 and 10).

As with ZI, the material is deposited serially in small volumes. But with ZP, the injection or flow is in the mid-dermis, below the level where ZI or ZII is placed.

ZP is injected at such a depth that minimal blanching and no beading are observed and the resistance of the dermal matrix is felt against the injecting hand. Indeed, the level of the skin should be seen to rise as the material is implanted, but only to the desired level of correction. It should be said here that some physicians prefer to inject ZP at a 90° angle. If a 90° angle is chosen, only the needle tip should penetrate the skin; again, numerous serial punctures should be utilized to deposit the material at the correct mid-dermal level. We have found it difficult to control the backflow through the injection sites using a 90° angle, particularly in porous sebaceous skin.

While some physicians massage or mold ZP after injection, the value of this practice has not been substantiated and might ultimately result in premature loss of correction as the material is forced into the subdermal space. Finally, the simultaneous-use or "layering" technique—that is, the immediate implanting of ZI over ZP injection sites—can improve both the aesthetic result and the longevity of the response (Figs. 11–14).

Lesions most amenable to correction with ZP include deep nasolabial folds, deep distensible acne scars, and deep drool grooves or "marionette" lines around the mouth. ZP is not recommended for use in the glabellar frown lines because of potential intravascular injection or extravascular compression of branches of the supraorbital/supratrochlear arteries, with resulting ischemia and slough (18).

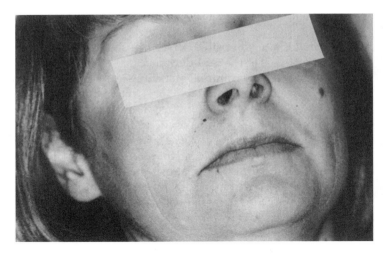

Figure 11
Zyplast® implanted in the right nasolabial fold.

MAINTENANCE OF CORRECTION AND FATE OF IMPLANT

Two to three treatment sessions are usually necessary to achieve an optimal correction. Most corrections will last about three to five months. Glabellar frown lines and acne scars appear to retain correction the longest. Specifically with regard to rhytides, correction appears to persist for period of three to six months.

The variation in longevity could possibly be explained by continued mechanical stress at the treatment site, lesion location, and the patient's

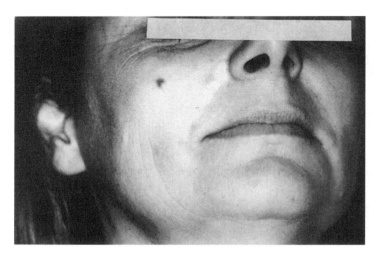

Figure 12
Zyderm® overlay of Zyplast® implanted in the right nasolabial fold.

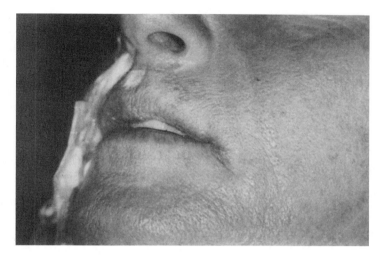

Figure 13
Zyplast® implanted in the right corner of the mouth.

individual response to ZC (10,19,20). Reports of animal studies using ZI and ZP have suggested recipient collagen production after implantation (21,22). This gradual colonization has been most marked with the use of ZP. Additionally, minimal inflammatory reactions and a high degree of biocompatibility have been noted. In humans, histologic studies with both ZI and ZP have also shown excellent biocompatibility with minimal inflammation at sites of implantation. It is interesting that, in humans, ZP implants have demonstrated infiltration of host fibroblasts and production of host collagen (23,24). Nevertheless, there is no convincing

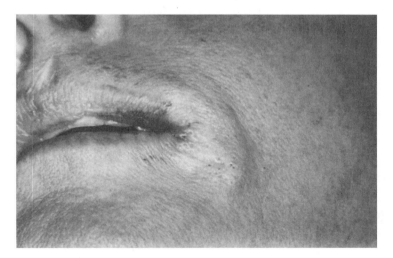

Figure 14
Zyderm® overlay of the Zyplast®-implanted right corner.

evidence in human studies that this collagen production contributes to longevity of either the correction or the interval between treatments. Indeed, correction in humans with all forms of bovine collagen appears to be lost as the material moves from its intradermal site of implantation into the subcutaneous space (25).

Adverse treatment responses of both the hypersensitive and non-hypersensitive variety do occur with bovine collagen implantation, and are fully discussed elsewhere in this text (5,9–12,16,26–32).

LIP AUGMENTATION

The aging process of the mouth is often associated with the development of circumoral radial grooves and a decrease in the volume of the lips themselves. Even a small volumetric increase in the size of the lips in selected individuals can produce a most pleasing cosmetic result. Thus, lip enhancement deals with the size of the lips and, by enhancing their size, the radial grooves. It should be remembered that, while injection into the glabrous skin surrounding the lips is an FDA-approved indication, mucosal injection is an off-label use of injectable collagen. Even though it is expensive, painful, and requires frequent maintenance, lip augmentation still remains the largest single indication for implantable collagen. If a patient is considering this procedure, the treating physician should carefully review the cost and the subject's expectations. While some authors advocate the use of lip blocks in association with injectable augmentation, the anesthesia creates some difficulty in monitoring the lip shape since the anesthetic interferes with the resting muscle tone of the orbicularis oris muscle and the volume of anesthetic used can alter the volume of the skin of the upper lip, making precise correction more difficult. Nevertheless, depending on the patient's pain tolerance, local blocks placed in the buccal mucosal gingival sulcus just at the third incisor on each side, using 0.5 mL of 1% plain lidocaine, will give almost complete anesthesia of the upper lip before significant edema begins to distort the lip architecture.

A review of the procedure of lip augmentation by six investigators revealed that the best results were achieved, by first injecting ZP in the potential space between the lip mucosa and skin (along the vermilion border) in the upper and lower lip (33). This was then followed by injections of ZI and- or ZP directly into the mucosa itself. It is to be remembered that the major vascular supply to the lips runs in the mucosa, and blind injections of ZP into this area will occasionally result in vascular occlusion or compression, especially after the lips are repeatedly treated.

TECHNIQUE OF LIP INJECTION

This is a less painful procedure. First, the ZP must be placed in the potential space of the lip. If submucosal blocks are not used, the patient gently

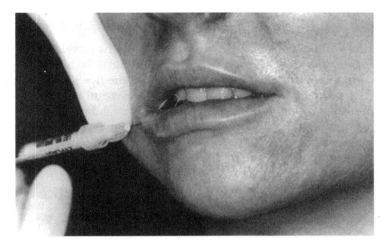

Figure 15
Initiation of a Zyplast® implantation of the right lower lip.

squeezes the nurse's hand, and initial injection is begun at the right corner of the lower lip. While injecting, the lip is held taut with the thumb of the opposing hand slightly stretching the lip posteriorly from the corner of the mouth. Anterior to the opposing thumb, the potential space at the right corner is entered with ZP, utilizing a 30-gauge needle at about 75° angle from the lip surface, with the syringe held perpendicular to the lower lip. Once the treating physician feels the needle tip drop into the potential space, the injection angle is changed to about 45° from the lip, and the flow of material is begun across the lower lip in the potential space (Fig. 15). If a spot is reached where the material will not easily

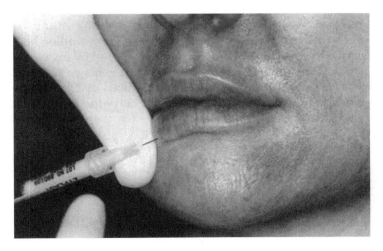

Figure 16
Injecting from a point of resistance with Zyplast®.

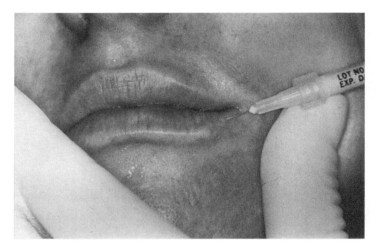

Figure 17
Injecting the left lower lip with Zyplast®.

advance, one should go to this spot and inject onward from this locale (Fig. 16). A smooth yellowish flow of ZP is desired in the potential space, not whitish lumps.

The vermilion potential space of the lower lip should be injected from the right corner to the center and from the left corner to the center (Fig. 17). It is very important to place sufficient ZP in the lateral sites of the lower lip, as this will "lift" the mouth (Fig. 18). In the upper lip, the potential space can be entered as in the lower lip, though some

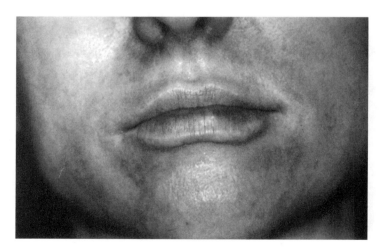

Figure 18
The lower lip immediately after Zyplast® augmentation.

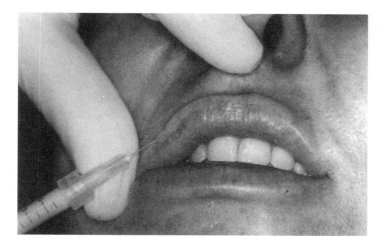

Figure 19
Injecting the right side of the upper lip with Zyplast®.

individuals prefer to enter the space centrally and inject from the center to the left corner and then from the center to the right corner. This latter approach will preserve the patient's natural cupid's bow (Figs. 19 and 20).

Once outlined, the lip can be further enhanced by placing ZP or ZI in the mucosa. Both are placed at this site in a manner similar to that used at other locales. It should be remembered that mucosal injection is an off-label use. It has been this author's experience that, after repeated injections, the augmentation process in the lip begins to "hold," and touch-ups are necessary only two or three times a year.

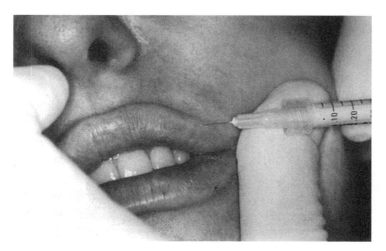

Figure 20
Injecting the left side of the upper lip with Zyplast®.

INJECTABLE BOVINE COLLAGEN (ALTERNATIVE FORMS)

Koken Atelocollagen™ and Resoplast™ are nonfibrillar forms of implantable collagen, but are not approved for use in the United States. While other investigators have found them quite beneficial, there is no experience of them in the United States.

INJECTABLE HUMAN COLLAGEN

The known 3% rate of allergy to bovine collagen implants prompted a search for alternative collagen materials that would perform with profiles similar to the bovine products. In March 2003 INAMED Corp. (which had absorbed Collagen Corporation as part of its acquisition of Mentor Corporation) received FDA approval to market two products, Cosmo-Derm and CosmoPlast, which are derived from a single human fibroblast cell culture line. The process is essentially tissue engineered, with extensive screening for viral and bacterial contamination, with the major advantages being nonanimal based, identical to host collagen, and therefore with no requirement of prior skin testing to eliminate delayed hypersensitivity reactions. The products are otherwise identical to the bovine products in terms of concentration of material. The CosmoDerm has 35 mg/mL of solubilized collagen. The CosmoPlast has 35 mg/mL of solubilized collagen cross-linked with glutaraldehyde, which is thought to slow normal degradation and immunogenicity.

CosmoDerm II, which has a higher concentration of solubilized collagen (65 mg/mL), is awaiting FDA approval at the time of this writing and is comparable to Zyderm II.

The CosmoDerm and CosmoPlast implants are used clinically the same way that Zyderm I and Zyplast are used. Essentially, the Cosmo-Derm is placed into the superficial or papillary dermis; CosmoPlast is placed into the deeper dermis. However, in the author's experience, there are some subtle differences between the comparable bovine and human products in the rheology or flow characteristics of the materials. In particular, the CosmoPlast flows much more readily through the small gauge needles than does Zyplast and, to some degree, appears to retain this malleability for a period of time after injection. Hence, when used in the lips or lip borders, with repetitive puckering some patients have noticed a greater tendency of the material to be massaged superficially into the high dermis. To avoid this, care is usually taken to place the CosmoPlast deep into the dermis or the dermis/subcutaneous junction and patients are cautioned about excessive puckering for the rest of the day. The advantage of the easier flow is that both CosmoDerm and CosmoPlast can be easily injected through 31- or 32-gauge needles, which offer a less traumatic puncture combined with greater control over flow of the material into the desired location.

Given the public's perception of the risk of bovine spongiform encephalopathy, it seems likely that CosmoDerm and CosmoPlast will

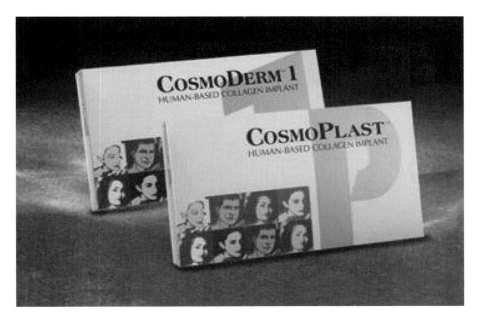

Figure 21
CosmoDerm® 1 and CosmoPlast®.

eventually supplant their bovine cousins, if for no other reason than to eliminate objections to the material in patients' minds. Except for the improved rheology, they will be used in exactly the same manner as their bovine-based analogs.

Other commercial sources of human collagen include cadaveric products such as Dermalogen (Collagenesis, Inc., Beverly, Massachusetts, U.S.), which was removed from the U.S. market for further study in 2003, and Cymetra (Lifecell Corporation, Branchburg, New Jersey, U.S., distributed by OMP, Long Beach, California, U.S.). Cymetra is micronized human collagen fibers harvested from cadaver skin. There is

(A)   **(B)**

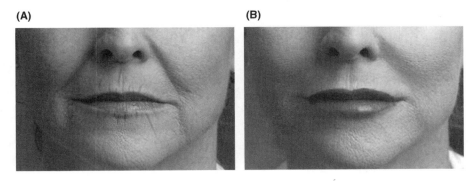

Figure 22
(A) Before and (B) after treatment.

no skin testing required, but the product is in powdered form and requires reconstitution with 1.0 mL of 1% lidocaine prior to injection. The material is injected through large gauge needles (0.5 inch and 1.0 inch 23-gauge needles are provided with the product), and a dermal pocket is usually created under local anesthesia with the needle to receive the implant. The postinjection erythema and edema can be significant. With the appearance of other fillers in the commercial market, the appeal of this cadaver-sourced product appears to be on the wane.

CONCLUSION

Injectable collagens (ZI, ZII, ZP, CosmoDerm, and CosmoPlast) are merely tools provided to a physician to resolve mild contour defects. They are a temporary, biocompatible solution to many, but certainly not to all, soft tissue deficiencies. The adverse reaction profile is of an acceptably low level and indeed only of local significance. Nevertheless, for both the physician and patient to benefit from these agents, effective reproducible implantation techniques must be developed by the treating physician (Figs. 21 and 22).

REFERENCES

1. Knapp TR, Kaplan EN, Daniels JR. Injectable collagen for soft tissue augmentation. Plast Reconstr Surg 1977; 60:398–405.
2. Bulletin Collagen Corporation. Bovine spongiform encephalopathy.
3. Wallace DG, et al. Injectable collagen for tissue augmentation. In: Nimni ME, ed. Collagen Biotechnology. Vol. 3. Boca Raton, Florida: CRC Press, 1988:117–144.
4. McPherson JM, Ledger PW, Sawamura S, Conti A, Wade S, Reihanian H, Wallace DG. The preparation and physiochemical characterization of an injectable form of reconstituted, glutaraldehyde cross-linked, bovine corium collagen. J Biomed Mater Res 1986; 20:79–92.
5. DeLustro F, et al. Immunology of injectable collagen in human subjects. J Dermatol Surg Oncol 1988; 14(suppl 1):49–56.
6. Elson JL. Clinical assessment of Zyplast implant: A year of experience for soft tissue contour correction. J Am Acad Dermatol 1988; 116:707–713.
7. Klein AW. Indications and implantation techniques for the various formulations of injectable collagen. J Dermatol Surg Oncol 1988; 14(suppl 1):27–30.
8. Elson ML. Corrections of dermal contour defects with the injectable collagens: Choosing and using these materials. Semin Dermatol 1987; 6:77–82.
9. Castrow FF II, Krull EA. Injectable collagen implant-update. J Am Acad Dermatol 1983; 9:889–893.
10. Cooperman LS, Mackinnon V, Bechlor G, Pharriss BB. Injectable collagen: A six-year clinical investigation. Aesthetic Plast Surg 1985; 9:145–151.
11. Kamer FM, Churukian MM. The clinical use of injectable collagen: A three-year retrospective study. Arch Otolaryngol 1984; 110:93–98.
12. DeLustro F, Smith ST, Sundsmo J, Salem G, Kincaid S, Ellingsworth L. Reaction to injectable collagen: Results in animal models and clinical use. Plast Reconstr Surg 1987; 79:581–594.
13. Klein AW, Rish DC. Injectable collagen: An adjunct to facial plastic surgery. Facial Plast Surg 1987; 4:87–89.
14. Klein AW. In favor of double testing. J Dermatol Surg Oncol 1989; 15:263.
15. Elson ML. The role of skin testing in the use of collagen injectable materials. J Dermatol Surg Oncol 1989; 15:301–303.
16. Klein AW, Rish DC. Injectable collagen update. J Dermatol Surg Oncol 1984; 10:519–522.
17. Klein AW. Implantation techniques for injectable collagen: Two-and-one half years of personal clinical experience. J Am Acad Dermatol 1983; 9:224–228.
18. Bailin PL, Bailin MD. Collagen implantation: Clinical applications and lesion selection. J Dermatol Surg Oncol 1988; 14(suppl 1):21–26, 74–75.
19. Robinson JK, Hanke CW. Injectable collagen implant: Histopathologic identification and longevity of correction. J Dermatol Surg Oncol 1985; 11:124–130.
20. Bailin MD, Bailin PM. Case studies: Correction of surgical scars, acne scars, and rhytides with Zyderm and Zyplast Implants. J Dermatol Surg Oncol 1988; 14(suppl 1):31–34.
21. Armstrong R, et al. Injectable collagen for soft tissue augmentation. Contemporary Clinical Applications, New Technology and Legal Aspects. Park Ridge, New Jersy: Noyes Publications, 1984:528–536.
22. McPherson JM, Sawamura S, Armstrong S. An examination of the biologic response to injectable, glutaraldehyde cross-linked collagen implants. J Biomed Mater Res 1986; 20:93–103.
23. Kligman AM, Armstrong RC. Histologic response to intradermal Zyderm and Zyplast (glutaraldehyde cross-linked) collagen in humans. J Dermatol Surg Oncol 1986; 12:351–357.

24. Kligman AM. Histologic response to collagen implants in human volunteers: Comparison of Zyderm collagen with Zyplast implant. J Dermatol Surg Oncol 1988; 14(suppl 1):35–38.
25. Stegman SJ, Chu S, Bensen K, Armstrong R. A light and electron microscopic evaluation of Zyderm collagen and Zyplast implants in aging human facial skin: A pilot study. Arch Dermatol 1987; 123:1644–1649.
26. Hanke CW, Higley HR, Jolivette DM, Swanson NA, Stegman SJ. Abscess formation and local necrosis after treatment with Zyderm or Zyplast collagen implant. J Am Acad Dermatol 1991; 25:319–326.
27. McGrew R, et al. Sudden blindness secondary to injection of common drugs in the head and neck, PT 1: Clinical experiences. Otolaryngology 1978; 86:147–151.
28. Siegle RJ, McCoy JP Jr, Schade W, Swanson MA. Intradermal implantation of bovine collagen: Humoral responses associated with clinical reaction. Arch Dermatol 1984; 120:183–187.
29. McCoy JP Jr, Schade WJ, Siegle RJ, Waldinger TP, Vanderveen EE, Swanson NA. Characterization of the humoral immune response to bovine collagen implants. Arch Dermatol 1985; 121:990–994.
30. Cooperman LS, Michaeli D. The immunogenicity of injectable collagen, Pt 2: A retrospective review of seventy-two tested and treated patients. J Dermatol Surg Oncol 1984; 10:647–651.
31. Ellingsworth LR, Delustro F, Brennan JE, Sawamura S, McPherson J. The human immune response to reconstituted bovine collagen. J Immunol 1986; 136:877–882.
32. DeLustro F, Dasch J, Keefe J, Ellingsworth L. Immune response to allogeneic and xenogeneic implants of collagen and collagen derivatives. Clin Orthop 1990; 260:263–279.
33. Klein AW, Brandt FD, Grekin DA, Harvey RA, Mittleman H. Collagen implants for lip augmentation. (Unpublished study).

5
Hylaform®

Ellen Gendler
Ronald O. Perelman Department of Dermatology,
New York University Medical Center, New York, New York, U.S.A.

INTRODUCTION

Physicians in many surgical specialties, including ophthalmology, orthopedics, dermatology, and plastic surgery, require space-filling substances for some of the procedures that they perform. Several materials have been used in the past in soft tissue augmentation procedures, including paraffin, silicone, and collagen (1,2). However, paraffin and silicone have been found to produce severe foreign body reactions and are known to migrate from the injection site. Collagen has several drawbacks when used as a filler material in these procedures, not the least of which is rapid degradation, leading to frequent reinjection to maintain the desired effect. Infrequent but significant hypersensitivity reactions have been noted with the use of collagen, requiring the physician to perform allergy testing prior to the use of this material in surgery (3,4). Physicians should be aware of the limitations of each of these materials when making decisions about augmentation procedures; these limitations also include product cost and longevity.

A new substance—hyaluronic acid (hyaluronan)—has been studied over the past ten years for its potential utility in these fields (5). A natural polysaccharide component of connective tissue, hyaluronic acid is produced by various cell types within the cell membrane. Hyaluronic acid is stored in the extracellular spaces; its functions include space filling, structure stabilization, and cell protection (6,7). It also has superb biocompatibility and interesting malleable physical properties because of the viscoelastic matrices and high water content (greater than 99%). There appears to be a direct correlation between the water content of the skin and the level of hyaluronic acid in dermal tissue; findings have suggested a relationship between youthful-looking skin and the presence of a hydrated, viscoelastic hyaluronic acid network in the dermal intercellular matrix (8,9).

Hyaluronan's biologic functions derive from the interaction between the linear, unbranched, polyanionic polysaccharide chains.

The high molecular weight (4–5 million) is reflected in its composition of repeating dimers of glucuronic acid and *N*-acetyl glucosamine (10,11). These complicated polysaccharide chains form random coils that entangle at low concentrations, creating the viscoelastic effects seen with hyaluronic acid products.

It is important to note that hyaluronan has the same chemical and molecular properties in all mammalian species; it is possible to use animal-derived hyaluronan in humans without the danger of foreign body reactions (12–14). Despite this favorable use profile, hyaluronan has a short half-life (1–2 days) in almost all connective tissues of the body. In this form, hyaluronic acid does not have sufficient resistance to breakdown for use in soft tissue augmentation procedures.

"Hylans," a group of substances produced by introducing sulfonyl-bis-ethyl cross-links between hydroxyl groups of the polysaccharide chains of hyaluronan, are viscoelastic, water-insoluble gels that retain the biocompatibility and biologic properties of hyaluronan. This network of complex cross-linked chains has a superior residence time in dermal tissue, with hylan B implants still evident at up to one year after the implant procedure (15). Various hylans are presently used for joint supplementation (16,17), to influence wound healing and regenerative processes in soft connective tissues (18,19), and as delivery vehicles for therapeutic agents (20). Hylans can be prepared as water-soluble solutions or water-insoluble gels, enabling design specificity for each intended indication.

One formulation of hyaluronan currently in use for soft tissue augmentation procedures is hylan B gel (Hylaform®; Genzyme Biosurgery, Cambridge, Massachusetts, U.S.). This product is under clinical investigation in the United States, but it is marketed in Europe, Canada, and Australia by INAMED Corporation (Santa Barbara, California, U.S.) as a dermal filler for the treatment of facial lines, wrinkles, and scars.

PRECLINICAL STUDIES

Immunologic Studies

The potential for hylan gel to generate an immunologic (humoral or cellular) response has been evaluated in experimental animals. Larsen et al. (12) studied the effects of hylan B gel injected intradermally or subdermally into mice, noting only minimal inflammation when tissue samples were evaluated at 24-hours postinjection. When additional mice were evaluated over a seven-week period, no significant cellular reaction was noted. Radioactive hylan gel was injected intradermally in guinea pigs, producing only a mild tissue reaction at seven days postinjection (12). Measurements at two and four weeks after injection showed only a slight decrease in radioactivity, indicating a low level of tissue reaction to the injected material.

Additional studies were performed to measure antibody production following Hylaform injection (12). Rabbits received repeated (over 12 weeks) intramuscular injections of Hylaform. Serum was collected from these animals periodically over the 12-week study period and was evaluated using an enzyme-linked immunosorbent assay procedure; the animals developed no antibodies to Hylaform during the study. Hylan gel was placed intravitreally in owl monkeys; over a three-year follow-up period, antihylan gel antibodies were not found when animals were tested using a passive cutaneous anaphylaxis assay.

In Vitro Studies

Hylaform has been found to be nonmutagenic, nontoxic, nonhemolytic, and nonthrombogenic when tested using in vitro methods (21).

In Vivo Studies

Hylaform has been found in several animal models to be nontoxic and biocompatible; a wide range of doses in several tissue compartments (intramuscular, intravitreal, intraperitoneal, intradermal, intra-articular, and subcutaneous) have been investigated (21–24). Study of the tissue sites of subcutaneous and intradermal injections of Hylaform indicates that there were no clinical or histologic differences from saline-injected sites, and that there were no associated inflammatory or fibrotic responses in the hylan-treated areas (21).

Animal reproductive studies, and evaluations of fetal and neonatal development indicated that Hylaform did not pose a hazard in terms of reproductive potential and development of offspring (documents on file, Genzyme Biosurgery, Cambridge, Massachusetts, U.S.).

DERMAL IMPLANT STUDIES

Preclinical investigation of the effect of hylan, specifically the determination of the product's residence time in dermal tissues, was pursued using a guinea pig model and radiolabeled Hylaform (25). Animals received intradermal injections of radiolabeled Hylaform; injection sites were harvested immediately after injection, or at 1, 4, 12, or, 24 weeks postinjection. Tissues specimens were analyzed for radioisotope concentration versus initial dose and a histological evaluation of the injection site was performed. Analysis of specimen radioactivity levels indicated that a mean of 77% of the original radiolabel was still present at the site of the injection when evaluated at 24 weeks postinjection. Linear regression analysis of the data indicated that Hylaform had an estimated half-life of 12.2 months in tissue. Radioactivity was not detected in the other organs of the animals at any point during the study, and histologic evaluation of the injection site showed no significant tissue reaction (no significant inflammation or fibrosis).

Additional guinea pigs were followed for up to 52 weeks after receiving intradermal or subcutaneous injections of Hylaform or collagen, with tissues collected periodically (25). At all evaluation times after the injection (from three days postinjection to 52 weeks postinjection), Hylaform was present in the tissue. This compared favorably with the findings from the collagen injection sites; most collagen had been digested at 26 weeks after the procedure, and all collagen was undetectable by the 52-week time point. The tissue reaction to Hylaform included minimal-to-mild inflammation that resolved by the 26-week time point, unlike the reaction to collagen, where the minimal-to-mild inflammation increased over time. These guinea pig dermal implant study results, with favorable biocompatibility and efficacy results, further reinforce the potential for use of Hylaform in soft tissue augmentation procedures.

SOFT TISSUE AUGMENTATION IN HUMANS

Plastic surgeons and dermatologists familiar with soft tissue augmentation procedures participated in a multicenter, open-label, 12-month study using Hylaform (21). Healthy patients with up to four cutaneous sites amenable to therapy were entered into the study. Wrinkles and folds in those facial areas that have responded to other agents, notably the glabellar lines, nasolabial folds, and other facial lines of expression, were chosen for treatment.

Intradermal Hylaform injections were performed to a maximum of four sites per patient. Touch-up injections were performed at the week 2 or week 4 visits at the discretion of the physician if the level of correction was less than 80%. At each follow-up visit (weeks 2, 4, 6, 12, 18, 24, 36, and 52), photographs were taken to document the changes in the injection sites. The physician assessed the degree of correction and the patient evaluated the overall impressions of improvement during each follow-up visit. Adverse local or systemic reactions not anticipated following typical soft tissue augmentation procedures were documented at each visit.

Of the 216 patients included in the trial, 39 discontinued study participation before the end of the 12-month follow-up period, leaving a long-term evaluable population of 177 study subjects with 724 sites that had been treated with Hylaform. Wrinkles and folds made up 86% of the treated sites, while the remaining sites included scars derived from acne, trauma, or other causes. The mean total volume of Hylaform injected per site was 0.32 mL. Touch-up injections were performed for 70% of the sites, with an average of 1.9 Hylaform injections per site.

Treatment success has been defined as 60% or more of the injection sites showing a 33% improvement over the baseline evaluation. Through week 18, all sites met this criterion (based on the physician evaluation of degree of correction). Significant improvements were still seen at 12 months after the initial Hylaform injection, with a more lasting positive effect seen for scars than for wrinkles or folds. Using linear regression analysis of the degree of correction by facial location and type of defect, treatment of wrinkles and folds showed mean effectiveness of 22 weeks versus 23 weeks for scar correction. This difference has been seen with other soft tissue augmentation materials, and it is thought that the effectiveness of the procedure is due to the superior retention matrix of scar tissue. Forehead and cheek augmentation lasted longer than nasolabial folds; it has been hypothesized that success with augmentation of these areas is because of the fact that they are not subject to the constant muscular action of facial expressions. Adverse reactions to the injections were minimal, transient, and were those typically seen with any soft tissue augmentation procedure, including mild erythema, swelling, and pain. More severe reactions occurred in less than 2% of the patient population and included persistent erythema, development of acneiform lesions, and ecchymosis. No immunologic responses were documented at any time during the study.

The published literature contains only a few references to the biocompatibility/immunologic response of patients to treatment using hyaluronic acid products in soft tissue augmentation procedures. Duranti et al. (26) reported their findings with Restylane® (Q-Med, Uppsala, Sweden), a hyaluronic acid gel produced by microbiologic engineering techniques. One hundred and fifty-eight patients underwent treatment for augmentation therapy of wrinkles, folds, or lip recontouring with markedly satisfying results. However, 12.5% of their patients had localized, transient adverse events reported postoperatively. Lowe et al. (27) reported a slight incidence of delayed inflammatory skin reaction to both Hylaform and Restylane, which started at eight weeks after injection; with 709 patients treated, only 0.4% of the patients developed a delayed reaction to the products. Lupton and Alster (28) described a granulomatous response to Restylane in one patient after the third injection to the nasolabial folds.

CONCLUSIONS

Preclinical and clinical studies have provided substantial evidence that Hylaform is a safe and effective material for use in soft tissue augmentation procedures. Patients do not require pretreatment skin testing, thus minimizing concerns regarding biocompatibility and allergy. Clinical results indicate that Hylaform performs as well as or better than soft tissue augmentation materials that are currently available. In addition, Hylaform Plus (with a larger particle size) is useful as a deeper filler in the nasolabial folds and in the vermilion border of the lip, with Hylaform or Hylaform Fine Line (smaller particle size) layered on top.

A new, double-blind study has recently been completed for submission to the Food and Drug Administration. In this study, only nasolabial folds were injected with either Hylaform or Zyplast. Because of its ease of injection, versatility, excellent safety profile, and high level of patient acceptance, Hylaform is poised to become a leader in the soft tissue augmentation market in the United States.

REFERENCES

1. Knapp TR, Kaplan EN, Daniels JR. Injectable collagen for soft tissue augmentation. Plast Reconstr Surg 1977; 60:398–405.
2. Selmanowitz VJ, Orentreich N. Medical-grade fluid silicone. A monographic review. J Dermatol Surg Oncol 1977; 3:597–611.
3. Fagien S. Autologous collagen injections to treat deep glabellar furrows. Plast Reconstr Surg 1994; 93:642.
4. Ford CN, Staskowski PA, Bless DM. Autologous collagen vocal fold injection: A preliminary clinical study. Laryngoscope 1995; 105:944–948.
5. Balazs EA, Denlinger JL. Clinical uses of hyaluronan. In: Evered D, Whelan J, eds. The Biology of Hyaluronan. Chichester, England: Wiley, 1989:265–280.
6. Balazs EA. Intercellular matrix of connective tissue. In: Finch CE, Hayflick L, eds. Handbook of the Biology of Aging. New York: Van Nostrand Reinhold, 1977:22–240.
7. Comper WD, Laurent TC. Physiological function of connective tissue polysaccharides. Physiol Rev 1978; 58:255–315.
8. Balazs EA, Gibbs DA. The rheological properties and biological function of hyaluronic acid. In: Balazs EA, ed. Chemistry and Molecular Biology of the Intercellular Matrix. Vol. 3. New York: Academic Press, 1970:1241–1254.
9. Yates JR. In: Eden NR, ed. Mechanism of Water Uptake by Skin. New York: John Wiley & Sons, 1971:485.
10. Balazs EA, Denlinger JL, Leshchiner E, Band P, Larsen N, Leshchiner A, Morales B. Hylan: Hyaluronan derivatives for soft-tissue repair and augmentation. Biotech USA 1988; 442–445.
11. Balazs EA, Leshchiner EA. Hyaluronan, its cross-linked derivative, hylan, and their medical applications. In: Inagaki H, Phillips GO, eds. Cellulosics Utilization: Research and Rewards in Cellulosics. New York: John Wiley & Sons, 1989:265–280.
12. Larsen NE, Pollak CT, Reiner K, Leshchiner E, Balazs EA. Hylan gel biomaterial: dermal and immunologic compatibility. J Biomed Mater Res 1993; 27:1129–1134.
13. Richter W. Nonimmunogenicity of purified hyaluronic acid preparations tested by passive cutaneous anaphylaxis. Int Arch Allergy Immunol 1974; 47:211–217.
14. Richter W, Ryde E, Zetterstrom EO. Nonimmunogenicity of purified sodium hyaluronate preparation in man. Int Arch Allergy Immunol 1979; 59:45–48.
15. Piacquadio D, Jarcho M, Goltz R. Evaluation of Hylan B gel as a soft-tissue augmentation implant material. J Am Acad Dermatol 1997; 36:544–549.
16. Adams ME, Atkinson MH, Lussier AJ, Schulz JI, Siminovitch KA, Wade JP, Zummer M. The role of viscosupplementation with hylan G-F 20 (Synvisc) in the treatment of osteoarthritis of the knee: a Canadian multicenter trial comparing hylan G-F 20 alone, hylan G-F 20 with nonsteroidal anti-inflammatory drugs (NSAIDs), and NSAIDs alone. Osteoarthritis Cartilage 1995; 3:213–225.
17. Goorman SD, Watanabe TK, Miller EH, Perry C. Functional outcome in knee osteoarthritis after treatment with hylan G-F-20: a prospective study. Arch Phys Med Rehabil 2000; 81:479–483.
18. Burns JW. Prevention of post-surgical adhesion formation with sodium hyaluronate-based products. Wound Healing III, Orlando, FL, January 20–21, 1992.
19. Weiss C, Dennis J, Suros JM, Denlinger JL, Badia A, Montane I. Sodium hylan for the prevention of postlaminectomy scar formation. Orthopedic Research Society 35th Annual Meeting, Las Vegas, Nevada, February 6–9, 1989.
20. Gurny R, Ibrahim H, Aebi A, Buri P, Wilson CG, Washington N, Edman P, Camber O. Design and evaluation of controlled release systems for the eye. J Control Release 1987; 6:367–373.

21. Piacquadio DJ, Larsen NE, Denlinger JL, Balazs EA. Hylan B gel (Hylaform) as a soft tissue augmentation material. In: Klein AW, ed. Tissue Augmentation in Clinical Practice: Procedures and Techniques. New York: Marcel Dekker, 1998:269–291.

22. Pozo MA, Balazs EA, Belmonte C. Reduction of sensory responses to passive movements in inflamed knee joints by hylan, a hyaluronan derivative. Exp Brain Res 1997; 116:3–9.

23. Auer JA, Fackelman GE, Gingerich DA, Fetter AW. Effect of hyaluronic acid in naturally occurring and experimentally induced osteoarthritis. Am J Vet Res 1980; 41:568–574.

24. Butler J, Rydell NW, Balazs EA. Hyaluronic acid in synovial fluid. IV. Effect of intra-articular injection of hyaluronic acid on the clinical symptoms of arthritis in track horses. Acta Vet Scand 1970; 11:139–155.

25. Larsen NE, Leshchiner E, Pollak CT, Balazs EA, Piacquadio E. Evaluation of Hylan B (hylan gel) as soft tissue dermal implants. In: Mikos AG, Leong KW, Radomsky ML, Tamada JA, Yaszemski MJ, eds. Polymers in Medicine and Pharmacy (Proceedings of the Materials Research Society Spring Meeting, San Francisco, CA, April 17–21, 1995). Pittsburgh: Materials Research Society, 1995:193–197.

26. Duranti F, Salti G, Bovani B, Calandra M, Rosati ML. Injectable hyaluronic acid gel for soft tissue augmentation. A clinical and histological study. Dermatol Surg 1998; 24:1317–1325.

27. Lowe JN, Maxwell CA, Lowe P, Duick MG, Shah K. Hyaluronic acid skin fillers: adverse reactions and skin testing. J Am Acad Dermatol 2001; 45:930–933.

28. Lupton Jr, Alster TS. Cutaneous hypersensitivity reaction to injectable hyaluronic acid gel. Dermatol Surg 2000; 26:135–137.

6

Subcutaneous Incisionless (Subcision) Surgery for the Correction of Depressed Scars and Wrinkles

David S. Orentreich and Anna-Sophia Leone
Orentreich Medical Group, LLP, New York, New York, U.S.A.

A complex problem confronts the skin surgeon who attempts to correct depressed scars and wrinkles. In light of the various causes, the anatomy of depressed areas, the type of patient, and the response of the patient to past or current trauma and/or surgery, it is unlikely that one treatment modality will successfully improve all depressions. Therefore, the greater the number of treatment options available, the more likely the surgeon will be in obtaining successful correction.

The use of injectable soft tissue–augmenting implants has grown in both frequency and type; however, there is no one ideal, readily available injectable augmentation agent. Existing materials have one or more disadvantages, including lack of persistence, risk of allergic reactions (1,2), localized tissue necrosis (1), and amaurosis (3,4). Other procedures, such as lipoinjection and autologous collagen injection require additional surgery at the harvesting sites. Other materials, such as liquid injectable silicone, are currently under U.S. Food and Drug Administration (FDA)- investigational study, as are hylauronic acid and polymethyl methacrylate.

The shortcomings of currently available materials coupled with the knowledge that bound-down defects will not respond ideally to fillers have spurred the ongoing development of techniques to correct depressed scars, wrinkles, and contours. The term "subcision" (5) describes a unique form of incisionless, local subcuticular undermining. The word subcision is a contraction of "subcutaneous incisionless" surgery; it is and a method that involves cutting under a depressed scar, wrinkle, or contour using a tri-beveled hypodermic needle (now standard on most disposable needles) inserted under the skin through a needle puncture. The procedure attempts to raise the base of the defect to the level of the surrounding skin surface. The integrity of the skin surface is minimally compromised, just as with a routine needle puncture.

The effectiveness of subcision for correcting various types of skin depressions depends on two distinct phenomena. First, the act of surgically releasing the skin from its attachment to deeper tissues results in skin elevation. Second, the introduction of a controlled trauma initiates wound healing with consequent formation of connective tissue, resulting in augmentation of the depressed site.

To the best of our knowledge, the use of subcuticular undermining to improve scars and wrinkles without the additional benefit of injectable augmenting agents was first reported by the authors in 1995 in the *Journal of Dermatologic Surgery* (6). In 1957, Spangler (7) reported using a Bowman iris needle to cut the fibrous strands beneath deeply depressed facial scars, prior to injecting fibrin foam into the resulting cavity. In 1977, Gottlieb (8) pursued this approach, eventually leading to the development of Fibrel® (Fibrel was purchased by Mentor Corporation in 1989 and was discontinued in 1996 for business reasons) (9). The Fibrel kit was equipped with a 20-gauge needle used to undermine fibrotic, depressed scars. Undermining created a pocket in the dermis into which the Fibrel was injected (10). However, the studies evaluating Fibrel's efficacy did not include positive controls, i.e., fibrotic scars treated by undermining alone (2,9). In 1989, Koranda (11) reported the treatment of bound-down, acne "crater" scars by inserting a No. 69 Beaver blade through a stab incision in the skin, sweeping through the scar tissue under the "crater," and allowing for clot formation followed by fibrosis to maintain the elevation. In 1992, Hambley and Carruthers (12) used an 18-gauge needle inserted through the skin to release depressed, bound-down, full-thickness skin grafts on the nose prior to microlipoinjection. Again, no positive controls were reported.

It is possible that a majority of the long-term benefits derived from fibrin foam (13), Fibrel (1), or lipoinjection (1) after undermining, may occur, not primarily as a result of the implant substance that is eventually absorbed, but rather as a consequence of connective tissue formation resulting from the preinjection undermining intended to create a pocket for the implant.

A review of the literature shows recommendations by physicians and at least one manufacturer (LifeCellMedical) to perform subcision prior to injection of augmenting agents, similar to Gottlieb's technique. Caution is urged in following such a approach, as there is potential for tissue necrosis when combining subcision with injectable fillers. The mechanism is not clear; however, it is possible that the filler acts as a barrier to oxygen and blood diffusion, thereby jeopardizing the viability of the skin overlying the subcised areas particularly in smokers. If subcision cannot be performed separately, it is prudent to avoid overcorrection with the injectable filler. By ensuring that there is no tension, pressure, or compression on the edge of the wound, the potential for tissue necrosis is decreased.

Subcision corrects depressed defects through two mechanisms. The first is the surgical act of cutting under and releasing the tethered, bound-down site; the second is the formation of new connective tissue.

The first mechanism is exemplified by cutting through the scar tissue under depressed, bound-down scars. In comparison, subcising facial wrinkles releases the skin from its fibromuscular attachments to deeper tissue. These attachments include those of the muscles of facial expression that insert into the overlying skin (14), unlike skeletal muscles that have no such attachments. In addition, numerous fibrous septa connect the superficial musculoaponeurotic system (SMAS), a broad, fibrous fascia enveloping and linking the muscles of facial expression to the overlying dermis (14). The SMAS transmits the mimetic muscular contractions that create facial expressions and, with repetition, result in facial wrinkles that form at right angles to the direction of muscle contraction.

The second corrective mechanism is the creation of controlled trauma to promote new connective tissue formation under the defect in the course of wound healing. After a subcision procedure, wound healing begins with a vascular response, then with subsequent phases of inflammation, granulation tissue formation, and fibroplasia. Surface re-epithelialization is essentially absent because subcision only minimally involves the epidermis. Ground substance is produced and collagen synthesis (peaking at 6–7 days) continues for two to four weeks (15). Finally, long-term collagen remodeling occurs. Collagen production is possibly influenced by physical factors such as location and tension (16). This, in part, may explain the occasional appearance of a localized hypertrophic reaction following subcision (see sequelae below). The degree of response to subcision varies with each patient's response to wounding.

The physiologic consequences of subcision demonstrate that the releasing action and the associated wound-healing process can, in many instances, be harnessed to correct distensile and bound-down skin depressions without the need for injectable augmentation agents.

TECHNIQUE

Subcision surgery uses standard, readily available, and inexpensive materials. A sterile, disposable, 1-inch, 22- or 27-gauge, hypodermic B-D® needle suffices for most cases; however, needles of different lengths and gauges are also useful. Close inspection reveals that these needles are tri-beveled to enhance their ability to puncture skin with minimal resistance (Fig. 1). During subcision, the sharp edges are manipulated while under the skin to cut subsurface tissue. Needles as large as 16-gauge may be used to treat cellulite and large, bound-down scars such as healed, surgical drain sites. Needles of 25- to 27-gauge (and even 30-gauge) can be used on particularly small, superficial facial scars and wrinkles, although care must be taken not to bend the finer caliber needles.

Areas to be subcised are first cleansed to remove dirt and cosmetic residue. Overhead lighting is adjusted to delineate, fully and precisely, the depressions, which are then outlined with a marking pen and subsequently anesthetized, typically with a 2% lidocaine with 1:100,000 epinephrine solution. Epinephrine is not used when contraindicated.

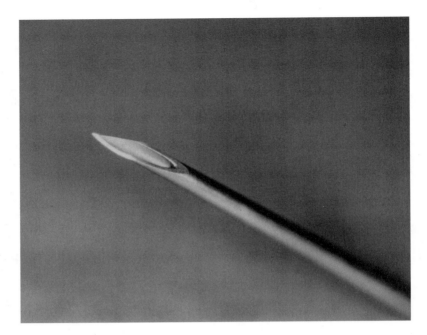

Figure 1
Tribeveled hypodermic needle. Note its sharp edges.

A eutectic mixture of local anesthetic (EMLA) cream may be used to produce topical analgesia prior to anesthetic injection. Local anesthesia should extend for several millimeters beyond the border of a marked area to ensure a pain-free entry of the subcision needle.

How one holds the subcision needle is a matter of personal preference, influenced by the needle size and the treatment site. Generally, one either grasps the needle by its hub, or clamps the needle in a needle holder.

After sufficient time has elapsed for maximal vasoconstriction, a needle of chosen gauge is inserted a few millimeters from the depressed site and advanced underneath it. The bevel is oriented upward on insertion, and the angle of insertion is acute. The entry point into the skin acts as a pivot about which the needle is moved. The sharp edges of the tribeveled needle tip are maneuvered to cut under the skin surface. The free hand acts as a guide to subcision and is used as and when needed to pinch, stretch, or stabilize the treatment site. If the needle is shorter than the full length of the wrinkle or scar, multiple puncture sites are chosen depending on the size and shape of the depression.

The term "lancing" subcision describes a simple, linear inserting and withdrawing movement of the needle; this technique may be used under "crows's feet" wrinkles or when subcising very fibrotic scars (Fig. 2A).

"Horizontal fanning" subcision involves moving the needle, bevel-side up, in a horizontal plane, from side to side, back and forth, while inserting and withdrawing it in a fan-like motion (Fig. 2B). After insertion,

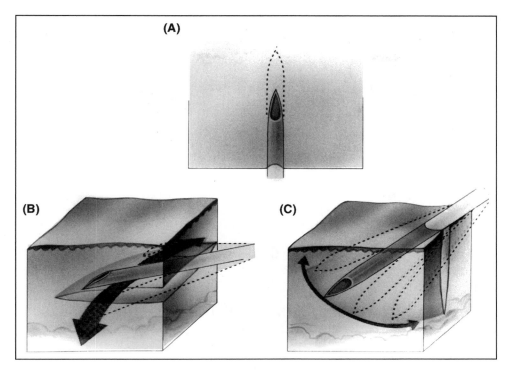

Figure 2
(**A**) Lancing subcision denotes inserting and withdrawing movements. (**B**) Horizontal fanning subcision denotes side-to-side movements. Note that the bevel is facing upward. (**C**) Vertical subcision denotes cutting in a plane that is perpendicular to the skin surface. Note that the bevel is oriented vertically.

the bevel may be turned vertically to cut in a plane that is perpendicular to the skin surface when withdrawing the needle. This is termed "vertical" subcision (Fig. 2C). When used on wrinkles, vertical subcision cuts at a right angle across superficially situated facial muscle fibers, thereby hampering the muscle's ability to wrinkle the skin.

Direct, manual pressure is applied by a medical assistant or the patient immediately after a site is treated, and pressure is maintained for several minutes to obtain hemostasis. Antibiotics are not usually prescribed unless there is a particular indication. Patients may apply makeup or Micropore® tape to camouflage bruised areas.

Subcision is performed at precise, predetermined depths to ensure optimal results. The depth chosen depends on the indication, the location of tethering structures, and the local microanatomy.

When treating depressed, bound-down scars, subcision is usually performed in the mid- to deep-dermis. Cutting through the fibrous bands of scar tissue permits the skin surface to elevate (Fig. 3). To correct distensile, depressed scars, subcision is usually performed in the deep dermis or subdermally.

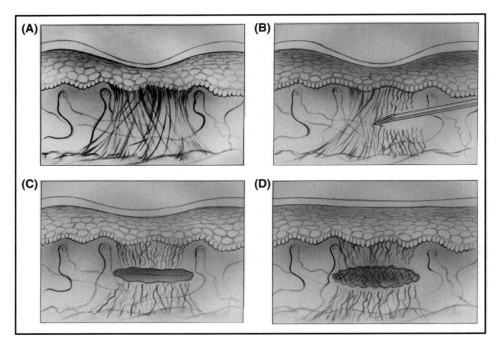

Figure 3
Treatment of bound-down scars. (**A**) Fibrous bands tether down scar surfaces. (**B**) subcision of the tethered scar releases the depressed area. (**C**) Extravasated blood collects in the subcision wound. (**D**) The wound heals with formation of new connective tissue, which further augments the depressed areas.

When treating facial expression lines, subcision is subdermal in order to release facial muscle fibers and SMAS insertions into the dermis (Fig. 4). Small, superficial wrinkles (such as those radiating from the lateral canthus or from the vermilion border) may be treated with upper-dermal, mid-dermal, or subdermal subcision depending on wrinkle morphology and the patient's response to previous subcision.

The dimpled appearance of skin on the upper legs and buttocks, commonly known as "cellulite," is partially caused by fibrous septa arising from the deep fascia investing skeletal muscles, traversing the adipose layer, and inserting into skin, thereby tethering it. These fibrous septa can be divided by subcision in the adipose layer.

Because the ability of individuals to form collagen varies, it is not possible to predict precisely how many subcision treatments will be needed for any given defect. In general, subcision is not a single treatment. The approximate number of subcision treatments required to correct a specific depression depends on variables such as the type of depression (Table 1), its location, the patient's wound-healing response, and the intensity of each treatment. Three to six visits suffice for the

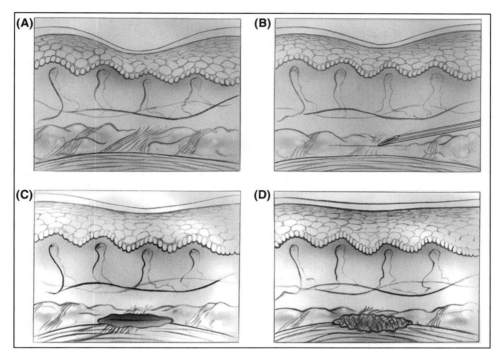

Figure 4
Treatment of wrinkles. (**A**) Mimetic muscle fibers and fibrous septa from the SMAS insert directly into the dermis. (**B**) The needle is maneuvered to release insertions from facial muscles and SMAS. (**C**) Extravasated blood collects in the subcision wound. (**D**) The wound heals with formation of new connective tissue, which further augments the depressed areas.

majority of cases of moderate wrinkling or scarring. Additional visits to treat other depressed sites and to re-treat partially elevated sites (or treat a hypertrophic site) are scheduled at intervals of about one month. Usually, a one-month interval between subcision treatments allows sufficient time for bruising and swelling to resolve and for connective

Table 1
Indications for Subcision

Depressed distensile scars	Depressed, bound-down scars
Acne	Acne (excluding deep, ice-pick scars)
Traumatic	Varicella
Surgical	Traumatic
Anetoderma	Surgical (e.g., healed drain site)
	Wrinkles
	Depressed contours (e.g., malar groove)
	Cellulite dimples

tissue formation to plateau. Longer intervals delay, but do not diminish, the quality of the end result.

During the first session, it is prudent to limit the number and intensity of the subcision until the patient's response is established. On subsequent visits, more or less intensive subcision may be performed, depending on the patient's previous response. Generally, deeply depressed sites require more intensive subcision carried out over more treatment sessions.

Certain anatomical locations, including areas of increased skin tension may have a greater propensity for fibroplasia (16); therefore, these areas are treated less intensively, particularly during initial sessions. The periorbital, glabellar, labial commissure, and upper lip areas are among those that appear to have a greater propensity for hypertrophic reactions in response to subcision.

Although scar correction is generally permanent, wrinkles may deepen or re-form with time. Patients are advised that follow-up treatments at 6- to 12-month intervals may be needed to correct either new or recurring areas of wrinkling.

While the majority of wrinkles and depressions are amenable to treatment with injectable fillers, a bound-down wrinkle such as a nasolabial fold or depression should be approached cautiously. Optimal correction with fillers depends on a variety of factors, including tissue distensibility. Nondistensible or minimally distensible depressions may result in tissue elevation, worsening the appearance of the depression.

The patient in figure (x) is shown with facial muscles relaxed. Upon palpation, it was determined that the nasolabial fold was bound down, with little tissue distensibility. This patient is a candidate for subcision rather than injectable fillers. If adequate correction is not achieved with subcision alone, the use of injectable fillers may be reconsidered once the fibrous connections have been released. This concept should also be applied to bound-down scars and depressions.

The appearance of muscle engagement is noted despite the facial muscles being relaxed, and the V-shaped appearance of the base of the fold, as opposed to a U-shaped curve. The V-shaped fold is more likely to indicate a bound-down wrinkle. A softer, U-shaped wrinkle is less likely to be bound down. When in doubt, a sterile saline solution may be injected to test distensibility.

CASES

Case 1

A 43-year-old man underwent subcision of horizontal forehead wrinkles (Fig. 5A). Three sessions were performed over a three-month period. The areas were prepared as described. A 22-gauge, 1-inch needle was used. Other than the expected bruising, there were no sequelae. Follow-up examination and a photograph four months after the last session revealed satisfactory improvement (Fig. 5B).

(A)   **(B)**

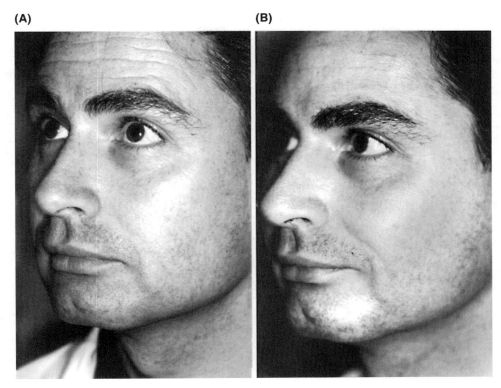

Figure 5
Case 1. (**A**) A 43-year-old man with forehead wrinkles before treatment.
(**B**) Follow-up examination four months after the last of three sessions of
subcision reveals satisfactory improvement.

Case 2

A 21-year-old woman presented with a depressed, bound-down, varicella
scar, approximately 4 mm in diameter, on the left tip of her nose (Fig. 6A).
The area was prepared as described, and a 22-gauge needle was used to
perform subcision. Follow-up at ten days showed one small comedo,
which was expressed, and one incipient acneiform lesion, which was
incised and drained. The photograph at one month post-subcision
shows nearly complete correction (Fig. 6B).

Case 3

A 42-year-old woman presented with three bound-down scars between
10 and 15 mm in length on the lower abdomen (Fig. 7A). The scars
resulted from drains inserted at the time of abdominal surgery five years
previously. The areas were treated with one session of subcision using a
22-gauge, 1-inch needle. Follow-up at ten weeks showed substantial
correction (Fig. 7B).

(A)   (B)

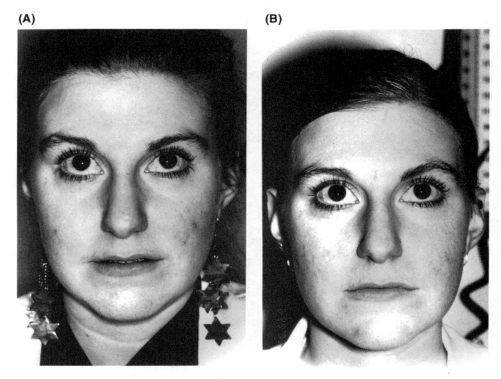

Figure 6
Case 2. (**A**) A 21-year-old woman before Subcision to correct a varicella scar on
left tip of nose. (**B**) One month after subcision with nearly complete correction.

CONTRAINDICATIONS AND SEQUELAE

The only known contraindication to subcision is active infection, at or
immediately adjacent to the site to be treated. Deep ice-pick scars will
not respond well to subcision; punch grafting is usually preferred (16).

There are three relative contraindications. Although depressed,
atrophic scars may be successfully raised to normal skin level but the
appearance of the surface remains atrophic. Nevertheless, correction by
subcision may be preferable to excision or grafting.

Patients with bleeding diathesis should be treated conservatively.

Any previous history of keloid scarring after trauma or surgery
should prompt the physician to consider the possibility of keloid
formation, and a carefully chosen test site may be subcised.

Sequelae. Ecchymosis, edema, erythema, and tenderness are normal
consequences.

Infection. Occasionally, localized acneiform, cyst-like lesions are
observed. It is likely that subcutaneous disruption of the pilosebaceous
apparatus is responsible for these lesions. These lesions respond to

(A)

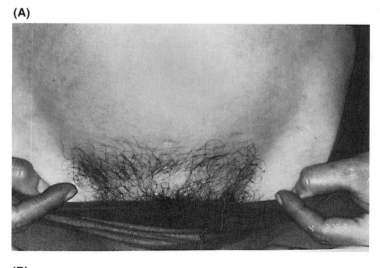

(B)

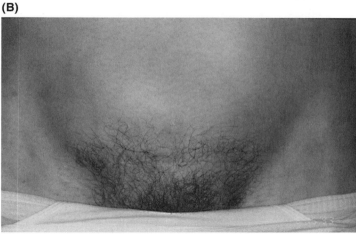

Figure 7

Case 3. (**A**) A 42-year-old woman with three bound-down scars of five years duration, developed after healing of abdominal surgical drain sites. (**B**) Follow-up examination at ten weeks after one session of subcision revealed satisfactory correction.

incision and drainage, intralesional corticosteroid injections (0.05–0.10 mL of triamcinolone acetonide, 1 mg/mL), and oral antibiotics, if needed.

Altered Physical Consistency of Treated Sites. The new connective tissue produced occasionally imparts a somewhat firmer skin texture. However, the improved overall appearance of the defect usually outweighs any change in physical consistency.

Discoloration. Temporary postinflammatory hyperpigmentation may appear in predisposed individuals. Patients are instructed to avoid sun exposure for at least one month after subcision.

Suboptimal Response. Partial elevation of the defect is a common occurrence after a single subcision. Prior to treatment, patients are advised that multiple sessions are usually required to correct a specific defect.

Excess Response. In approximately 5% to 10% of cases, excess fibroplasia develops and an elevated or hypertrophic response results about two to four weeks postoperatively. These elevations usually have normal skin surface markings in contrast to hypertrophic scars that appear after scalpel surgery. They respond favorably to intralesional corticosteroid injections (0.05–0.10 mL of triamcinolone acetonide, 1–5 mg/mL).

Keloid Scarring. See relative contraindications earlier.

CONCLUSION

The advantages of subcision are long-lasting scar correction and reasonably persistent correction of wrinkles. The materials required to perform subcision are readily available and inexpensive. Furthermore, subcision is not associated with the risk of allergic reactions (1,2) or amaurosis (3,4).

In our experience, the combination of surgical release and spontaneous fibroplasia induced by subcision is effective in treating cutaneous depressions, such as scars, wrinkles, depressions, and cellulite. We find subcision a valuable addition to the cutaneous surgeon's armamentarium of rehabilitative techniques.

REFERENCES

1. Hanke CW, Higley HR, Jolivette DM, Swanson NA, Stegman SJ. Abscess formation and local necrosis after treatment with Zyderm® or Zyplast® collagen implant. J Am Acad Dermatol 1991; 25:319–326.
2. Millikan L, Banks K, Purkait B, Chungi V. A 5-year safety and efficacy evaluation with Fibrel in the correction of cutaneous scars following one or two treatments. J Dermatol Surg Oncol 1991; 17:223–229.
3. Teimourian B. Blindness following fat injections [Letter]. Plast Reconstr Surg 1988; 82:361.
4. Zyplast® Implant Physician Package Insert. Collagen Corporation, Palo Alto, CA. 1985, 1987.
5. U.S. Trademark for "Subcision®." Registration No. 1,841,017 Date granted: 6/21/94.
6. Orentreich D. Punch grafting. In: Moy RL, Lask G, eds. Principles and Techniques of Dermatologic Surgery. MCGraw-Hill, In Press.
7. Spangler AS. New treatment for pitted scars. Arch Dermatol 1957; 76:708–711.
8. Gottlieb S. GAP repair technique [Poster Exhibit]. Annual Meeting of the American Academy of Dermatology, Dallas, TX, December 1977.
9. Multicenter Study. Treatment of depressed cutaneous scars with gelatin matrix implant. J Am Acad Dermatol 1987; 16:1155–1162.
10. Cohen IS. Fibrel®. Semin Dermatol 1987; 6:228–237. Fibrel® is a registered trademark of the Mentor Corporation.
11. Koranda FC. Treatment modalities in facial acne scars. In: Thomas JR, Holt GR, eds. Facial Scars: Incision, Revision & Camouflage. St. Louis: The C.V. Mosby Co., 1989:285.
12. Hambley RM, Carruthers JA. Microlipoinjection for the elevation of depressed, full-thickness skin grafts on the nose. J Dermatol Surg Oncol 1992; 18:963–968.
13. Spangler AS. Treatment of depressed scars with fibrin foam: seventeen years of experience. J Dermatol Surg Oncol 1975; 1:65–69.
14. Salasche J, Bernstein G, Senkarik M. Surgical Anatomy of the Skin. Norwalk: Appleton & Lange, 1988.
15. Zitelli SA. Wound healing and wound dressings in dermatologic surgery. In: Roenigk RK, Roenigk HH Jr, eds. Dermatologic Surgery: Principles and Practice. New York:Marcel Dekker, 1989:98–101.
16. Ketchum LD, Kelman CI, Masters FW. Hypertrophic scars and keloids: a collective review. Plast Reconstr Surg 1974; 53:140–154.

7

ePTFE Augmentation of Facial Soft Tissue

Corey S. Maas and Howard D. Stupak
Division of Facial Plastic Surgery, Department of Otolaryngology–Head and Neck Surgery, University of California, San Francisco, California, U.S.A.

INTRODUCTION

The search for the ideal facial soft tissue augmentation material continues. While injectable and implantable tissue-derived and synthetic biologic materials are effective, soft, and reliable, the materials have transient and unpredictable half lives in vivo (1,2). Purely synthetic injectable fillers have the capacity to maintain long-term persistence but have a generally higher rate of inducing foreign body response (3,4). In the event of complication, these materials may require wide tissue excision for removal. Solid implantable materials (e.g., silicone) are easily removed, but do not closely match soft tissue features. They are poorly stabilized with high rates of extrusion (5).

The characteristics of biocompatibility, soft and natural feel, and ease of insertion and removal were not available in any single implant material until the introduction of expanded polytetrafluoroethylene (ePTFE) as a facial filler in the 1980s. ePTFE is a synthetic polymer that has been expanded and fibrillated to form a micoporous material. The material has been in clinical use for over 30 years with safety and efficacy demonstrated in several million vascular grafts, abdominal wall reconstructions, and hernia repairs (6,7). ePTFE has also been successfully utilized as a facial skeletal augmentation material.

SURGICAL TECHNIQUES

A number of techniques for the placement of ePTFE material have been reported as successful for augmentation of folds and wrinkles in the face. These techniques, performed under local anesthesia, generally employ a retrograde "dragging" technique of ePTFE strips, cords, or sutures via a passing needle or hollow cannula. Proper placement of the implant is

105

(A)   **(B)**

(C)

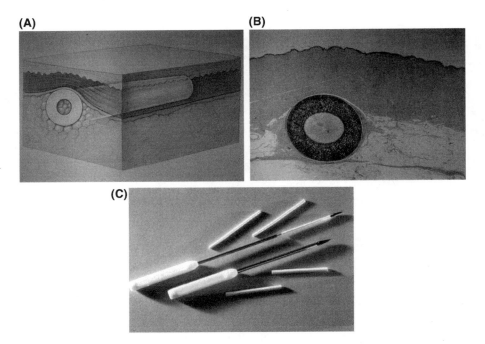

Figure 1
(**A**) The tubular ePTFE implant in its subdermal location, tenting-up its overlying dermis. (**B**) Low-powered hematoxylin and eosin stained micrograph of a thick-walled tubular ePTFE implant with extensive luminal fibrous ingrowth and absent inflammatory reaction. (**C**) The SoftForm® implant, trocar, and delivery system.

ensured by careful tunneling of the cannula at the deepest point of the fold or wrinkle, which may be marked before placement with the patient in the upright position.

Such techniques provided satisfactory results with moderate correction or augmentation in areas of anatomic deficiency. However, variable rates of extrusion or exposure of the ends of the material were reported when these techniques were used, presumably the result of migration of the insufficiently stabilized material (8–15).

Animal studies evaluated a series of shapes of the ePTFE implants for subcutaneous augmentation of tissues. When compared to strips, rolls, and cords, a tubular form of the material demonstrated the lowest extrusion rates with enhanced long-term stability while maintaining ease of removal. These findings were accepted because of the fibrous ingrowth into the lumen of the tube, anchoring the implant in place (Fig. 1A and B) (16,17).

The thick-walled tubular ePTFE implant with an associated trocar delivery system was approved by the Food and Drug Administration (FDA) for facial soft tissue augmentation in 1997 and was distributed

(A) **(B)**

(C) **(D)**

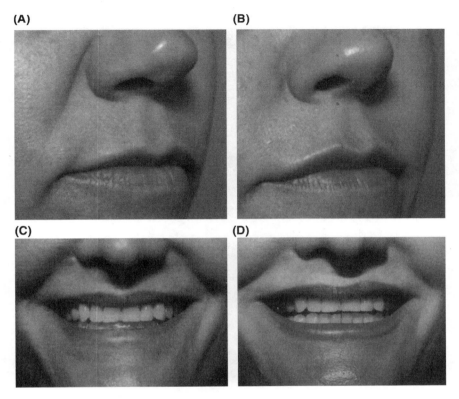

Figure 2
SoftForm® patients. Patient 1: (**A**) Preoperative. (**B**) Six months postoperative after implantation of bilateral nasolabial folds and upper lips. Notice the incomplete augmentation of nasolabial folds at the alar–facial junction. Patient 2: (**C**) Preoperative. (**D**) Eight months after upper and lower lip augmentation. Notice the slight assymmetry at cupid's bow.

under the trade name SoftForm® (Collagen Corp., Palo Alto, California, U.S.).[a] The delivery system employs a small cutting trocar and shaft, which is placed in an outer cannula (Fig. 1C). The procedure is performed in the office setting under local anesthesia after careful marking of the patient's soft tissue defect, wrinkle, or fold with the patient in the upright position. Although technically easy to perform, precise tunneling of the trocar cannula in the subcutaneous tissues beneath the defect is essential for proper correction.

Clinical trials of SoftForm, conducted at the University of California at San Francisco, demonstrated excellent short-term results, but more variable long-term results. Implantation indications in this trial included

---

[a] This product is no longer produced. It has been replaced by the UltraSoft™ implant, described later in the text.

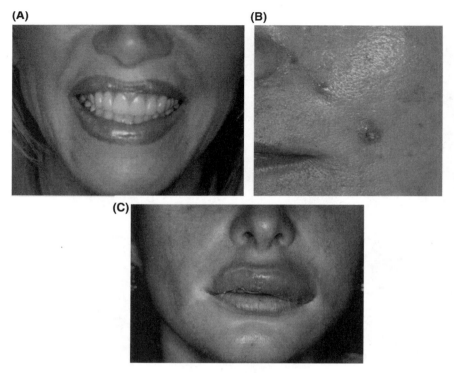

Figure 3
(**A**) A patient one year after SoftForm® implantation, with bilateral protruding ends and shortening of upper lip implants. (**B**) Another patient with extrusion of SoftForm® within two months of nasolabial fold augmentation. (**C**) A patient with an infected upper lip implant one month after implantation.

thin or atrophic lips, deep facial creases, depressed scars, and tissue deficiencies. Upon evaluation of patients at 30- to 90-days postprocedure, high satisfaction rates were noted by both physicians and patients (Fig. 2). However, in 34 patients (106 implants) for whom long-term (three to six years) follow-up data were available, there was a significant decline in patients' perception of the implant efficacy and the natural appearance and feel of the implants. There appeared to be several issues with SoftForm that led to this decline (Fig. 3). The most commonly reported problems with the implant were shortening or contraction of the implant with time and implant stiffening. The implant shortening appears to be due to the inherent nature of the thick-walled device, which can collapse upon itself like an accordion along its longitudinal axis and may remain as such (Figs. 3A, 6A and C). Thus, mobility of surrounding tissues, before full luminal anchoring of the implant may generate compressive forces that may cause the implant to contract. For this reason, patients were advised to avoid excessive lip mobility for three weeks postimplantation (18).

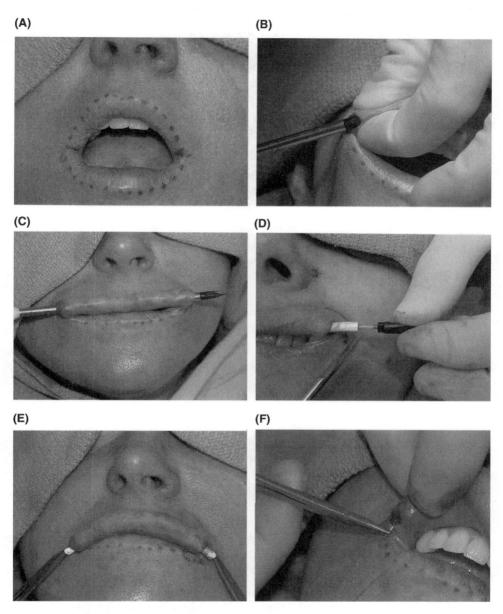

(A)   **(B)**

(C)   **(D)**

(E)   **(F)**

Figure 4

UltraSoft™ implantation to the upper lip. (**A**) The red lip margin is marked prior to local anesthetic infiltration and infraorbital nerve block. (**B**) After completion of small stab entry and exit incisions, the lip is pinched and the loaded UltraSoft trocar is passed along the vermillion border (**C**), through the entire upper lip, and out the exit incision. (**D**) Gentle pressure on the plunger releases the interference at the device tip. The cannula is withdrawn, leaving the trocar implant in place. Subsequently, the trocar tip is grasped and advanced as pictured. (**E**) The tube is gently adjusted, the exposed ends are trimmed to a taper using scissors, and the ends are tucked into the wounds. (**F**) Wound closure is achieved with one or two absorbable sutures, removed in three to five days.

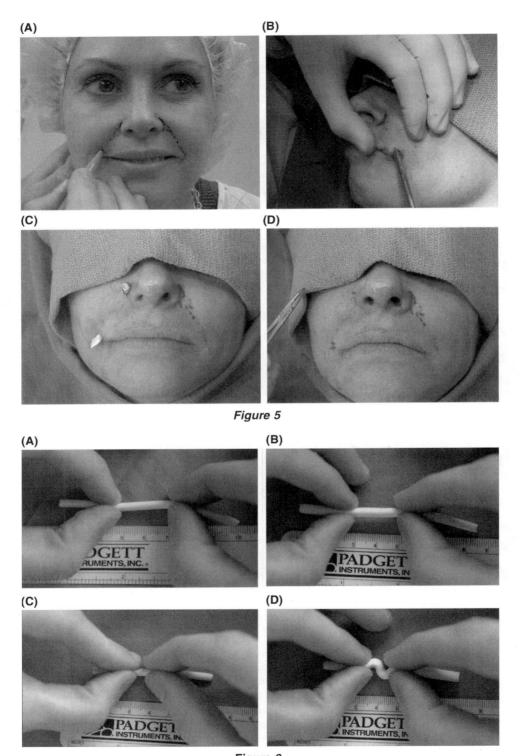

Figure 5

Figure 6

Figure 5
UltraSoft™ implantation of the nasolabial fold is similar to the procedure for upper lip implantation. (**A**) Marking of the nasolabial fold in the upright patient before anesthetic infiltration. (**B**) After completion of exit and entrance stab incisions, the UltraSoft trocar is introduced in its precise subdermal position. (**C**) After removal of the cannula and trocar tip, the ends of the implant are tapered and tucked below the skin. (**D**) The wounds are closed with one or two nonabsorbable sutures, removed in three to five days.

Increasing implant palpability or stiffening seems to be a separate issue. This problem is due to fibrocytic ingrowth *into the interstices* of the implant walls over time. Thicker walled implants would permit more interstitial fibrous ingrowth and become more firm over time than a thinner walled implant.

Technique changes have also been implemented. Initially, two tubular ePTFE implants were used for the upper lip (Fig. 3A), neither reaching midline, theoretically to preserve the natural appearance of cupid's bow. The 7-cm implants were too short for a single pass through the upper lip. This resulted occasionally in an unnatural-appearing bulge of the implant at cupid's bow (Fig. 3A). The short implants also occasionally led to incomplete augmentation of a defect (Fig. 2). Some patients complained of inadequate augmentation with SoftForm, which in some cases was due to incorrect positioning of the tube, and in others to insufficient amounts of augmentation material (18).

On long-term follow-up of the 106 patients, there was a low rate of extrusion (two implants), infection (two implants), and noticeable scar formation (two implants). However, 15 of the 34 patients required at least one revision procedure for the problems described above (18). Other studies found similar complication rates (19). Despite problems with the SoftForm implants, patient satisfaction over the long term remained moderately high, with 72% of respondents willing to repeat the implantation process in this long-term study (18).

After an in-depth analysis of SoftForm's design flaws, an improved tubular ePTFE facial soft tissue implant was introduced in 2001 by the manufacturer. The new thin-walled implant marketed under the name UltraSoft® retains the basic SoftForm delivery system but with several modifications (Figs. 4 and 5). The implant is larger in diameter but with a thinner wall. It is longer, allowing single pass augmentation of the lip and full augmentation of long defects. The larger lumen is more compliant, and resists contracture (Fig. 6) and stiffening. This results in an enhanced augmentation, with a softer, more natural feel and higher

Figure 6
Compression of thick-walled tubed ePTFE (SoftForm®) implant (**A**) results in accordion-like collapse (**C**). Compression of the thin-walled tubed ePTFE (UltraSoft™) implant (**B**) results in bending, *not* collapse (**D**).

(A)   (B)

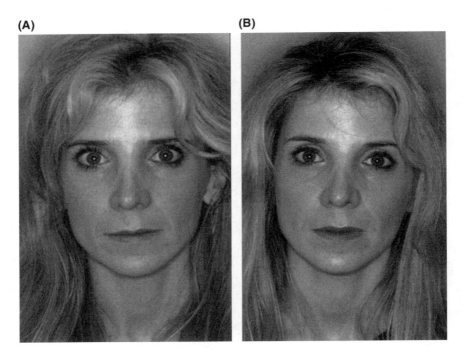

Figure 7
UltraSoft™ implantation. (**A**) Preoperative. (**B**) Four months after nasolabial
fold and upper and lower lip UltraSoft™ implantation.

satisfaction rates (Figs. 7–12). Long-term clinical trials of the UltraSoft
system are underway at the University of California at San Francisco.
Follow-up data from eighteen months of follow-up have shown no
increase in palpability or shortening of the implant.

Studies and clinical experience with ePTFE material for soft tissue
augmentation have demonstrated the following three key design features
of the implants: (i) they should be tubular to provide *controlled* ingrowth

(A)   (B)

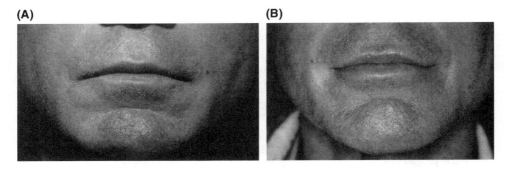

Figure 8
UltraSoft™ implantation. (**A**) Preoperative. (**B**) Three months after upper and
lower lip UltraSoft™ implantation.

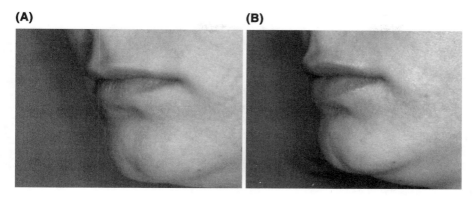

Figure 9
UltraSoft™ implantation. (**A**) Preoperative. (**B**) Four months after upper and lower lip UltraSoft™ implantation.

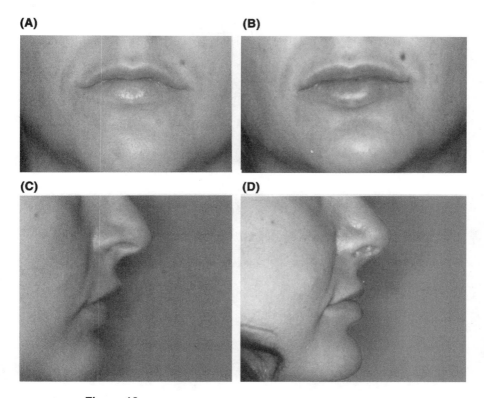

Figure 10
UltraSoft™ implantation. (**A** and **C**) Preoperative. (**B** and **D**) Five months after upper and lower lip UltraSoft™ implantation.

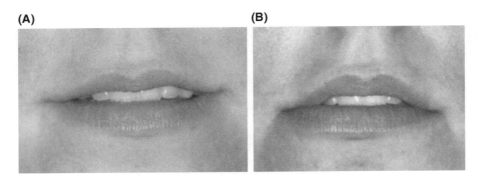

Figure 11
UltraSoft™ implantation. (**A**) Preoperative. (**B**) Three months after upper and lower lip UltraSoft™ implantation.

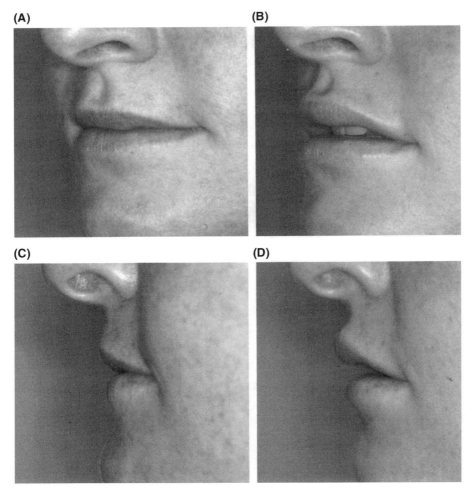

Figure 12
UltraSoft™ implantation. (**A** and **C**) Preoperative. (**B** and **D**) Two months after upper lip UltraSoft™ implantation.

for stabilization; (ii) the amount of ePTFE material should be minimized (thin-walled) to prevent stiffening due to interstitial ingrowth; and (iii) the implant must be fully removable. In essence, the implant material should act as a framework for fibrous ingrowth and collagen deposition, creating an environment for *bioreactive autologous augmentation.*

SUMMARY

Correction of soft tissue defects has been a perplexing clinical problem for physicians seeking persistent results. The SoftForm implantation system, although troubled by problems of shortening, stiffening, and high revision rates, demonstrates a promising future as a facial augmentation material. The thin-walled UltraSoft device is designed to overcome the structural flaws of SoftForm, improving both the stability and softness of the implant over the long term. Trials of UltraSoft are underway.

REFERENCES

1. Kligman AM, Armstrong RC. Histologic response to intradermal Zyderm and Zyplast (glutaraldehyde cross-linked) collagen in humans. J Dermatol Surg Oncol 1986; 12:35.
2. Billings E, May JW. Historical review and present status of free fat autotransplantation in plastic and reconstructive surgery. Plast Reconstr Surg 1989; 83:368–381.
3. Wilkie TF. Late development of granuloma after liquid silicone injections. Plast Reconstr Surg 1977; 60(2):179–188.
4. Denton AB, Maas CS. Synthetic soft tissue substitutes 2001. Facial Plast Surg Clin North Am 2001; 9(2):219–227.
5. Davis PK, Jones SM. The complications of silastic implants. Br J Plast Surg 1971; 23:405–411.
6. McAuley CE. Seven year follow-up of expanded polytetrafluoroethylene in femoropopliteal bypass grafts. Ann Surg 1984; 199:57–60.
7. Bauer JJ, Salky BA, Gelernt M, Kriel I. Repair of large abdominal wall defects with expanded polytetrafluoroethylene. Ann Surg 1987; 206:765–769.
8. Sherris DA, Larrabee. Expanded polytetrafluoroethylene augmentation of the lower face. Laryngoscope 1996; 106:658–663.
9. Sclafani AP, Thomas JR, Cox AJ, et al. Clinical and histologic response of subcutaneous expanded polytetrafluoroethylene (Gore-Tex) and porous high-density polyethylene (Medpor) implants to acute and early infection. Arch Otolaryngol Head Neck Surg 1997; 123:328–336.
10. Petroff MA, Goode RL, Levet Y. Gore-Tex implants: Applications in facial paralysis rehabilitation and soft-tissue augmentation. Laryngoscope 1992; 102:1185–1189.
11. Conrad K, MacDonald MR. Wide polytef (Gore-Tex) implants in lip augmentation and nasolabial groove correction. Arch Otolaryngol Head Neck Surg 1996; 122:664–670.
12. Robertson KM, Dyer WK. Expanded polytetrafluoroethylene (Gore-Tex) augmentation of deep nasolabial creases. Arch Otolaryngol Head Neck Surg 1999; 125:456–461.
13. Mole B. The use of Gore-Tex implants in aesthetic surgery of the face. Plast Reconstr Surg 1992; 90(2):200–206.
14. Linder RM. Permanent lip augmentation employing polytetrafluoroethylene grafts. Plast Reconstr Surg 1992; 90:1083–1090.
15. Courtiss EH, Glicksman CA. Discussion of "Permanent lip augmentation employing polytetrafluoroethylene grafts." Plast Reconstr Surg 1992; 90:1091–1092.
16. Greene D, Pruitt L, Maas CS. Biomechanical effects of e-PTFE implant structure on soft tissue implantation stability: A study in the porcine model. Laryngoscope 1997; 107:957–962.
17. Maas CS, Eriksson T, McCalmont T, et al. Evaluation of expanded polytetrafluoroethylene as a soft-tissue filling substance: An analysis of design-related implant behavior using the porcine skin model. Plast Reconstr Surg 1998; 101:1307–1314.
18. Ramirez AL, Stupak HS, Maas CS. SoftForm implant for soft tissue augmentation of the face (Parts I and II). Archives of Facial Plast Surg 2002. Submitted.
19. Brody HJ. Complications of expanded polytetrafluoroethylene (e-PTFE). Facial Implant. Derm Surg 2001; 27:792–794.

8

Use of Botulinum Toxin A for Facial Enhancement

Alastair Carruthers
Division of Dermatology, University of British Columbia, Vancouver, British Columbia, Canada

Jean Carruthers
Department of Ophthalmology, University of British Columbia, Vancouver, British Columbia, Canada

INTRODUCTION

Five years have passed since this chapter was published in the last edition of this book; in this short time, there has been a remarkable expansion in the amount of clinical data on the use of botulinum toxins for cosmetic purposes. Two of the biggest milestones since the last edition have been the approval by the U.S. Food and Drug Administration (FDA) of botulinum toxin type A (BTX-A; BOTOX®) for the treatment of glabellar lines, and the introduction into clinical use of an additional neurotoxin alternative—botulinum toxin type B (BTX-B, MYOBLOC). In addition, the use of cosmetic BTX has moved beyond simple clinical efficacy to what is now called an art, shaping and sculpting the face into more pleasing contours without scalpel or other invasive procedures.

With BTX injections becoming one of the most common cosmetic procedures performed, it is increasingly important for treating physicians to understand not only when, where, and how much to inject, but also the science behind what has been called the most potent biological toxin known to man (1). This chapter, then, will review the biochemical activity and history of this unique biological agent before focusing specifically on the clinical application of BTX-A—primarily the BOTOX and BOTOX Cosmetic formulations—for the treatment of hyperfunctional facial lines.

HISTORY OF COSMETIC BOTULINUM TOXIN

The anaerobic bacterium *Clostridium botulinum*—implicated over 100 years ago as the cause of muscle paralysis secondary to food poisoning

117

(2)—produces seven distinct serotypes of BTX (A to G). Pure BTX-A was first isolated in its crystalline form in 1946, and its mechanism of action identified in the 1950s (3). Two decades later, Dr. Alan Scott (Smith-Kettlewell Eye Research Foundation, San Francisco, California, U.S.) began to study BTX-A for the treatment of strabismus in both monkeys and humans; he first described its safety and efficacy in humans in 1980 (4). Dr. Scott believed that BTX-A could become useful for a number of conditions caused by muscle spasms or hyperactivity (4). Subsequently, the FDA approved BTX-A for the treatment of strabismus and blepharospasm in 1989, which was followed by approval for the use of both BTX-A and BTX-B in cervical dystonia in 2000.

We first noted improvement in the appearance of glabellar lines with BTX-A in patients treated for blepharospasm in 1987, although we have been using BOTOX since 1983 (5). Prior to our first published report in 1992, Dr. Scott used BTX-A for cosmetic purposes, as did other clinicians, convinced of its safety and efficacy in reducing facial wrinkles and bolstered by reports of aesthetic benefits in patients treated for facial dystonias (6,7). Following a number of publications, two randomized, placebo-controlled studies involving 537 patients confirmed the impressive safety and efficacy of BTX-A, leading to the FDA approval of BTX-A (BOTOX Cosmetic®) for the treatment of glabellar lines in 2002 (8). Since then, its use has rapidly expanded to include many other cosmetic problems that result, at least in part, from muscular overactivity.

BOTULINUM NEUROTOXINS

Of the seven identified *C. botulinum* neurotoxin serotypes, BTX-A is the most potent in producing muscular paralysis in humans (2), followed by types B and F (9). Although all subtypes block neuromuscular transmission, the precise mechanism of action and the clinical effects of each are different.

Pharmacology and Mechanism of Action

BTX causes profound, transitory muscular paralysis through a selective blockade of the regulated exocytosis of acetylcholine (10). All BTX subtypes vary in biosynthesis, size, cellular mechanism of action, methods of purification and formulation, and clinical usefulness. The commercially available subtypes, BTX-A and BTX-B, are both 150 kD dichain polypeptides composed of heavy and light chains linked by disulfide bonds (11). During biosynthesis, BTX-A and BTX-B form neurotoxin–protein complexes (900 and 700 kD complexes, respectively), with different properties (12). Following successful binding of the heavy chain to the motor nerve terminal, the toxin is internalized via receptor-mediated endocytosis, a process in which the plasma membrane of the nerve cell invaginates around the toxin receptor complex, forming a toxin-containing vesicle inside the nerve terminal. The neurotoxin molecule is released into the cytoplasm and cleaved into heavy and light chairs. Finally, the light chain of BTX-A cleaves a 25 kD synaptosomal-associated protein (SNAP-25), a protein integral to the successful docking and release of acetylcholine from vesicles situated within nerve endings. The light chain of BTX-B cleaves the vesicle-associated membrane protein (VAMP or synaptobrevin). These differences may be responsible for some of the varying clinical effects reported between the subtypes.

The process of cellular recovery after injection of BTX is only partially understood. Initial recovery of muscle contraction after BTX-A and BTX-B is accompanied by collateral sprouting of active terminal buds near the parent terminal. However, research suggests that these new sprouts are only transitory, with neurotransmission eventually restored at the original nerve ending and the sprouts eliminated (10).

Manufacturing and Storage

BTX-A (BOTOX®, BOTOX Cosmetic) and BTX-B (MYOBLOC®) are currently the only botulinum neurotoxins commercially available in North America. However, Dysport® (BTX-A) is available in Europe and will likely seek FDA approval in the near future.

Each vial of BOTOX contains 100 mouse units of vacuum-dried *C. botulinum* type A neurotoxin complex. The vacuum-dried product is stored in a freezer at or below $-5°C$, or in a refrigerator between $2°C$ and $8°C$. The manufacturer's guidelines recommend reconstitution with sterile, nonpreserved 0.9% saline solution and discarding the vial after four hours (11). However, some physicians report no significant differences in efficacy when used within six weeks of reconstitution (13,14). Moreover, recent data suggest that reconstitution with preserved saline does not impair the stability of BTX-A (13,15) and is considerably less painful on injection (16).

MYOBLOC is available in a liquid formulation containing BTX-B 5000 U/mL and is available in 0.5, 1.0, and 2.0 mL vials containing BTX-B, saline, human serum albumin, and sodium succinate, with a pH of approximately 5.6 (accounting for the stinging sensation reported on injection). Reconstitution is not required and is hampered by "overfill" of the vials. Clinicians with the desire to add saline are advised to do so in the syringe. The unopened vial is stable for months or years; once opened, the labeling is similar to BTX-A (17).

Dysport is available as a lyophilized vial containing 500 U of BTX-A, as well as sodium chloride, lactose, and human serum albumin. The smaller amount of albumin in Dysport compared to BOTOX may account for some of the difference in effectiveness between the units of the two products. In Europe, Dysport is labeled for transport at ambient temperature and storage at $2°C$ to $8°C$, and the guidelines for reconstitution and use are similar to those of BOTOX (18).

Comparative Clinical Efficacy

There is a wide range of potency among the different serotypes in humans. The gold standard for assessing potency of BTX is the mouse lethality assay (MLA), in which 1 U is defined as the murine LD_{50} of intraperitoneal-injected BTX. For reasons that are not clear, the potencies of 1 U of BOTOX, Dysport, and MYOBLOC are vastly different in humans. The literature describes a BOTOX:Dysport potency ratio of 1:2 to 1:6 (19,20) and a BOTOX:MYOBLOC potency ratio of 1:50 to 1:100 (21,22). Obviously, doses of one formulation cannot be substituted for another formulation, and precise dosage conversion factors have not been established.

Although the clinical efficacy and safety of BTX-A has been well documented (5,8), fewer data exist on the use of BTX-B. However, the cosmetic clinical trials in existence show key differences: BTX-B has more rapid onset of action and diffuses more widely, has a shorter duration of action, and is associated with greater pain and other side effects, compared to BTX-A (23–28). Overall, BTX-A has demonstrated greater therapeutic success with longer lasting results and fewer side effects.

SPECIAL CONSIDERATIONS

Sources of BTX-A

There are currently two commercially available sources of BTX-A: BOTOX and Dysport. The majority of our clinical experience resides with BOTOX, and all references in this chapter refer to the BOTOX or BOTOX Cosmetic formulations, unless otherwise specified. However, the clinician should be aware of the significant clinical differences between the two sources of BTX-A and adjust dosages accordingly.

Dilution

The appropriate diluent volume must be selected based on the desired concentration of the injection solution. Evidence indicates that higher doses of BTX-A delivered in smaller volumes (50 or 100 U/mL) keep the effects more localized and allow for the precise placement of the toxin with little diffusion, while smaller doses in larger volumes (5–10 U/mL) may cause more widespread effects (9,29). We find that it is more efficient to apply low-volume, concentrated toxin (100 U/mL), although other clinicians use dilutions as high as 10 U/mL to smooth crow's feet and the brow area (30).

Immunogenicity

Botulinum toxins are proteins capable of producing neutralizing antibodies and eliciting an immune response, causing patients to not respond to treatment any longer (9). These individuals, who initially respond but then fail to respond completely, are referred to as "secondary nonresponders" and are considered to have neutralizing antibodies to BTX. The rate of formation of neutralizing antibodies has not been well studied, nor have the crucial factors for neutralizing antibody formation been well characterized (11). However, the total protein concentration and number of units injected are critical in determining potential immunogenicity, and some studies suggest that BTX-A injections at more frequent intervals or at higher doses may lead to a greater incidence of antibody formation (11). The protein concentration in the current lots of BOTOX is significantly lower than in the previous lots and has been shown to be less antigenic than the original product. Secondary lack of effectiveness to BTX-A (due to the development of immunologic resistance) is exceedingly rare in cosmetic patients and must be distinguished from a much more common degree of resistance, associated with the need for increased doses, which is probably not due to immunologic mechanisms.

CONTRAINDICATIONS AND PRECAUTIONS

BTX-A is contraindicated in the presence of any neuromuscular disorder that could amplify the effect of the drug, such as myasthenia gravis, Eaton–Lambert syndrome, myopathies, or amyotrophic lateral sclerosis. Other contraindications include the presence of infection at the injection site or a known hypersensitivity to any of the product contents. Caution should be used in disorders that produce a depletion of acetylcholine (11). The safety of BTX-A in pregnant or nursing women has not been evaluated in any study.

Patients with an inflammatory skin problem at the injection site, marked facial asymmetry, ptosis, excessive dermatochalasis, deep dermal scarring, thick sebaceous skin, or glabellar lines that could not be lessened by physically spreading them apart were excluded from the phase 3 safety and efficacy trials. Theoretically, caution should be used when administering BTX-A with aminoglycosides or other agents that interfere with neuromuscular transmission (11), but the use of these agents is rare in cosmetic patients.

GLABELLAR FROWN LINES

BTX-A injections for glabellar rhytides are rapid, can be performed on an outpatient basis, and do not require a lengthy recovery period, unlike more invasive procedures (8). Treatments can be individually tailored and given serially to produce optimal—and reversible—results.

Anatomy

Muscles producing the frown include the corrugator and orbicularis oculi, which move the brow medially, and the procerus and depressor supercilii, which pull the brow inferiorly (Fig. 1). Clinical techniques should take into account the variation in location, size, and use of the muscles among individuals.

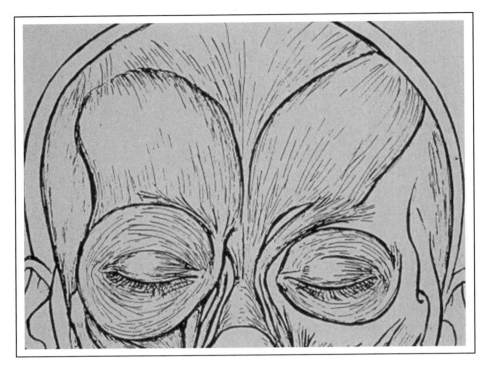

Figure 1
The anatomy of the muscles of facial expression.

Procedures

Before treatment, standardized, same-magnification, color photographs of the glabellar region when the muscles are at rest and during maximal frowning determine the individual characteristics of the patients. The type of brow arch, brow asymmetry, whether the brow is ptotic or crosses the orbital rim, and the amount of regional muscle mass are important factors in determining injection sites and dosages. For example, the male brow is associated with greater muscle bulk and requires more toxin to produce paresis. Data show that women achieve the greatest reduction in glabellar lines with 30 and 40 U BTX-A, whereas men require larger doses of 60 or 80 U to achieve the same effect (31,32). We find it useful to halve the volume of saline used to reconstitute the vial when treating males, as this technique reduces the injected volume while simply doubling the injected dose. Our initial doses are 30 U (for women) and 60 U (for men), diluted to 1 U/0.01 mL. If the patient has an insufficient response after the first treatment, we will increase the dose to 40 U in women and 80 U in men.

The appropriate dose of BTX-A is drawn into the syringe and air is expressed. In our clinic, we use the Beckton, Dickinson Ultra-Fine II short needle 0.3 insulin syringe, which has an integrated 30-gauge, silicone-coated needle, minimizing both patient discomfort and drug

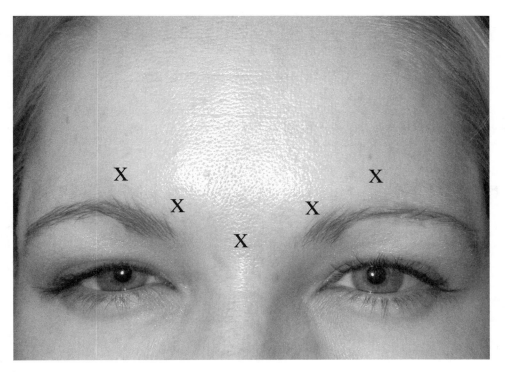

Figure 2
Glabellar injection technique.

wastage compared to traditional syringes with a needle hub (33). The needle dulls after approximately six injections and should then be discarded. We use a bottle opener to gently remove the rubber stopper so that the injecting needle remains sharp.

We seat the patient chin down with the head slightly lower than ours, and insert the needle just above the eyebrow, directly above the caruncle of the inner canthus. The injection site is always placed above the position of the bony supraorbital ridge, regardless of the eyebrow position. The needle insertion point, located near a vascular area, should be at a site where it is safe to apply postinjection pressure; the supratrochlear vessels are located immediately medial to the site of injection, and minor bleeding commonly occurs.

After injecting 4 to 6 U, the needle is slowly withdrawn (with its tip kept superficially beneath the skin), repositioned, and advanced superiorly and superficially to at least 1 cm above the previous injection site in the orbicularis oculi, where an additional 4 to 5 U of toxin are injected. The procedure is repeated on the opposite side of the brow to obtain a balanced appearance. We inject another 5 to 10 U into the procerus in the midline, at a point below a line joining the brows and above the crossing point of the "X" formed by joining the medial eyebrow to the contralateral inner canthus (Fig. 2). Finally, we inject an additional 4 to 5 U into a point 1 cm above the supraorbital rim in the midpupillary line in those with horizontal brows. It is critical to check that excessive eyebrow ptosis is not present by feeling the supraorbital rim with the thumb of the nondominant hand.

Patients are advised to remain vertical during the immediate post-injection period and told to frown as much as possible within the next two to three hours (while the toxin is binding), but not to press or manipulate the treated area.

Follow-Up

We ask patients to return in two to three weeks for a follow-up examination to take photographs and assess treatment responses. For patients who still have deep furrows at two weeks, one may consider adding a filler. Consideration should be given to the amount of time between the initial treatment and any touch-ups. Because of the theoretical risks of an immunological response, a cautious approach would be to re-inject no earlier than two weeks postinjection. We recommend further injections at three- to four-month intervals over a period of one year in those with deep glabellar frown lines, which keeps the musculature paralyzed and allows the glabellar furrows to drop out (34). At higher doses, many patients experience clinical benefits lasting three to four months, and some continue to benefit for as long as six to eight months. After one year, the patients return when they desired. All patients are instructed to contact their physician if anything unexpected occurs.

CROW'S FEET

"Crow's feet" are wrinkles extending laterally from the periorbital area and are usually a sign of aging, particularly photoaging. By relaxing the relevant muscles, treatment of crow's feet is successful, even in severely photoaged skin (35).

Anatomy

The muscle group involved in the production of crow's feet in the lateral periorbital area is the orbicularis oculi that rings the orbit. The lateral fibers of the orbicularis oculi are arranged in a vertical, circular pattern around the eyes. Contraction of the fibers produces forceful closure of the eyelids. Therefore, the goal of treatment of these muscles is relaxation or weakening, rather than paralysis. The lateral radiation of wrinkles from the area of the lateral canthus occurs at right angles to the muscle group, although variations in anatomy can produce different patterns.

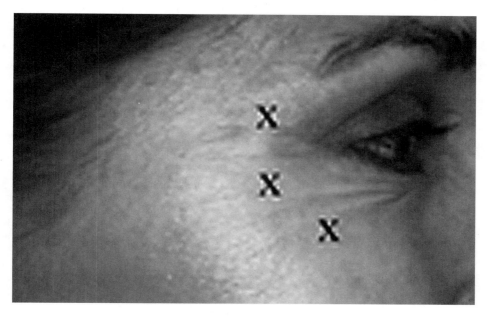

Figure 3
Injection of crow's feet using the three-spot technique.

Procedures

In general, two to three injection sites lateral to the lateral orbital rim are used (7,30,36,37), and equal doses of toxin are injected into each of the sites (approximately 4–7 U/site; 12–20 U/side). The dosage used in the lateral orbital region can vary. A recent dose-ranging study found no significant difference in efficacy between 6 U/side and 18 U/side (37). Total dose ranges used by others include 5 to 15 U (38) and 4 to 5 U per eye over two or three injections sites (30). We use 12 to 15 U/side, distributed in equal parts over two to four injection sites, and recommend using as few and as superficial injections as possible to minimize bruising (36).

To identify the injection sites, the patient is asked to smile maximally and the center of the crow's feet is noted. The first injection site is in the center of the area of maximal wrinkling, approximately 1 cm lateral to the lateral orbital rim. The second and third injection sites are approximately 1 to 1.5 cm above and below the first injection site, respectively (Fig. 3). In some cases, crow's feet are distributed equally above and below the lateral canthus, while in others, they are primarily below the lateral canthus. In these individuals, the injection sites may be in a line that angles from anteroinferior to superoposterior. In any case, the most anterior injection should be lateral to a line drawn vertically from the lateral canthus. The injection should not be made while the subject is still smiling, as the BTX-A then may affect the ipsilateral zygomaticus complex, causing upper lipoptosis.

Follow-Up

Results generally last from three to six months, with few adverse effects noted. A recent study that compared the treated side to the placebo side reported a notable drop in effect three months following the first injection, but interestingly, a duration greater than four months was noted after the second injection (37).

HORIZONTAL FOREHEAD LINES

The cosmetic treatment of horizontal forehead lines with BTX-A requires a more cautious approach than treatment of the glabellar or the lateral periorbital region.

Anatomy

The forehead musculature includes a large, vertically oriented muscle (frontalis) underlying the forehead that inserts into the galea aponeurotica superoposteriorly and inferiorly into the skin of the brow, the procerus, orbicularis oculi, corrugator supercilii, and the depressor supercilii. Although most figures depict the frontalis in two sections, it may span across the forehead from one temporal fusion line to the other and may be thicker in certain portions of the forehead. The frontalis raises the eyebrows and skin over the root of the nose and draws the scalp forward, with the lower 2 cm largely responsible for eyebrow elevation. Contraction of the frontalis produces horizontal forehead lines.

Procedures

An excessive weakening of the frontalis muscle without weakening of the depressors will result in unopposed action of the depressors, producing a lowering of the brow and an angry expression. Thus, the clinician should be conservative and allow some functional areas to remain intact to permit brow elevation. Softening the horizontal forehead rhytides can be accomplished by a careful weakening of the muscles, keeping injection sites well above the brow to avoid ptosis or a complete lack of expressiveness. Patients with a narrow brow (defined as less than 12 cm between the temporal fusion lines at mid-brow level) should receive fewer injections (four sites, compared to five) and lower doses than patients with broader brows (Fig. 4). We previously injected a total of 10 to 20 U in four to five sites horizontally across the mid-brow, 2 to 3 cm above the eyebrows (9). However, recent dose-ranging data show that a total of 48 U in the procerus, frontalis, lateral orbicularis oculi, and depressors gives the greatest improvement in the response and in its duration, although adverse effects such as headache, eyelid swelling, and brow ptosis, are dose-related (39).

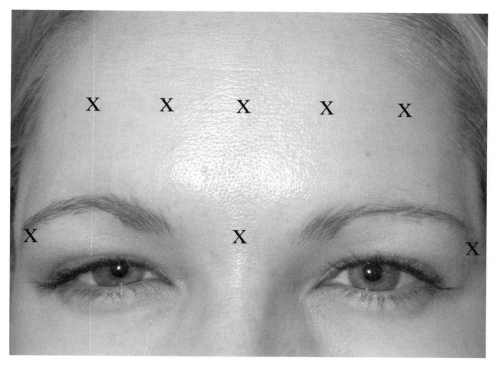

Figure 4
Injection sites for horizontal forehead lines showing injection of both frontalis and the brow depressors.

Follow-Up

With the higher doses used, BTX-A in the forehead lessens undesirable horizontal forehead lines for a period of four to six months (9).

BROW SHAPING

Clinicians can use the knowledge and understanding of how BTX-A works in the glabellar region to change the appearance of the brows in patients who desire a more aesthetically pleasing look.

Brow Elevation

Several clinicians have reported an elevation of the brow resulting from treatment of the glabellar lines (40–42), and our own objective dose-ranging study, using 30 and 40 U BTX-A in the glabella, showed a lateral and mid-pupil elevation as a beneficial result (31). Until recently, we believed this to be due to the action of the toxin on the medial (corrugator supercilii, procerus, and the medial portion of the orbicularis oculi) and lateral (the lateral portion of the orbicularis oculi) brow depressors. In a more complete analysis, we found that a total of 10 U BTX-A injected into the glabella produced mild, medial brow ptosis that disappeared after two months (43). However, injections of 20 to 40 U produced an initial lateral eyebrow elevation, followed by central and medial eyebrow elevation that peaked at 12 weeks but was still significantly present at 16 weeks. This is the first time in our experience that the effects of BTX-A injections into skeletal muscle have peaked at 12 weeks, rather than the usual four weeks. Based on these results—specifically, that the primary effect is lateral, an area not injected—we now presume that this brow lift is owing to the partial inactivation of the frontalis and not to the action on the brow depressors, as previously thought. The subsequent central and medial eyebrow elevation could be owing to the frontalis muscle "resetting," leading to a gradual lift.

Eyebrow Asymmetry and Shaping

Eyebrow asymmetry may result from a number of scenarios, and injections of BTX-A into (or overlying) the frontalis muscle, approximately 1 cm above the eyebrow, can be an alternative to surgery in patients who desire a more symmetrical appearance. As discussed, injection of BTX-A for glabellar frown lines can cause a mild medial brow ptosis, a lateral brow elevation, and a more pleasing contour to the eyebrow. Understanding that the lateral, orbital aspect of the orbicularis oculi muscle above the lateral retinaculum serves as an antagonist muscle to the lateral frontalis muscle will aid clinicians in improving the shape and position of the eyebrows (44).

MID AND LOWER FACE

The use of cosmetic BTX-A in the mid and lower face and neck has increased drastically over the past few years. There are now a number of wider applications that push BTX-A toward an "art," rather than a clinical procedure. It is important to remember that each patient has individual features and musculature requiring an expert approach. Only clinicians with a large base of clinical experience and those with a thorough understanding of facial anatomy (both dynamic and resting) and vasculature should attempt more advanced procedures, since incorrect application can result in catastrophic impairment of function and expression. We recommend the use of electromyographic (EMG) guidance in some patients (36).

Hypertrophic Orbicularis

The act of smiling can transiently diminish the perceived size of the palpebral aperture, particularly in Asian patients. We have found that

(A)

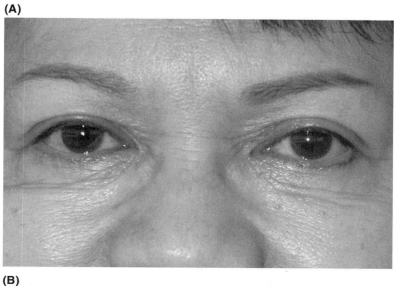

(B)

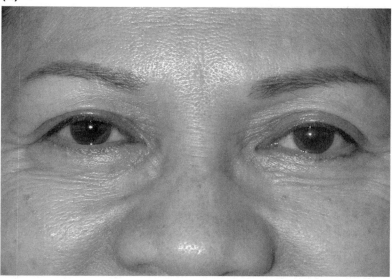

Figure 5
Before (**A**) and after (**B**) injection of the infraorbital orbicularis oculi with BTX.

injecting 2 U into the lower pretarsal orbicularis will relax the palpebral aperture at rest and while smiling (36). Flynn et al. reported mean palpebral aperture increases of 1.8 mm (at rest) and 2.9 mm (at full smile) after injection of 2 U subdermally, 3 mm inferior to the lower pretarsal orbicularis, and three 4-U injections placed 1.5 cm from the lateral canthus, each 1 cm apart (Fig. 5) (45).

Nasalis

BTX-A injections into the nasalis can significantly weaken the appearance of "bunny lines" (radial rhytides that fan obliquely across the radix of the nose) and repeated nasal flare, caused by involuntary dilation of the nostrils. For bunny lines, we inject anterior to the nasofacial groove on the lateral wall of the nose, well above the angular vein, and massage gently after injection to help diffuse the toxin. Care is taken to avoid injecting the nasofacial groove, which can affect the levator labii superioris and levator labii superioris aleque nasi. In patients with repeated nasal flare, we inject into the lower nasalis fibers, which drape over the lateral nasal ala.

Nasolabial Folds

In patients who have a naturally shorter upper lip, 1 U BTX-A into each lip elevator complex in the nasofacial groove will collapse the upper aspect of the nasolabial fold but also elongate the upper lip. However, weakening the lip levator, zygomaticus, and risorius muscles may not be desirable in every patient and will flatten the mid face and elongate the upper lip muscles. Patients must understand the aesthetic result of the procedure and its long-lasting ($\pm$6 months) effects.

Perioral Lip Rhytides

The orbicularis oris is the sphincter muscle that encircles the mouth, lying between the skin and mucous membranes of the lips and extending upward to the nose and down to the region between the lower lip and chin, and causes the lips to close and pucker. Overactive orbicularis oris causes vertical perioral rhytides radiating outward from the vermilion border. Small doses (1–2 U per lip quadrant) are usually sufficient to weaken the orbicularis oris without causing a paresis that could interfere with elocution and suction, especially when used in combination with a soft-tissue augmenting agent. We increase the dilution and inject a total of 6 U into eight injection sites (0.75 U in 0.03 mL/injection), carefully measuring the sites to balance on either side of the columella or the lateral nasal ala. Appropriate patients must be chosen carefully, as those who play wind instruments or professional singers/speakers are not ideal candidates.

Depressor Anguli Oris

The depressor anguli oris (DAO) is an important cosmetic muscle, extending inferiorly from the modiolus to attach into the inferior margin of the mandible on the lateral aspect of the chin. Contraction of the DAO causes a downward turn to the corner of the mouth and a negative appearance. Since the DAO overlies the depressor labii inferioris, direct injections lead to usually asymmetrical paresis. Instead, we inject 3 to 5 U at the level of the mandible but at its posterior margin, close to

(A)

(B)

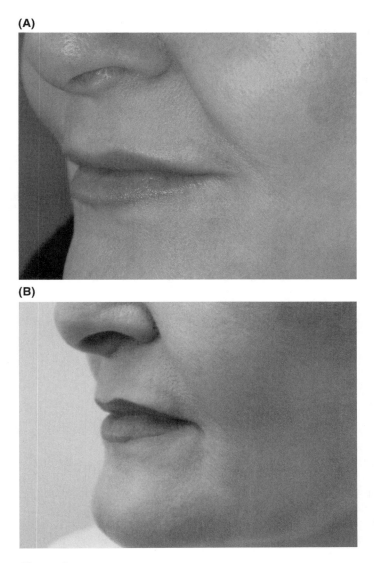

Figure 6
Before (**A**) and after (**B**) injection of depressor anguli oris with BTX showing upturn of the corner of the mouth.

the anterior margin of the masseter, which will significantly weaken, rather than paralyze, the muscle (Fig. 6).

Melomental Folds

Melomental folds are deep skin folds that extend from the depressed corner of the mouth to the lateral mentum and have traditionally been treated with soft-tissue augmentation alone. However, the combination of soft-tissue augmentation and BTX-A injected into the DAO will lengthen the duration of the augmentation and prevent the repeated molding and contortion of the soft-tissue augmenting agent.

Mental Crease

Softening of the mental crease can be achieved by injecting the mentalis, just anterior to the point of the chin. We inject 3 to 5 U into each side of the midline under the point of the chin, just anterior to the bony mentum, rather than injecting centrally. Care is taken not to inject at the level of the mental crease, since this will also weaken the lower lip depressors and orbicularis oris and cause serious adverse effects that can persist for six months or more, depending on the dose. Again, as in the perioral area, weakening, rather than paralysis, is the aim of treatment.

Peau d'Orange Chin

When the mentalis and depressor labii muscles are used in speech that requires cocontraction of the orbicularis oris, an apple-dumpling appearance (or "peau d'orange" chin) can occur due to a loss of subcutaneous fat and dermal collagen. A combination of soft-tissue augmentation and BTX-A in the mentalis (or BTX-A alone in patients who do not require augmentation) will soften this effect.

Mouth Frown

It is important to remember that the effect of BTX-A on one muscle often has an effect—positive or negative—on another. A good example of this is the "mouth frown," the permanent downward angulation of the lateral corners of the mouth, which is caused by the action of the DAO and the upward motion of the mentalis. We have found that attempts to weaken the DAO or mentalis alone, while appropriate in some individuals, is ineffective or associated with unacceptable side effects in others. We currently inject both muscles at the same time—3 U of BTX-A into each DAO and into each side of the mentalis, to a total of 12 U in a female patient—which produces a subtle, synergistic effect. However, this technique should only be used in patients who have experienced the effects of BTX-A injections elsewhere, and who are aware of the aim of treatment and its possible outcomes.

Facial Asymmetry

We have used BTX-A with success to treat facial asymmetry owing to surgical or muscular causes. In hemifacial spasm, for example, repeated clonic and tonic facial movements draw the facial midline toward the hyperfunctional side. Relaxation of the hyperfunctional zygomaticus, risorius, and masseter will allow the face to be centered at rest. Likewise, hypofunctional asymmetry, such as that following the VII nerve paresis, requires injection of 1 to 2 U of BTX-A into the zygomaticus, risorius, and orbicularis on the normofunctional side, and 5 to 10 U in the masseter. In patients who experience asymmetry of jaw movement, 10 to 15 U BTX-A injected intraorally into the internal pterygoid can relax the jaw and relieve discomfort when chewing and speaking.

Decentration of the mouth can occur in patients who have experienced surgical or traumatic section of the orbicularis oris or risorius muscle, and is caused by the unopposed action of the partner muscles in the normally innervated side. BTX-A injected into the overdynamic risorius, immediately lateral to the lateral corner of the mouth and in the mid-pupillary line, will re-center the mouth when the face is in repose. Likewise, some patients have congenital or acquired weakness of the DAO, resulting in the inability to depress the corner of one side of the mouth; chemodenervation of the partner muscle restores functional and aesthetic balance.

Masseteric Hypertrophy

The use of BTX-A for contouring in the lower face may be a simple alternative method of shaping the mandible with a short recovery period. Although most of the studies reported have been small (46,47), a larger study demonstrated a gradual reduction in masseter thickness (average 1.5–2.9 mm reduction) with 25 to 30 U BTX-A injected into five to six sites, evenly, at the prominent portions of the mandibular angle (48). Clinical effects lasted for six to seven months following injection, and side effects (mastication difficulty, muscle pain, and verbal difficulty during speech) lasted from one to four weeks.

CHEMODENERVATION OF THE NECK

Chemodenervation with BTX-A can be useful in the aging neck, reducing the appearance of necklace lines and platysmal bands.

Necklace Lines

In our clinic, we have found that the simplest way to treat horizontal necklace lines is to inject along the lines with 1 to 2 U at each site in the deep intradermal plane, avoiding the deeper venous perforators that can bleed and the underlying cholinergic muscles of deglutition. Not more than 10 to 20 U is injected in one treatment session, and after injection, the neck is gently massaged to prevent bruising.

Platysmal Bands

Although traditional rhytidectomy (49) remains the gold standard for most aging necks, BTX-A can be used alone or as adjunctive therapy for residual postoperative banding. However, BTX-C can worsen the appearance of platysmal bands in patients with accompanying jowl formation and bone resorption. Ideal candidates for BTX-A are those with obvious platysmal bands, good cervical skin elasticity, and minimal fat descent. When injecting the neck, the cautious approach is best; the vertically oriented platysmal bands are external to the muscles of deglutition and neck flexion. We use no more than 30 to 40 U/treatment, as more can result in profound dysphagia (36).

ADJUNCTIVE THERAPY

Adjunctive BTX-A can produce a more polished result, can prolong the effects of other cosmetic procedures, and is becoming an increasingly important aspect of facial rejuvenation (44).

Surgery

Since the constant action of facial muscles can interfere with or reverse the results of cosmetic surgery, weakening the muscles with BTX-A before surgery may make it easier to manipulate tissues, allowing for greater surgical correction or better concealment of the surgical incisions. In addition, some experts report that BTX-A during or after the procedure prevents or slows the return of the wrinkles by reducing the action of the responsible muscles (9). Beneficial effects have been noted in many surgical procedures, including brow lifts, periorbital rhytidectomy, blepharoplasty, and lower eyelid ectropion and "roundeye" repair (9,50).

Soft-Tissue Augmentation

We use BTX-A routinely as adjunctive therapy with soft-tissue augmentation to achieve more effective, longer lasting results, especially in certain facial areas (i.e., deep glabellar furrows or lip augmentation). BTX-A often eliminates or reduces the muscular activity responsible for the wrinkles, improves the response, and increases the longevity of the filling agent (44,51).

Laser Resurfacing

Several studies have demonstrated superior and longer lasting outcomes of BTX-A in conjunction with laser resurfacing (9,44,52–54). The adjunctive use of BTX-A aids the healing of newly resurfaced skin long enough to effect a more permanent eradication of wrinkles. Regular postoperative injections, given every 6 to 12 months, prolong the effects of resurfacing (52), especially for the improvement of forehead, glabellar, and canthal rhytides, compared to laser resurfacing alone (53,54).

COMPLICATIONS

Most complications are relatively uncommon and are related to poor injection techniques (55). We have been treating patients with BTX-A for more than 20 years, with dosages ranging from 2.5 to 400 U/injection (with an average of 40 U), and none of our patients has suffered a serious, irreversible complication.

Brow Ptosis

One of the most undesirable adverse events, brow ptosis, occurs when the injected toxin affects the frontalis during glabellar or brow treatment, is related to poor technique, and underscores the necessity of understanding the effects of BTX-A on facial musculature. Avoiding brow ptosis begins with proper patient selection and pre-injecting the brow depressors in patients with low-set brows, mild brow ptosis, and patients over the age of 50 years (55). A higher concentration allows for more accurate placement, greater duration of effect, and fewer side effects, since there is an area of denervation associated with each point of injection owing to toxin spread of about 1 to 1.5 cm (diameter, 2–3 cm). Injecting the glabella and the whole forehead in one session is also more likely to produce brow ptosis (55). Patients must be advised to remain upright for two hours, exercise the treated muscles as much as possible for the first four hours, and strictly avoid rubbing or massaging the injected area for two hours following treatment. Mild brow ptosis responds to apraclonidine (Iopidine® 0.5%) alpha-adrenergic agonist ophthalmic eye drops.

Eyelid Ptosis

Ptosis of the upper eyelid occurs when the injected toxin migrates to the upper eyelid levator muscle, producing a weak paralytic effect as early as 48 hours or as late as 14 days after injection, and persisting for 2 to 12 weeks. The incidence of ptosis in our clinic is low (0–1.0%) and is technique-related. We recommend accurate dose dilution and injecting the toxin no closer than 1 cm above the central eyebrow. Patients should remain vertical for two to three hours after injection and should refrain from manipulating the injection site. Bothersome ptosis can be treated with alpha-adrenergic eyedrops, which causes the contraction of Muller's muscle, situated beneath the levator muscle of the upper eyelid (55).

"Mr. Spock" Eyebrow

A quizzical or "cockeyed" appearance can occur in the brow when the lateral fibers of the frontalis muscle have not been injected appropriately and the untreated lateral fibers of frontalis pull upward on the brow. To rectify this, a small amount of BTX-A is injected into the fibers of the lateral forehead that are pulling upward; overcompensation can lead to an unsightly hooded brow that partially covers the brow (55).

Periorbital Complications

Bruising, diplopia, ectropion, or a drooping lateral lower eyelid and an asymmetrical smile (caused by the spread of toxin to the zygomaticus major) are all reported complications of BTX-A in the periorbital area. BTX-A is injected laterally at least 1 cm outside the bony orbit or 1.5 cm lateral to the lateral canthus. Ecchymoses is reduced by injecting superficially and avoiding blood vessels by placing each injection at the advancing border of the previous one. Patients with a significant degree of scleral show pre-treatment, dry eye symptoms, significant previous surgery under the eye, a great deal of redundant skin beneath the eye, or a slow snap test of the lower eyelid are not good candidates for infraorbital orbicularis injections (55).

Lower Face and Cervical Complications

Complications in the lower face and neck, such as drooling or asymmetry, are usually owing to the overenthusiastic use of BTX-A in large doses (55). Starting with low doses and injecting more superficially rather than deeply, limits the potential for complications, as do symmetrical injections, to ensure uniform postinjection movement. Injections are avoided in singers, musicians, or other patients who use their perioral muscles with intensity. When injecting the DAO, areas too close to the mouth, the mental fold, and interaction with the orbicularis oris are avoided, all of which can result in a flaccid cheek, incompetent mouth, or asymmetric smile. Large doses (greater than 100 U) of BTX-A in the platysma have resulted in reports of dysphagia and weakness of the neck flexors.

CONCLUSION

In the last five years, the role of BTX-A in facial rejuvenation has exploded to include many previously unheard of applications, such as facial contouring, which pushes its use to a new form of art. Since 1988, when we first used BTX-A for cosmetic applications, our clinical experience has rapidly widened and now features prominently as either stand-alone or adjunctive therapy. As with any cosmetic procedure, a solid knowledge of the variability and synergy of facial anatomy is mandatory to understand the effects of BTX on the musculature, avoid possible complications, and provide the best possible patient care.

REFERENCES

1. Gill DM. Bacterial toxins: A table of lethal amounts. Microbiol Rev 1982; 46:86–94.
2. Scott AB, Collins CC. Pharmacologic weakening of extraocular muscles. Invest Ophthalmol 1973; 12:924–927.
3. Schantz EJ. Botulinum toxin: the story of its development for the treatment of human disease. Persp Biol Med 1997; 40:317–327.
4. Scott AB. Botulinum toxin injection into extraocular muscles as an alternative to strabismus surgery. Ophthalmology 1980; 87:1044–1049.
5. Carruthers JDA, Carruthers JA. Treatment of glabellar frown lines with C. botulinum-A exotoxin. J Dermatol Surg Oncol 1992; 18:17–21.
6. Borodic GE. Botulinum A toxin for (expressionistic) ptosis overcorrection after frontalis sling. Ophthal Plast Reconstr Surg 1992; 8:137–142.
7. Blitzer A, Brin MF, Keen MS, et al. Botulinum toxin for the treatment of hyper-functional lines of the face. Arch Otolaryngol Head Neck Surg 1993; 9:1018–1022.
8. Carruthers JA, Lowe NJ, Menter MA, et al. A multicentre, double-blind, randomized, placebo-controlled study of efficacy and safety of botulinum toxin type A in the treatment of glabellar lines. J Am Acad Dermatol 2002; 46:840–849.
9. Carruthers A, Carruthers J. Botulinum toxin type A: history and current cosmetic use in the upper face. Semin Cutan Med Surg 2001; 20:71–84.
10. Meunier FA, Schiavo G, Molgo J. Botulinum neurotoxins: from paralysis to recovery of functional neuromuscular transmission. J Physiol Paris 2002; 96:105–113.
11. Product monograph: BOTOX Cosmetic (botulinum toxin type A for injection) purified neurotoxin complex. Markham, Ontario: Allergan Inc., 2001.
12. Sakaguchi G. Clostridium botulinum toxins. Pharmacol Ther 1982; 19:165–194.
13. Klein AW. Dilution and storage of botulinum toxin. Dermatol Surg 1998; 24:1179–1180.
14. Hexsel DM, De Almeida AT, Rutowitsch M, et al. Multicenter, double-blind study of the efficacy of injections with botulinum toxin type A reconstituted up to six consecutive weeks before application. Dermatol Surg 2003; 29:523–529.
15. Huang W, Foster JA, Rogachefsky AS. Pharmacology of botulinum toxin. J Am Acad Dermatol 2000; 43:249–259.
16. Alam M, Dover JS, Arndt KA. Pain associated with injection of botulinum A exotoxin reconstituted using isotonic sodium chloride with and without preservative: a double-blind, randomized controlled trial. Arch Dermatol 2002; 138:510–514.
17. Package insert. MYOBLOC™ (botulinum toxin type B) injectable solution. San Francisco, CA: Elan Pharmaceuticals, Inc.
18. Package insert. Dysport®: Clostridium botulinum type A toxin-haemagglutinin complex. Maidenhead, Berkshire, UK: Ipsen Limited.
19. Nussgens Z, Roggenkamper P. Comparison of two botulinum-toxin preparations in the treatment of essential blepharospasm. Graefes Arch Clin Exp Ophthalmol 1997; 235:197–199.
20. Odergren T, Hjaltason H, et al. A double blind, randomized, parallel group study to investigate the dose equivalence of Dysport and Botox in the treatment of cervical dystonia. J Neurol Neurosurg Psych 1998; 64:6-12.
21. Brashear A, Lew MF, et al. Safety and efficacy of NeuroBloc (botulinum toxin type B) in type A-responsive cervical dystonia. Neurology 1999; 53:1439–1446.
22. Brin MF, Lew MF, et al. Safety and efficacy of NeuroBloc (botulinum toxin type B) in type A-resistant cervical dystonia. Neurology 1999; 53:1431–1438.
23. Ramirez AL, Reeck J, Maas CS. Botulinum toxin type B (Myobloc) in the management of hyperkinetic facial lines. Otolaryngol Head Neck Surg 2002; 126:459–467.
24. Sadick NS. Botulinum toxin type B (Myobloc) for glabellar wrinkles: a prospective open-label response study. Dermatol Surg. In press 2003.

25. Sadick NS. Prospective open-label study of botulinum toxin type B (Myobloc) at doses of 2400 and 3000 units for the treatment of glabellar wrinkles. Dermatol Surg. In press 2003.

26. Alster TS, Lupton JR. Botulinum toxin type B for dynamic glabellar rhytides refractory to botulinum toxin type A. Dermatol Surg. In press 2003.

27. Lowe N, Lask G, Yamauchi P. Efficacy and safety of botulinum toxins A and B for the reduction of glabellar rhytids in female subjects. Presented at the American Academy of Dermatology 2002 Winter Meeting, New Orleans, LA, February 22–27, 2002.

28. Matarasso SL. Comparison of botulinum toxin types A and B: a bilateral and double-blind randomized evaluation in the treatment of canthal rhytides. Dermatol Surg 2003; 29:7–13.

29. Carruthers A, Carruthers J. Dose dilution and duration of effect of botulinum toxin type A (BTX-A) for the treatment of glabellar rhytids. Presented at the American Academy of Dermatology 2002 Winter Meeting, New Orleans, LA, February 22–27, 2002.

30. Garcia A, Fulton JE Jr. Cosmetic denervation of the muscles of facial expression with botulinum toxin: a dose–response study. Dermatol Surg 1996; 22:39–43.

31. Carruthers A, Carruthers J, Said S. Dose-ranging study of botulinum toxin type A in the treatment of glabellar lines. Presented at the 20th World Congress of Dermatology, Paris, France, July 1–5, 2002.

32. Carruthers A, Carruthers J. Botulinum toxin type A for treating glabellar lines in men: A dose-ranging study. Presented at the 20th World Congress of Dermatology, Paris, France, July 1–5, 2002.

33. Flynn TC, Carruthers A, et al. Surgical pearl: The use of the Ultra-Fine II short needle 0.3-cc insulin syringe for botulinum toxin injections. J Am Acad Dermatol 2002; 46:931–933.

34. Carruthers A, Kiene K, et al. Botulinum A exotoxin use in clinical dermatology. J Am Acad Dermatol 1996; 34(5 Pt 1):788–797.

35. Glogau R. Chemical peeling in aging skin. J Geriatr Dermatol 1994; 2:30–35.

36. Carruthers J, Carruthers A. BOTOX use in the mid and lower face and neck. Semin Cutan Med Surg 2001; 20:85–92.

37. Lowe NJ, Lask G, et al. Bilateral, double-blind, randomized comparison of 3 doses of botulinum toxin type A and placebo in patients with crow's feet. J Am Acad Dermatol 2002; 47:834–840.

38. Keen M, Kopelman JE, Aviv, et al. Botulinum toxin: a novel method to remove periorbital wrinkles. Facial Plast Surg 1994; 10:141–146.

39. Carruthers A, Carruthers J, Cohen J. Dose dependence, duration of response and efficacy and safety of botulinum toxin type A for the treatment of horizontal forehead rhytids. Presented at the American Academy of Dermatology 2002 Winter Meeting, New Orleans, LA, February 22–27, 2002.

40. Huilgol SC, Carruthers A, Carruthers JDA. Raising eyebrows with botulinum toxin. Dermatol Surg 2000; 25:373–376.

41. Ahn MS, Catten M, Maas CS. Temporal brow lift using botulinum toxin A. Plast Reconstruct Surg 2000; 105:1129–1135.

42. Huang W, Rogachefsky AS, Foster JA. Brow lift with botulinum toxin. Dermatol Surg 2000; 26:55–60.

43. Carruthers A, Carruthers J. Glabella BTX-A injection and eyebrow height: a further photographic analysis. Presented at the Annual Meeting of the American Academy of Dermatology, San Francisco, CA, March 21–26, 2003.

44. Fagien S, Brandt FS. Primary and adjunctive use of botulinum toxin type A (Botox) in facial aesthetic surgery: beyond the glabella. Clin Plast Surg 2001; 28:127–148.

45. Flynn TC, Carruthers JA, Carruthers JA. Botulinum-A toxin treatment of the lower eyelid improves infraorbital rhytides and widens the eye. Dermatol Surg 2001; 27:703–708.

46. To EW, Ahuja AT, Ho WS, King WW, Wong WK, Pang PC, Hui AC. A prospective study of the effect of botulinum toxin A on masseteric muscle hypertrophy with ultrasonographic and electromyographic measurement. Br J Plast Surg 2001; 54:197–200.

47. von Lindern JJ, Niederhagen B, Appel T, Berge S, Reich RH. Type A botulinum toxin for the treatment of hypertrophy of the masseter and temporal muscle: an alternative treatment. Plast Reconstr Surg 2001; 107:327–332.

48. Park MY, Ahn KY, Jung DS. Botulinum toxin type A treatment for contouring of the lower face. Dermatol Surg 2003; 29:477–483.

49. Kane MA. Nonsurgical treatment of platysmal bands with injection of botulinum toxin A. Plast Reconstr Surg 1999; 103:656–663.

50. Guerrissi JO. Intraoperative injection of botulinum toxin A into orbicularis oculi muscle for the treatment of crow's feet. Plast Reconstr Surg 2000; 105:2219–2228.

51. Carruthers J, Carruthers A. A prospective, randomized, parallel group study analyzing the effect of BTX-A (BOTOX) and nonanimal sourced hyaluronic acid (NASHA, Restylane) in combination compared with NASHA (Restylane) alone in severe glabellar rhytides in adult female subjects: treatment of severe glabellar rhytides with a hyaluronic acid derivative compared with the derivative and BTX-A. Dermatol Surg 2003; 29:802–809.

52. Carruthers J, Carruthers A, Zelichowska A. The power of combined therapies: Botox and ablative facial laser resurfacing. Am J Cos Surg 2000; 17:129–131.

53. West TB, Alster TS. Effect of botulinum toxin type A on movement-associated rhytides following CO_2 laser resurfacing. Dermatol Surg 1999; 25:259–261.

54. Lowe N, Lask G, Yamauchi P, Moore D, Patnaik R. Botulinum toxin type A (BTX-A) and ablative laser resurfacing (Erbium: YAG): A comparison of efficacy and safety of combination therapy vs. ablative laser resurfacing alone for the treatment of crow's feet. Presented at the American Academy of Dermatology 2002 Summer Meeting, New York, NY, July 31–August 4, 2002.

55. Klein AW. Complications and adverse reactions with the use of botulinum toxin. Dermatol Surg. In press 2003.

9

Liquid Silicone for Soft Tissue Augmentation: Histological, Clinical, and Molecular Perspectives

David M. Duffy
Department of Dermatology, University of Southern California, Los Angeles, California, and Department of Dermatology, University of California, Los Angeles, California, U.S.A.

INTRODUCTION

A Nottingham chemist, F. S. Kipping, introduced the term "silicone" during the early 1900s, when he synthesized the crude precursors to the 60,000 silicone-containing compounds now available. Kipping was not much impressed with silicone's potentiality, concluding that the materials were scientifically interesting, but had no practical applications. Modern processes for the synthesis of silicones followed the research carried out by Hyde, Warrick, and McGregor during the 1930s (1). In 1943, the exigencies of war lead to the production of Dow–Corning's first silicone product, DC-4, a greasy material used to waterproof bomber electrical systems and permit flight at higher altitudes (1).

Silicones, versatile and easily fabricated, have long been considered biologically nontoxic, chemically nonreactive, and structurally unaltered by exposure to a wide range of environmental conditions. These compounds, whose density is a function of polymerization and cross-linkage, can exist as solids (elastomers), liquids, gels, and foams. Technologically advanced societies employ a veritable cornucopia of silicones by the ton. Antiflatulents and cosmetics contain silicone. It is also present in paint thinners, lubricants, scar dressings, cardiac valves, joint prostheses, contact lenses, and breakfast food. Silicone is used for penile, testicular, breast and vocal cord implants, implantable binding matrices for drug releasing capsules, artificial urethras, catheters, drains, tubing, and as a coating for sutures and hypodermic needles, insuring that the average American has at least five grams of silicone in his body (2). Despite such widespread industrial and medical use of all types

Terms in boldface are further defined in the glossary at the end of this chapter.

of silicone products, in one American state (Nevada), injection of small amounts of liquid silicone into the human skin, or its possession for that purpose, is a felony. If these laws are challenged, silicone issue may again take its place among the major legal controversies of our time, potentially pitting the federal government against the state of Nevada, to wit: the U.S. Food and Drug Administration (FDA) Modernization Act of 1997, which allows any legally marketed FDA-approved device to be prescribed or administered for any condition or disease within the doctor/patient relationship (off-label use). A letter by a colleague addressed to the FDA discussing the use of Ada-toSil^{TM} (silicone) for the treatment of a cutaneous defect received the reply "You state you've never advertised the product and it was an individual physician's decision based upon the unique needs of one of your patients. The situation you described has always been viewed by the FDA as a practice of medicine, and therefore this off-label use is considered legal" (3). Bureaucratic uncertainty regarding the legality of "off-label applications" of approved drugs and devices is embodied in a letter to a colleague from the Medical Board of the State of California, which contains the admonition: "Most physicians do not use injectable silicone for lips (below accepted standards of care?), and that its' use for that purpose is an off label use." The physician involved contacted Alcon Laboratories (the manufacturers of silicone) and confirmed the fact that "Hundreds of physicians throughout the US are using silicone." In his reply to the state board, he notes that the board is "Out of touch" with what is being used for lip enhancement" (4).

PHYSICAL CHARACTERISTICS AND TERMINOLOGY

Silicones are synthetic polymers based upon the element silicon, atomic number 14, the second most abundant element in the earth's crust. Kipping referred to the materials he prepared as "silicones" because simple elemental analysis indicated they might be analogs of organic ketones. Further reactions, using elemental silicon, produced a class of compounds referred to as "siloxanes." This term is a mnemonic acronym derived from *sili*con, *oxy*gen, and meth*ane*. Siloxanes consist of chains of silicon and oxygen atoms, with hydrocarbon groups or single hydrogen atoms bound to the silicon, corresponding to the general formula $(R_{1-3} SiO)_x$, with the subscript "x" designating the viscosity or chain length of the polymer (1,5). The structure of the *liquid* silicones most commonly used for tissue augmentation is illustrated in the figure below:

Note the placement of trimethyl siloxane units at each end and repetitive dimethylsiloxane units in between. Viscosity is directly related to chain length indicated by the value of "X" in the above formula.

Viscosity

The viscosity of silicone fluids is measured in "centistokes." One *stoke* (100 *centistokes*) is the viscosity of water. Three hundred and fifty centistokes is the viscosity of mineral oil (paraffin), as well as the viscosity of non-FDA–approved silicone oils, which were frequently used for tissue augmentation in the past.

Chemical Reactivity

Several features of the silicon/oxygen bond are believed to account for its lack of chemical reactivity. The bond angle between silicon and oxygen is more obtuse than the bond angle between carbon and oxygen (5). This allows freer rotation of the organic groups, providing a somewhat inaccessible environment for chemical reactivity. For biological systems, many of the unique properties of silicone *fluids* are due to the electronic structure of the silicone atom. The atomic orbitals used to form the silicon/oxygen bonds in the siloxane backbone permit a wider range of bond angles with virtually no energy barrier to rotation (1,5,6).

Protein Denaturation

In the case of liquid silicones, organic side chains experience minimal interfascial surface energy with water and, therefore protein solutions resulting in the smallest possible driving force for protein absorption and denaturation (6). Another possibly important feature for biological applications is the fact that silicone oils have the highest permeability coefficient for oxygen and nitrogen hitherto discovered (7,8).

THEORETICAL BENEFITS

For use in soft tissue augmentation, liquid silicone appears to fulfill most of the criteria for an ideal implantable substance. Its viscosity remains constant in the range of body temperature; it is clear, colorless, tasteless, nonvolatile, insoluble in alcohols, and soluble in ether and certain other solvents (2,9). It is unaffected by exposure to air, sunlight, and most chemicals. It does not support bacterial growth, and it can be safely heat sterilized. Liquid silicone can be stored without refrigeration, but it can be contaminated upon contact with certain rubbers from which it absorbs bleaches and other chemicals. It should not be gas-sterilized for this reason.

THEORETICAL DRAWBACKS/THE PERMANENCE PENALTY

The possibility of unforeseen complications as a consequence of infectious processes, or pharmacologic, surgical or heat-mediated therapies must be considered before using permanent implants of any type.

BIOCOMPATIBILITY: CHEMICAL AND BIOLOGICAL INERTNESS

As World War II ended, it became apparent that silicones had many potential uses. Toxicological studies carried out before commercial production indicated that certain classes of silicone, particularly those in nonvolatile compounds containing methyl and mixed methyl and phenyl groups as a class, were nontoxic. It was also noted that finished silicone resins were also found to be "physiologically inert and presented no hazards." With the publication of this toxicological information in 1948 (10), interest grew within the health community because of the need for biocompatible medical and surgical materials.

Silicon, the elemental precursor of silicones, is normally found in human tissues as a component of mucopolysaccharides. It may function in the connective tissues by bridging polysaccharides or by linking polysaccharides to protein.

Indications

Injected silicone carries the same indications of "fillers," such as injectable bovine collagen, in adding tissue volume, but it is much less forgiving. Problems with dispersion of filler material into the periphery of inelastic scars or wrinkles (doughnutting) will not, as in the case of collagen or other temporary fillers, disappear with the passing of time. Liquid silicone works best for atrophic and soft, flexible cutaneous depressions, which can easily be effaced by stretching. The injection of local anesthetic or temporary fillers (although their viscosity makes them act somewhat differently from liquid silicone) will permit a "preview" of the results, which might be obtained using a permanent filler. Silicone works particularly well for thumbprint-like depressions, broad, distensible scars caused by acne, excoriation, trauma, varicella, microbial infections, and surgery, including skin grafting. Certain types of rhytides resulting from aging or photo-damage, glabellar frown lines, nasolabial folds, and the labial commissures respond well, as do groove-like depressions that surround permanent implants, or areas where osseous atrophy has occurred. Atrophy of the skin following corticosteroid injections, linear scleroderma, neurotrophic or diabetic ulcers, and painful corns or callosities can also be treated effectively. Postrhinoplasty irregularities and atrophic deformities of the ears (age-related lobular atrophy) respond well. Silicone can also be used to correct congenital and atrophic facial asymmetries. It is of particular value in treating lipoatrophic defects (Figs. 1–10) (2,11–16).

Technique

Early practitioners, using large (25- to 18-gauge) needles, utilized a fanning technique in which the needle was inserted subcutaneously and rotated to be parallel with the skin's surface. Enormous (by contemporary standards) volume of silicone, up to 4 ml in each injection site or 10 to 12 ml at one

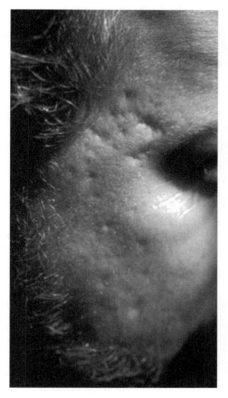

Figure 1
Patient A (6/21/84): These pliable acne scars are suitable for soft tissue augmentation.

sitting, were also employed. In at least one case, a total volume of 95 ml of silicone was used for the correction of severe hemifacial defects (17,18).

In contrast to these earlier injection methods, the preferred contemporary microdroplet serial puncture technique employs 27- to 30-gauge needles (depending on the viscosity of the silicone injected) to deposit tiny microdroplets of silicone at multiple injection sites in the deep dermis, spaced 2 to 10 mm apart. Unlike bovine collagen and earlier silicone injection techniques, where the skin is literally stretched by the volume of implanted material, advocates of microdroplet technique stress the need for undercorrection and the necessity of waiting at least for four weeks while new collagen forms around these minuscule volumes of silicone, before carrying out further injections. It is worth remembering that no one knows the exact volume of silicone that is tolerable for any patient, but it is generally agreed that the use of large volumes leads to more problems[a] (19). These problems may also occur when patients

---

[a] Possibly by increasing potential antigenic burden.

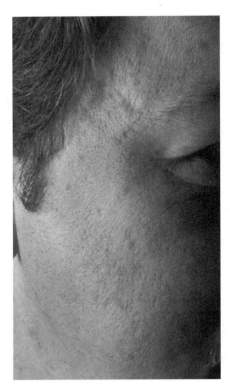

Figure 2
Patient A (6/25/85): Note the appearance after three treatments of liquid silicone at one year.

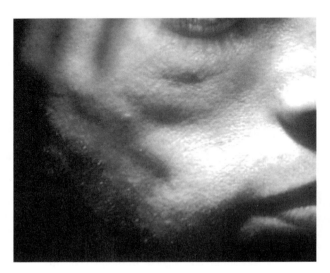

Figure 3
Patient B (6/24/86): Facial atrophy in this case followed severe weight loss before treatment.

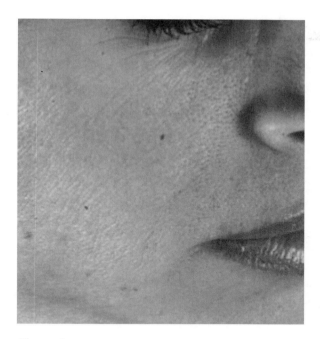

Figure 4
Patient B (2/24/88): At two years, three treatments of liquid silicone, note results.

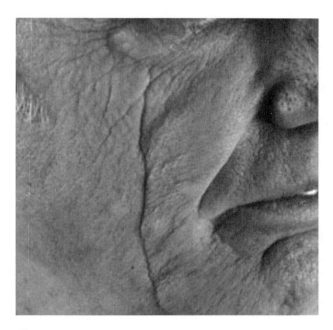

Figure 5
Patient C (1/11/84): In this pretreatment picture, a deep groove is noted.

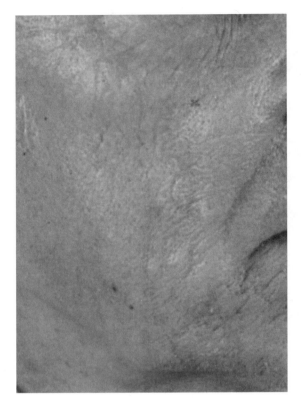

Figure 6
Patient C: This picture demonstrates results achieved with liquid silicone six months after the 2nd treatment. As a general rule rhytides, which are oriented cephalad to caudad, are more easily correctable than those oriented horizontally on the face.

receive small amounts of silicone at each sitting, but repeat these multiple injections over many years. The fine points of injection technique are beyond the scope of this paper but have been exhaustively detailed in several publications (2,9,12).

Contraindications

Liquid silicone is not a suitable agent for breast augmentation. The large volume needed for this purpose may migrate along tissue planes or induce the formation of esthetically unacceptable thick-walled cystic accumulations of injected material. For patients who have received both injectable silicone and breast implants, problems with the former (encapsulation contractures, or replacement) may increase the risk of complications developing at the sites where liquid silicone was injected, possibly on the basis of memory T cell-activation (20). Liquid silicone should

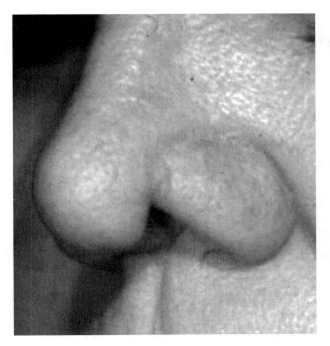

Figure 7
Patient F (8/5/87): This notch-like deformity in the ala nasi followed resection of a basal cell carcinoma.

not be injected into cysts; it can produce elevation of the overlying skin. Injection into vessels showing abnormalities carries a risk of embolism. Ridging or beading, and overcorrection often follow the injection of *horizontal* creases on the face, such as the creases in the forehead, the mental

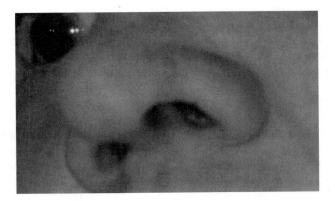

Figure 8
Patient F (10/7/87): At two months, two treatments with liquid silicone produced the above results.

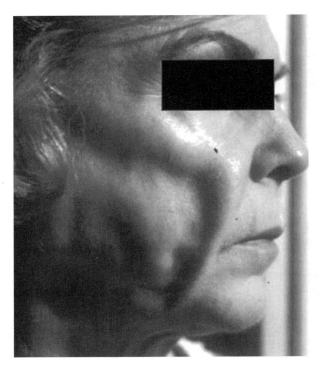

Figure 9
Patient G (6/11/84): Pretreatment photograph revealing facial atrophy, which
followed an unspecified illness.

line and the fine horizontal crease, which traverses the philtrum. Injection
of shallow V-shaped rhytides, particularly those which bridge the vermillion border, can also lead to overcorrection or "doughnutting," while
injecting the easily distensible wrinkles surrounding the eyes can result
in "beading" and overcorrection. These areas are best treated with resurfacing. Several immune processes may play an important role in
infectious and granulomatous silicone complications, including T cell–
activation, foreign body processing abnormalities, infections, and cytokine abnormalities (20). Accordingly, patients with systemic infections
or other conditions associated with these processes, particularly elevations in tumor necrosis factor alpha (TNF-α; 21), may be at greater risk
to develop complications following any type of permanent implant. These
conditions include psoriasis, rheumatoid and psoriatic arthritis, inflammatory bowel disease, Weber–Christian disease, erythema nodosum,
and tuberculosis. Patients with sarcoidosis, and HIV who have developed
"immune restoration syndromes" consisting of an exaggerated response
to previously subclinical foreign materials that follows effective human
immunodeficiency virus therapy (HIV therapy), may also be at greater
risk for complications. Patients with rosacea, granulomatous cheilitis

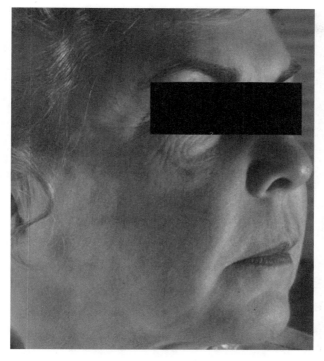

Figure 10
Patient G (1986): Results obtained after one year of treatment with liquid silicone (approximately 30 cc), demonstrated in this photograph taken two years after the initiation of treatment, have persisted over 20 years.

(22), and those whose lifestyle subjects them to repeated trauma may be at greater risk to develop complications following silicone injections. Patients with localized *infections* such as sinus infections, carious teeth, and labial herpes simplex, should not receive glabellar, central facial, or perioral injections. Personal experience suggests that the treatment of patients, who have received silicone injections of unknown purity, and in unknown volumes, from another practitioner carries with it the onus of blame for complications unrelated to the proper use of small volumes of silicone by the second practitioner.[b]

Patients who engage in contact sports may be in danger of traumatically induced excessive fibrosis. In addition, those who carry out strenuous exercise immediately after implantation run the risk of vasodilatory induced nodule formation (Figs. 11–13). Those with histories of keloidal

[b] Patients who are determined to receive more silicone are sometimes less than honest in admitting previous silicone treatments carried out by another practitioner; particularly so, if they believe that they may be excluded from further treatment on the basis of their honesty.

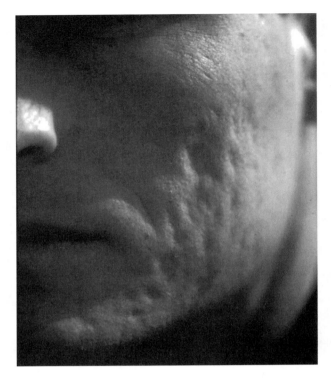

Figure 11
Patient I: This photo reveals pretreatment scarring, due to severe acne in this
33-year-old semi-professional athlete.

scarring may be at greater risk for excessive fibrosis, following the treatment of scars. Patients with familial or personal histories of immune disease are not at risk for systemic complications. However, if active
systemic immune disease presents itself after treatment, silicone may be
indicted as a causative agent. The physician who used it might face subsequent litigation, which might not be settled on the basis of scientific
merit. Patients with severe seasonal rhinitis and multiple allergies may
be at greater risk for inflammatory reactions following the use of any permanent implant, during allergy flare-ups.

RELATIVE CONTRAINDICATIONS

The ability of silicone oils to retain heat has led to their widespread use as
insulators in a variety of industrial applications. This property may have
important clinical implications following the use of therapies which
employ heat, on skin previously treated with liquid silicone. It has been
suggested that the presence of silicone may be a contraindication for CO_2
resurfacing (23). Other permanent agents such as Artecoll®, may also
interact negatively with heat generating therapies.

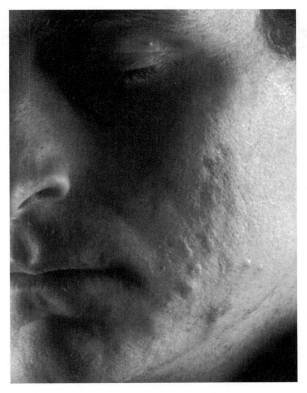

Figure 12
Patient I: After one treatment with liquid silicone, a partial elevation of the depressed scars is seen. This patient ran a 10K run and about eight hours after finishing, he noted these nodules, which appeared at the sites of injection.

CUTANEOUS SURGERY

Although patients who have received liquid silicone have routinely undergone surgical procedures involving the treated areas without adverse sequelae, at least one anecdotal report documents the occurrence of granulomata in silicone-treated tissues, following blepharoplasty. Traumatic or infectious activation of T cells may play a role in this process (case number 12).

SILICONE FLUID TYPES

Dow–Corning Medical Grade 360 Liquid Silicone

This 350-centistoke fluid is widely used as a lubricant for needles, syringes, and IV tubing. It is estimated that a diabetic taking daily injections with disposable syringes receives five milliliters of liquid silicone yearly (24). When used in small volumes for soft tissue augmentation, excellent results have been reported. However, silicone was sold in gallon

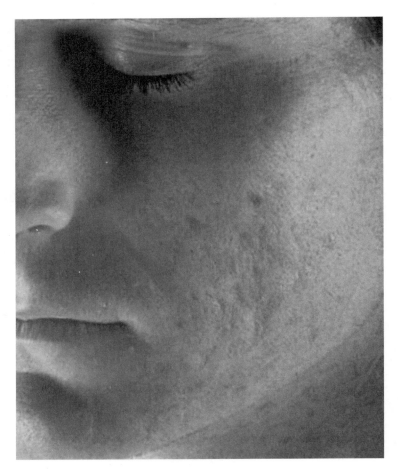

Figure 13
Six months after three treatments with liquid silicone, complete resolution of these nodules was observed. Patient I demonstrates an excellent example of the effect of vasodilatory activities upon the production of what are probably transient granulomas.

and stored in open containers, unsterilized and subject to contamination. Moreover, it was injected in enormous quantities, "As much as a pint, or 500 cc, taken from 55 gallon drums" and deposited, in some cases, under great pressure with caulking gun–like equipment into a single site at one time (25). Under these circumstances, 360-fluids produced horrific complications following its use for breast and facial injections (26–29). The shedding or spallation of this material from damaged hemodialysis pump tubing has also resulted in severe hepatitis and pancytopenia, as silicone particles were engulfed by macrophages throughout the reticuloendothelial system (30–32).

MDX-4-4011

This highly purified 350-centistoke DMPS fluid was filtered to remove heavy metals, short-chain polymers, and other "impurities." It was developed in 1965, specifically for use in clinical investigations for soft tissue augmentation, supervised by the U.S. FDA. It was used successfully in 1400 patients over a 20-year period (33,34).

Dow–Corning 200 Silicone Fluid

This industrial grade "electrical" silicone is unfiltered and unfit for medical use.

FDA-Approved Silicone Fluids (AdatoSil 5000™ and Silikon 1000™)

The approval by the U.S. FDA of two liquid silicones, whose viscosity is designated by their trademarks, removed all legal obstacles for their use in soft tissue augmentation. Both fluids were FDA approved for production of prolonged retinal tamponade for proliferative vitreoretinopathies and complicated retinal detachments for which no other treatment exists (35).

For soft tissue augmentation, Silikon 1000, which can be injected through relatively small needles, will probably become the agent of choice.

INTENTIONALLY ADULTERATED SILICONE FLUIDS (HINDSIGHT IS 20/20)

In a misguided attempt to create a more vigorous fibroblastic response and inhibit fluid migration when large volumes of fluid were injected at one sitting, a wide variety of irritants were added to silicone, some bearing the names of their creators. Adulterants varied from region to region and from country to country. Some are being used to this day. Under normal circumstances, hydrophobic materials such as silicone elastomers, are coated with host proteins within a few hours of implantation. Inflammatory cells that enter the tissues do not respond to the foreign material itself, but to a surface layer of partially denatured plasma proteins. Adulterants may very well promote an inflammatory response by converting the haptenic potential of silicone into an adjuvant state. Kagan (36) noted that "Silicone polymers alone did not remain in situ when injected, and they have a tendency to migrate, or drift, into dependent areas." This statement reflects both the unsophisticated understanding of implant host interactions and the willingness of practitioners to use enormous volumes of liquid silicone (750 cc to 2 L/patient, for breast and body contouring). Kagan's article, appearing as it did in a highly respected peer reviewed journal, helped lay the groundwork for the disrepute and suspicion, which disparages the use of liquid silicone to this day. Even more optimistically, Kagan

(36) proclaims that "Our experiments have given no indication that silicone oils and silicone preparations will cause toxicosis of any kind." The idea that fibroplasia can be induced beneficially in human tissues without granulomatous penalties has resurfaced in the form of silica injections as part of cellulite treatment protocols (37).

Sakurai "Formula" and Other "Macro" Use

No one can agree exactly what combination of adulterants were added to this material, named after the Japanese researcher who developed it, and who claimed to have treated over 72,000 patients with it in Japan. A number of authors have reported the presence of ricinoleic acid, animal and vegetable fatty acids, mineral and vegetable (perhaps castor oil, olive oil, croton oil, peanut oil), concentrated vitamin D, snake venom, talc, and paraffins (2,9,33,38, pg. 23). This material was often used in large volumes, over 100 cc at one sitting, for facial and breast augmentation. Silicones adulterated with sesame oil or 1% oleic acid were also used in the United States west Coast, and may currently be used in Mexico. In addition, a number of chemicals, chemically unrelated to silicone, are indiscriminately injected into the skin. These chemicals are commonly mislabeled as silicone, but in reality include a great variety of substances, including linseed oil. For about three decades, beginning in the early 1900s, paraffin (mineral oil) was used to elevate facial and nasal contour deformities, and for breast enlargement (2). During the 1940s, physicians in Los Angeles injected paraffins and flax oil as a baldness cure, into balding scalps, in an attempt to "increase circulation by loosening an excessively tight scalp."

Months to years later, nodules, plaques, and ulcerations developed at the injection sites. Hypersensitivity reactions also occurred, sometimes accompanied by systemic toxicity and fevers (2). Histologically, these nodules were characterized by granuloma formation. They were often followed by cellulitis and extensive fibrosis. Migration of large volumes of paraffin and/or silicone have occurred, when gravity and muscular activity forced them along tissue planes.

HISTORY OF LIQUID SILICONE USE

The use of liquid silicone to improve body contours became popular first in Germany, Switzerland, and Japan during the 1940s, when thousands of patients were treated with it.

In the United States during the early 1960s, several investigators, using more refined techniques, reported excellent results following the injection of small volumes of liquid silicone for cutaneous defects (34). However, horrific complications resulting from the gross misuse of adulterated liquid silicone, used in massive volumes for breast augmentation, lead to emergency legislation criminalizing its use in the state of Nevada and by 1964, the FDA declared silicone to be a "new drug." Its major manufacturer, Dow–Corning, encouraged by excellent anecdotal results from investigators, who had been informally provided with Dow–Corning 360 fluid, obtained authority from the FDA to investigate a more refined liquid silicone, MDX-4-4011. By 1974 Dow–Corning had a trademark, and planned to market this injectable form of silicone. Despite results which seemed to have clearly established the safety and efficacy of the silicone used in this study, Dow–Corning decided to drop its efforts to gain FDA approval because it could not "Effectively prevent misuse of its products" (39).

In 1978, another study began in which patients with severe atrophic deformities in four specific categories could be treated. The results of this study were favorable. By 1987, the Ortho Pharmaceutical Corporation planned an open study to determine the safety and efficacy of microdroplet injections of "siloxane" to correct minor facial contour defects (40). This protocol was abandoned when "Insurmountable regulatory obstacles were encountered" (41). Despite its eclipse as a manufacturer-sponsored–investigative drug, silicone was used continually (often by those who received it from authorized sources before it was declared a new drug) with great success for over 40 years, in the treatment of over 100,000 patients for scars, rhytides (29,42), postrhinoplastic defects (43), and decubitus ulcers. The podiatric literature unequivocally supports the use of silicone, citing results following the treatment of over 800 patients in a 30-year period, for treatment of diabetic neurotrophic ulcers, and plantar callosities. A recent double-blind, randomized placebo controlled trial confirmed the efficacy of plantar silicone injections in reducing recognized risk factors associated with diabetic foot ulcerations (44–51).

A substantial number of publications have presented carefully researched studies confirming the usefulness of injectable silicone for scars, scleroderma, and a variety of atrophic conditions. Liquid silicone's safety, lack of carcinogenicity, and long-term biocompatibility have also been presented (13,29,33,52–54). By 1989, practitioner interest in the use of injectable silicone was spurred by a growing belief in its intrinsic safety when used properly. This opinion was articulated in a study published by highly respected researchers, which stated, "Although controlled studies are difficult to establish, it appears that silicone is both safe and effective when used in small amounts for appropriate indications" (55). Several years later, when the silicone breast implant controversy was at its hight, CBS News "60 Minutes" (56) presented a blistering attack upon the use of liquid silicone, replete with pictures of several horribly disfigured patients, and a melodramatic comment by FDA chief Dr. David Kessler, who averred that the FDA was investigating doctors who were "Buying industrial grade silicone in garages and injecting it into people" (56,57). Once again, the value and future of liquid silicone was in doubt. The resulting publicity led to the creation of a Soft Tissue Augmentation Task Force by the American Academy of Dermatology (AAD) and the American Society of Dermatologic Surgery (ASDS). The report published by this group in 1993 concluded that "There was a wealth of clinical experience in dermatology with the use of liquid injectable silicone by the microdroplet technique, which demonstrated its efficacy and safety, in many individuals, over many years." However, it was noted that there were no published long-term clinical trials establishing safety, and until a placebo controlled double-blind trial could be carried out, the concern about possible autoimmune reactions could not be responded to scientifically (58). At the time of this publication, the AAD/ASDS Soft Tissue Augmentation Force requested two manufacturers to support such clinical trials; neither company agreed to support such an effort.

In 1996, Rapaport et al. (59) once again raised the specter of the Jekyll and Hyde character of liquid silicone when they presented 54 patients with problems following "Medical grade silicone injections." The authors sarcastically noted that "Dermatology has recently blossomed with the wonderment of silicone injections into the face for the correction of wrinkles and acne scarring." They suggested that severe problems occurred despite employing good technique, good material, and small amounts of injected material. They also cautioned that "further studies must be performed to insure silicone safety." In a more recent article, Rapaport (60) reaffirmed his concerns about liquid silicone and at a recent lecture (61), added about 20-odd patients to his original list of 54 patients with complications ascribed to liquid silicone. Unfortunately, statistical, histological, and clinical evidence supporting the incidence and etiology of these complications was not presented.

The Dispute—Passionate Advocates

Advocates are certain that pure liquid silicone, used in small volumes, in properly selected anatomical sites, is extraordinarily safe and effective. They are quick to point out that the misuse of silicone in large volumes, particularly when combined with adulterants, creates a formula for disaster. It is, they contend, the chronicling of disasters resulting from absolute misuse of silicone, or other materials masquerading as silicone, which has created reams of sensationalized negative publicity, almost all of which can be refuted if carefully evaluated.

Dr. Norman Orentreich, liquid silicone's most ardent supporter, characterizes silicone as "The safest material I have ever used, in the treatment of over 100,000 patients." The basic record, he contends, is "One of safety essentially without serious flaw" in approximately 1400 patients under continuous study (9). Other authors have shared Dr. Orentreich's belief that silicone is intrinsically safe, in accounts involving thousands of patients. Aronsohn, who treated 4862 patients over a 22-year period, concluded, "There was absolutely no evidence that shows that subcutaneous injections of minute amounts of pure medical-grade silicone into suitable areas spaced over a long interval of time leads to any systemic physiological problems." He also notes that liquid silicone must "Rank as one of the most remarkable adjuncts ever to emerge in the field of cosmetic surgery" (62).

Webster and associates report favorable results obtained in 17,000 facial treatments over a 26-year period (42). In several other articles, he describes a favorable outcome in over 347 patients following rhinoplasty (43), and recommends that silicone be released in a controlled fashion for medical use (25,43,63,64). Greenberg reports excellent results following the treatment of 14,000 patients by dermatologists, who responded to an informal poll carried out in 1991 (65). Others have joined Dr. Webster in supporting the use of liquid silicone, among them Stegman, Auerbach, Yarborough, and Waxman (54,66–68). Barnett has treated over 10,000 patients during a 26-year practice, with excellent results and minimal problems (personal communication). Duffy reported good results following the treatment of 2500 patients over a 13-year period (2,33,53).

The Adversaries: Shrill Critics

In stark contrast to the advocates' claims that pure liquid silicone, used properly, is incapable of provoking serious or untreatable local complications, adversaries of silicone present patients, who, in their opinion, develop "Massive, deforming and sometimes absolutely untreatable granulomas, despite good technique, good materials, and small amounts injected" (59). Two recent editorials summarize the nature of the current dispute (60,69). Silicone's adversaries are absolutely convinced that liquid silicone is intrinsically unpredictable and that the complications resulting from its use are sometimes horrific, almost never reported, and often untreatable, occurring many years after the injections were carried out. They note the advocates' position that side effects seen in the past were due to "Bad contaminated material" or "Too much material injected" and "Poorly trained physicians injecting silicone" (59) would not explain the problems that they were seeing in patients who were "As best as can be determined treated with unadulterated sterile silicone (volume unspecified)." They note that "Medical-grade silicone" was made available and used or misused in an estimated 20,000–40,000 people during the 1960s in Las Vegas. The complications of this use resulted in the state criminalization of liquid silicone. The same authors advance the theory that reactions to the use of pure silicone occur 5 to 20 years after injection whereas "Experience with adulterated preparations show problems occurring very quickly, often within 6 months." This delay in the appearance of complications is theorized as a method of distinguishing reactions following pure silicone from those which occur after adulterated forms of silicone are used. They suggest that it is the nature of these "fixer chemicals (croton oil, paraffin) to cause reactions almost immediately." They ask, "Why does silicone migrate? Why does it insinuate itself into the depths of skin and infiltrate into local vessels? Is this infiltration the cause of recurrent cellulitis?" They feel that the "collective clinical evidence demonstrates a propensity for major problems to occur when silicone is injected into the face" and suggest that because of the long latency period before problems occur, any studies concerning safety need to be performed over many years. They do concede that the incidence of complications is low but that these complications can be devastating and cannot generally be resolved satisfactorily. Despite what appears to be credible scientific studies exonerating all forms of silicone as contributory, systemic immunopathologic agents, (38, pg. 512) a variety of opponents including litigants and consumer groups are still convinced that silicone breast implants are associated with collagen vascular disease. Critics of liquid silicone wonder openly whether advocates of its use reveal the whole truth about their experiences. They point out that until 1997, the use of silicone was excluded by name by many malpractice insurance carriers, while some of silicone's prime supporters were ordered to cease and desist by the FDA. Other critics of silicone have categorized certain ambiguities and contradictions affecting basic issues, such as the number of patients treated, the nature and incidence of certain side effects, and the ease with which they are treated (9,27,29,39,59,66,70). They note that the favorable outcome presented by advocates of silicone never seemed to include any important side effects. All issues involving injectable liquid silicone crystallize around Dr. Norman Orentreich, whose claim to have treated 100,000 patients published in a 1983 publication shrank to 75,000 patients in a later interview (34). Orentreich's claim that "Except possibly for rare idiosyncratic reactions to medical grade silicone of which I have no personal experience" (9,10) was followed six years later in another text claiming that such reactions occur "with an approximate incidence of 1 in 10,000 patients" (2). These reactions are reported to "respond within days to intralesional corticosteroid injections and oral antibiotics." This simplistic dismissal of potentially serious reactions is negated by several FDA reports (71), at least one successful lawsuit (34) and later studies, which accurately describe the difficulty of treating silicone granulomas (59).

SILICONE AND THE MEDIA (GOOD NEWS DOESN'T SELL NEWSPAPERS)

"Americans have a fascination with newly discovered mass health hazards and a penchant to assume a cover up in any disaster" (72), indeed, the cosmetic use of liquid silicone for scars, wrinkles, and aging has all the elements, which make editorial mouths water. The occasional publication, which documents excellent results with minimal complications, is more than counterbalanced by reports, which gleefully describe the occurrence or possibility of physical disfigurement, disgusting complications, and disastrous misuse. In this setting various "experts" and pundits get a chance to do what they like best, assume a position of self-righteous moral outrage while presenting intimidating predictions of impending doom (73). The public is assaulted with a cacophony of conflicting and sensationalist silicone reportage (57,74). Advocates rarely speak out, and other than studies regarding its use for treatment of podiatric disorders (not melodramatic enough for the media), formal studies, which clarify the benefits and risks of this modality, simply do not exist. A recent article (75) provides a wonderful example of the kind of soap opera summaries, which appear regularly in the popular press. A famous New York dermatologist characterizes silicone as the gold standard of wrinkle fillers. An equally famous Beverly Hills dermatologist calls it a time bomb, and suggests, "that there are women who would stuff a Vuitton bag in their face if someone said it was permanent." He predicts that the widespread availability and use of permanent fillers will be a disaster. Lurid horror stories, "Silicone Kills Eight" (76), "Pumping Parties" (77), are followed by articles that describe the ability of plasma drawn from three women whose implants had been in place for more than a decade to kill cancer cells (78). The dramatic removal of silicone breast implants in 1992 provoked a "tidal wave" of litigation, involving some 16,000 lawsuits, brought by over a thousand lawyers on behalf of women with breast implants (72, pg. 69) which, by the time of a class action settlement (unsupported by scientific evidence), had swollen to over 30,000 lawsuits. Many of these lawsuits were "clones" because they contained the same typographical errors (72, pg. 70). The unscientific settlement of these claims for hundreds of millions of dollars provoked an even wider frenzy of litigation, involving real or imagined complications following the implantation of anything containing silicone, including penile implants (72, pg. 82), and Norplant, provoking a ripple of legal liability concerns among manufacturers who are anxious that their products not be used for any biomedical purposes. This includes Teflon and other types of products with possible biologic applications, all of which could be pilloried in the lottery of tort trials. Dow–Corning, a corporation with assets estimated at US 948 million dollars, declared bankruptcy to protect its ability to function. Although extensive and unbiased clinical and theoretical studies appear to exonerate unadulterated silicone as causative factors for systemic disease (38), authorities (and juries) persist in giving opposite and equally convincing opinions regarding risks associated with silicone use.

A New Round of Horror Stories and Another Class Action Suit

Reports in the press and on the Internet document the practice of non-trained lay personnel injecting "Silicex," a material that has not been structurally identified. Similar epidemics of misuse have been reported in Mexico, and in Thailand. In Florida, where at least 50 cases of illegal usage have been reported, this practice has resulted in severe disfigurement, deformity, and death (79–83). A Canadian physician (84) is facing a hundred million dollar class action suit brought by one hundred patients, which attempts to link silicone injections into the face with hair loss, fatigue, migraines, and numbness of the legs. The U.S. FDA is quoted as noting that the substance can "shift to other parts of the body, cause inflammation and discoloration into surrounding tissues, and form nodules of granulated or inflamed tissue." The plaintiffs' attorney notes that his clients are "stuck with a time bomb forever."

LABORATORY EVALUATIONS OF SILICONE

Early Investigations

Rees (85) utilized more than 1000 animals to determine the local and systemic effects of liquid silicone. Injections employing massive volumes of silicone, which made it difficult for the animals to move, were not followed by systemic toxicity. These early studies indicated that silicone injected in small volumes was secured with a delicate self-limited fibroblastic response without significant inflammation or foreign body reaction. With the injection of larger volumes, fibroplasia was increased, producing thicker capsules similar to those seen surrounding breast implants. Silicone was found to be nontoxic and noncarcinogenic in humans (10). Studies relating tumors in rats to liquid silicone proved to be related to a biopeculiarity of rodents: i.e., in these animals, cancerous changes can be induced by the implantation of any smooth substance, including glass or metal balls (86,87). Dimethylpolysiloxane polymer (DMPS) has been shown to undergo phagocytosis and incorporation into the reticuloendothelial systems in small quantities without adverse effects (2,85). This phenomenon has been compared to the process that occurs following injection of tattoo pigments into the skin (9).[c]

Effect of Volume

When large volumes of silicone were used, vital structures were compromised. Death occurs when large volumes of silicone have been administered intravenously or intra-arterially (2,9,26).

Carcinogenicity

Although current studies conclude that there is no credible scientific evidence to support an association of silicone or silicone breast implants with carcinogenesis (38), more intriguing is the observation that plasma drawn from three women whose implants have been in place for more than a decade, killed cancer cells, whereas plasma drawn from two women whose implants have been in place for less time and from patients without breast implants failed to kill the cancer cells (78).

Neurologic Disease

Although silicone does not appear to cause human neurologic disease (38), local problems may occur owing to the physical presence of silicone and compression of nerves. One report documents the occurrence of peripheral neuropathy in a 40-year-old patient, whose retinal detachment was treated with injectable silicone. Silicone oil was found to have migrated into the lateral ventricles of the brain, presumably along the intracranial portion of the optic nerve (90).

---

[c] Although the incorporation of tattoo pigments and silicone into the reticuloendothelial system is sometimes associated with less than desirable clinical effects (88,89).

DETECTING SILICONE IN TISSUES

Histopathology, energy dispersive X-ray elemental analysis, and transmission electron microscopy, which have been used to study the effects of silicone in living subjects, are not chemically specific, and cannot distinguish between silica, silicon, and silicones: various degrees of chemical functionality. They can neither provide a direct measurement of the metabolic activity involving silicone nor reveal alterations in the chemical nature of this complex polymeric material. More advanced techniques used to study the effects of breast implant gel in living tissues using nuclear magnetic resonance (NMR) and combinations of in vivo ^{1}H NMR localized spectroscopy and in vitro Si NMR have demonstrated that polysiloxanes are not metabolically inert or biostable, and undergo oxidization by the activity of macrophage-like cells in vitro and monocyte/macrophages in vivo (91). These reports clearly support the hypothesis that silicones can degrade to silica and elemental silicon. Silica has been shown to be associated with granuloma formation (92). The number and kind of these degradation products depends on the tissue where the silicone has metabolized (93). Recently, Haycox et al. described the technique of quantitative detection of silicone in skin using electron spectroscopy, also known as X-ray electron spectroscopy, for chemical analysis (94; ESCA). In this article, the authors report what may be the "First *quantitative* detection of silicone in the human skin." The authors also suggest that this technique appears to be highly sensitive. They further note that ESCA analysis of biologic tissues may be useful for clarifying the ongoing dispute regarding the role of injectable or implantable silicones and inflammatory or systemic disease. Whether this technique can detect and quantify adulterants, or their role in producing these complications, is yet to be seen.

Skin Tests

Orentreich reported a negative reaction to an intradermal skin test (2) involving a patient who developed a granuloma. Pearl (95) performed a skin test with liquid silicone, which "became inflamed".

Silicone Tests

A variety of diagnostic testing profiles have been offered by commercial laboratories for evaluating silicone breast disease. These tests measure chemical constituents of the implant, silicone (methyl, polysiloxane) or its breakdown products. Other tests measure circulating serum antibodies to silicone or autoantibodies, to silicone-modified host proteins. Whether or not these tests truly reveal antibodies, which are involved in the production of silicone induced systemic disease, is extremely controversial.

John Nagle, consumer safety officer in the Center for Devices and Radiological Health Diagnostics Devices Branch noted, "The tests themselves may be harmless but they sure are expensive," "somewhere between \$500–\$1000," adding that "a lot of them are being done for litigation purposes rather than to help the patient medically" (96). "Detecsil," an expensive ELISA-based test, was offered (for profit) by its inventor as a means of detecting the denaturation effects of breast implants. The importance of this test in diagnosing a true generalized reaction to silicone, has been criticized by both the FDA, who regard it as experimental, and by lay publications, which note that some of the evidence supporting this test was presented in garbage cans following its destruction after an earthquake in California. At the time of writing, the British government considers silicone tests scientifically unsound (97). Most importantly, for the purpose of this presentation, *small amounts of pure liquid silicone have never been implicated* in the production of systemic disease or associated with antibodies (98).

IMMUNOLOGIC INVESTIGATIONS

Most of the conclusions regarding the immunoreactivity of silicone were based on studies carried out before anyone had the slightest notion regarding the complexity and number of immunologic variables affecting foreign implants in biological systems. Later studies using more advanced techniques revealed more detailed information. Although no antibodies to pure liquid silicone have been discovered, Nosanchuk (99), using liquid silicone mixed with complete Freund's adjuvant, produced granulomas and commented, "under different conditions and in a different species, antibodies might be detectable". Nineteen years later, Kossovsky, using complete Freund's adjuvant, produced data suggesting that "silicone protein complexes are potentially immunogenic." Further studies suggested that all forms of silicone may act as hapten-like incomplete antigens. Further confirmation of this concept appeared in several other articles (100–103). Unlike the case of liquid silicone, for which true antibody formation is only postulated, silicone elastomers (solid silicones) used in ventriculoperitoneal shunts have been demonstrated by some investigators to elicit antibodies. Reilly et al. describe immunoreactivity with silicone gels and tubing resulting from biodegradation of the polymer in which macrophages are activated and present antigen (104). He noted that experimental animals could mount granulomatous responses to these elastomers and gels, which resembled cellular mediated immunity (CMI) granulomas. While these studies were the first to demonstrate that certain forms of silicone were capable of provoking antibodies, they did not prove that the antibodies themselves caused the reactions. Moreover, other investigators have attempted to immunize animals to silicone gels, elastomers, or fluids using powerful adjuvants, and have failed to observe any differences in tissue reactions to subsequent silicone implants in normal or immune deficient animals. It is worth remembering that most of the modern techniques developed for exploring the mechanism of immune response to both foreign bodies and microbes have never been used to determine the mechanics of successful or unsuccessful cutaneous integration of liquid silicone. There are several reasons for this (i) These techniques are expensive. (ii) Many of them are of relatively recent origin and available only as investigational modalities. (iii) Complications following use of liquid silicone are rare, cosmetic in nature, and their treatment may never generate significant revenue for companies that would have to invest millions of dollars in understanding their mechanics. An application for funding to explore the immunologic basis for silicone complications was "reluctantly rejected" because of other more compelling priorities (105).

TOXICITY AND IMMUNOGENICITY—THE FINAL VERDICT

In her book, *Science on Trial* (72), Marcia Angell, an executive editor for the *New England Journal of Medicine*, presents a compelling thematic summary of the political, economic, and scientific forces, which led to the creation of a federally appointed committee to explore the relationship between silicone breast implants and immune disorders. Their findings, presented in a comprehensive publication (38), suggested that there was "insufficient evidence to support an association between breast implants and immune-related health conditions." Had the results of this study (which passed unnoticed by the dermatologic community) concluded differently, I would not be writing this chapter and all forms of silicone, including liquid silicone would have disappeared both from the armamentarium of legitimate physicians and from a broad range of products with biological applications. In point of fact, it was the migration of liquid silicone, which was first injected into the breasts, coupled with horrific complications when adulterants were added to "anchor" large volumes of liquid silicone, which lead to the creation of modern day, envelope type breast implants (72, pg. 39).

THE COMMITTEE'S CONCLUSIONS: INSUFFICIENT EVIDENCE, PLUSES, AND MINUSES FOR SILICONE

The committee concluded that (i) "Silicones are not biologically inert, some silicones have clear biological effects." (ii) "Silicone toxicology has focused on short-term studies and there is a proportionate dearth of chronic lifetime and immunologic studies." (iii) "Silicone of various types implanted into tissues in ways that are 'relevant to the human experience are reassuring'. These materials tend to stay in place and do not appear to have long-term *systemic* toxic effects." (iv) "No significant toxicity has been uncovered by studies of individual compounds found in breast implants" (38, pg. 92, 93, 112, 197). (v) "There is no convincing evidence to support clinically significant immunologic effects of silicone or silicone breast implants." "This includes insufficient evidence for an association to a particular HLA type in women with breast implants and health conditions; insufficient evidence for silicone as a superantigen; insufficient or flawed evidence that silicone produces immune activation in cells of the immune system, silicone antibodies, delayed-type hypersensitivity (DTH) to silicone, cytokines as an immune response, antigen specific immune cellular infiltrate; and insufficient evidence for autoantibodies or T cell self antigen activation." It is suggested that the "paucity of significant, well-controlled studies examining these questions is responsible for these conclusions." "There is conclusive evidence that some silicones have adjuvant activity but there is no evidence that this has any clinical significance" (38, pg. 6).

READING BETWEEN THE LINES

Although the committee found no evidence of clinically significant *systemic* immune effects following breast implants was found, what it did discover and/or allude to may help explain localized complications, which occur following cutaneous injections of liquid silicone. (i) Although certain authors (19) believe that the intensity of granulomatous and fibrotic reactions to silicone are unaffected by location and are proportional to quantity, most authoritative publications suggest that permanent implants cause reactions that may vary as a function of size, shape, surface texture, and porosity, as well as a function of other surface physical characteristics, such as charge energy, chemical characteristics of the implant, location of the implant site, and animal species. (ii) Silicone products are not chemically identical or generically equivalent. Each type of silicone may have a differing potential for biological mobility and activity. It is mandatory to evaluate each product, individually, for safety, and avoid inappropriate extrapolations among differing chemical entities (6). (iii) *All* implants may provoke foreign body inflammatory reactions (38, pg. 141–142). (iv) These reactions are considered to be a "normal" part of the body's intrinsic (innate) defense mechanisms. (v) All types of silicone may provoke an immune response.

Hydrophobic materials such as silicone elastomers (and possibly liquid silicones) are coated with host proteins within a few hours of implantation. Inflammatory cells that enter tissues may not respond to the silicone itself, but to a surface layer of partially denatured adsorbed plasma proteins for which there are specific receptors. Responding macrophages may secrete two-fold more IL-1B, IL-6, and TNF-α than macrophages exposed to naked silicone (38, pg. 191).[d]

INFECTION AND IMPLANTS

There is a growing awareness that infections, overt or occult, will adversely affect permanent implants (33). Kossovsky et al. (107) noted

---

[d] The influence of these proteins on the intensity of macrophage activity has been cited as a rationale for complications following Artecoll® injections (106, pg. 18).

that local infections accelerated the process of capsule formation around implanted silicone prostheses. Virden et al. (108) noted infections with *Staphylococcus epidermidis* or *Propionibacterium acnes* in up to 56% of explanted breast implants (108). Other authors have noted that antibody formation, including that of anti-DNA antibodies, occurs naturally against *S. epidermidis*, while bacterial infection has been used to explain the production of interleukins (IL-2 and IL-6) within fibrous breast capsules (109).

Indolent infections around implants have also been used to explain a zone of T lymphocytes surrounding breast capsules (110). It may be that the relief from symptoms of a variety of immunologic ailments achieved via explantation of silicone implants is due to the removal of "a nidus of infection" (2), rather than that of the silicone implant itself. FDA protocols permitting silicone gel implants to be used for reconstructive purposes specifically exclude patients who have an abscess or infection anywhere in the body (111). These studies unquestionably have relevance for liquid silicone implantation as well. Indeed, the use of liquid silicone in the presence of overt (even distant) clinical infections is contraindicated in all authoritative publications (2,58). Inflammatory and granulomatous complications following the implantation of liquid silicone are most frequently seen in association with infectious processes (2,20,29,33,52,53,61,112,113).[e]

Sources of Infection

Although a variety of bacterial species can be cultured from the surface of, or from around the breast tissue, in implants without clinical signs, there is suggestive evidence that the presence of bacteria correlates with contracture, a feature that may have implications for the development of excessive fibrosis surrounding injectable silicone implants. The tissue of the breast is open to the environment through the lactiferous ducts, leading to the colonization of the breast by a variety of commensal and potentially pathogenic organisms. Over 90% of female breasts are colonized by bacteria, which may lead to the development of an infection in an otherwise well-tolerated breast implant many years after implantation, without an apparent inciting event (38, pg. 167–172). In a similar fashion, a conduit for bacterial contamination of liquid silicone injected into the face (and the production of granulomatous and nongranulomatous inflammation) may be related to the proximity of sinus and oral cavities, which are often colonized by potentially pathogenic bacteria, as well as to the number and distribution of sebaceous glands that contain *P. acnes*, a known stimulus for the development of granulomata (114–116).

---

[e] Perhaps on the basis of molecular mimicry.

CYTOKINES AND T CELL ACTIVATION—THE NEW INFECTION CONNECTION

Although studies relating silicone breast implants to T cell activation and cytokine production revealed the levels of these compounds to be below the range of detection of the various assays, and did not provide sufficient evidence for immune system activation, it was suggested that (i) Changes in **cytokine**[f] concentrations were a general response to biomaterial implantation (38, pg. 183). (ii) Studies by several groups of workers suggesting that silicone induces IL-1, TNF-α, or IL-6 production may have been linked to the possibility of microbial contamination with endotoxin, lipopolysaccharides (LPS), lipoteichoic acid, or similar molecules. Bacterial products such as these are known to stimulate immune activation (117, pg. 476).

RELEVANCE TO COMPLICATIONS FOLLOWING THE USE OF LIQUID SILICONE

It is reasonable to assume from the information assembled that although all forms of pure silicone are biocompatible materials, prolonged tissue exposure provides an interface for possible bacterial and viral infectious processes with these potentially haptenic compounds. This rare event may lead to the localized activation of both innate and adaptive immune systems and the subsequent production of cytokines, particularly TNF-α. This paradigm would provide both an immunopathogenetic mechanism for the development of silicone granulomas, and a good explanation for their successful treatment, using immunosuppressive agents such as corticosteroids, and antibiotics, whose anti-inflammatory effects may also be immunosuppressive and completely separate, and distinct from their antimicrobial action (114,115,119–121). Agents such as biologic response modifiers and other immunosuppressants used to treat diseases, which share similar immunopathogenetic mechanisms, provide a rational alternative treatment resource for granulomata that do not respond to "first line agents." Baumann and Halem (121) has reported successful treatment of "silicone granulomas" using the biological immune response modifier imiquimod—a therapeutic strategy that has also proved successful for the treatment of certain types of granulomas, which followed the use of cosmetic tattoos (122). The tantalizing therapeutic possibilities inherent in understanding the immunologic processes underlying silicone complications will be discussed in more detail later in this chapter.

---

[f] Terms in bold appear in a glossary of immunologic terms, processes, and definitions at the end of this chapter.

COMPLICATIONS

The future of all permanent implants, including liquid silicone (Artecoll) and others yet to be discovered or employed, will be determined by a factual, understanding of the incidence, etiology, and treatment of complications, which might follow their proper use. Accordingly, any meaningful presentation dealing with the use of liquid silicone must be accompanied by a thorough presentation and analysis of extraordinarily rare, but highly publicized complications associated with their use.

EVALUATING REPORTS OF SILICONE COMPLICATIONS

What makes an honest evaluation of liquid silicone so difficult is the fact that both lay and scientific journals constantly proffer an extraordinary variety of conflicting information in the form of anecdotal opinions unsupported by statistical proofs. It is agreed upon that liquid silicone is permanent, has been abused, will migrate when large volumes are employed, but complicationsshould not be used in specific areas, such as the penis or glandular tissue of the breast. Serious complications are extremely rare when small volumes of sterile, pure liquid silicone are employed, but complications are much more common and severe following the use of large volumes of adulterated silicone. All types of complications can occur immediately or many years after treatment. Formal studies and clinical observations have clearly implicated infection, usually but not always, coupled with large volumes of silicone, pure or adulterated, as a contributory or causative factor in the development of severe localized granulomatous/inflammatory complications. There is general agreement that the use of adulterants, particularly when coupled with large volumes of silicone, creates a true formula for disaster. What has not been determined, and what is most important in assessing the true usefulness of liquid silicone, is the incidence or etiology of serious complications following the use of small volumes of pure liquid silicone in appropriate anatomical areas. To date, there has been no retrospective method to determine how much liquid silicone was employed or to determine its purity.

Moreover, no one has looked for occult infectious agents using DNA polymerase technology, employed modern immunohistochemical techniques to determine the specifics of immune system activation, or considered the use of immunosuppressive drugs (some of which were not previously available, i.e., antipsoriatic medications) other than corticosteroids and antibiotics. No one has compared silicone complications to other conditions, which exhibit similar histopathologic or clinical features. The logic of using therapies, which have worked for related diseases, is beginning to be applied in the United States for the treatment of sarcoidosis (123), and in Europe for the treatment of complications that follow other types of permanent implants (106). A 1996 monograph (59), which compiles complications in 54 patients following the use of "Medical-grade" silicone, suffers from the same inadequacies characterizing other horrific reports, which appear sporadically in the world literature. No attempt is made by the authors to determine the incidence of such complications, or to address the possibility that liquid silicone may provide extraordinary good results for the vast majority of properly selected patients. The notion that small volumes of silicones were employed was supported by the recollection by a single patient that minute quantities were given through "a tiny needle"(59). The purity of the silicone used was documented only by the comment: "As best as can be determined, unadulterated sterile silicone of 350 centistokes was used in the overwhelming majority of our cases." Implicit in this answer is the fact that the authors really do not know how much silicone was used, how often the patients were treated, and whether the silicone used was pure or adulterated. It might also be fair to ask whether any of these patients had received treatments from experienced clinicians, who because of the numbers of patients they claim to have treated, would be at greater statistical risk for such complications.

One patient reportedly treated using good technique and sterile silicone was, in fact, treated by the same physician whose handiwork was presented in the example of his patient, ElaineYoung. Her grotesquely disfigured face was presented on National Television (56). These same authors also note that many patients who received silicone injections had no problems, while others who were injected during the same period by the same physician with the "same material" did develop complications. Their puzzlement is most easily addressed by postulating an infectious etiology for these complications and/or by attributing their occurrence to the use of both pure liquid silicone and adulterated silicone by the same clinician at different times. Kagan (36) used the Sakurai formula to inject at least 300 patients before switching over to pure liquid silicone while Aronsohn (62) treated 538 patients with oleic acid or sesame oil before going on to treat 4324 patients with pure liquid silicone.

FORMAL CLINICAL STUDIES

Only two localized, serious, cutaneous complications have been reported following the use of liquid silicone under FDA authorization for the treatment of over 1400 patients, during a 20-year period. During the first phase of the study in which over 1300 patients were treated, migration occurred in the leg of one polio patient treated with large volumes (34,39,71). In the second phase of this study, which followed 144 patients, another serious reaction was reported to occur in a woman with Weber–Christian Disease, rheumatoid arthritis, and atypical mycobacterial infection,[g] who received a large (25 cc) volume of liquid silicone for facial

---

[g] All of which are united by TNF-α, LPS, and T cell activation.

atrophy. In this case, massive facial necrosis and inflammation unresponsive to systemic steroids or antibiotics occurred about 11 years after her last injection of silicone. In his review of this patient's history, Achauer noted the occurrence of two similar reactions reported by other researchers not involved in the formal study. One patient was diagnosed with Weber–Christian disease and the other had no specific diagnosis (95,124). In 1996, a similar severe granulomatous reaction occurred periorally, 12 years after the injection of an unknown volume of silicone of undetermined purity (125). Histologic examination in all these cases revealed a chronic inflammatory reaction with foreign body giant cells. In his analysis of the single case, which occurred during the FDA study, Achauer notes that it was impossible to be certain whether this condition was a reactivation of Weber–Christian disease, or a reaction to silicone (124). To date, no immunologic or immunohistochemical studies or PCR evaluations have ever been employed epidemiologically for the evaluation of silicone granulomas.

Clinical Features

Complications to liquid silicone injection can be asymptomatic (noninflammatory) or symptomatic (inflammatory), and of early or late onset. The most common cause of these problems is improper technique. Silicone is permanent, unforgiving, and extraordinarily technique sensitive. Patients must be carefully selected and slowly treated. The intrinsic safety experienced by established practitioners in the use of silicone is summarized by Robert Auerbach, "I am embarrassed to say," Dr. Auerbach remarked, "that in more than 20 years of using and following silicone I have never had a bad reaction." "The whole trick as well as the whole disadvantage of using this material is to proceed *slowly* with small amounts injected into numerous sites over a number of sessions" (66). David Orentreich concurs (12), noting that he has "Not experienced granulomatous reactions to liquid injectable silicone administered by the microdroplet serial puncture technique." He attributes "granulomatous reactions to purported silicone" to overinjection, injection into contraindicated sites, or injection of impure silicone or substances of unknown composition. He does report that "idiosyncratic" (nongranulomatous) inflammatory reactions to liquid silicone, characterized by well-demarcated areas of moderate swelling with or without erythema, can appear months or years after injection, at an incidence of 1:5000 to 1:10000 treatment sessions. These "are frequently proceeded by an infection at a distant site" and respond within days or weeks to "intracorticoid steroid injections and oral antibiotics." These reactions are attributed to "silicone acting as a nidus for infection, proliferation of bacteria on the surface of an inert substance, and chemicals present in living tissues which may become concentrated on silicone, provoking a reaction of these sites" (12). No histologic or immunologic evaluation of these complications was presented in this paper.

Pain during injection, transient edema, ecchymosis, and erythema are routine, following injection. Dyschromia, consisting of a bluish tinge resulting from superficial deposition of fluid, and temporary brownish-yellow pigmentation of the skin, have been reported. Textural changes consisting of a firm, rubbery consistency on palpation have been noted. Peau d'orange appearance may occur possibly on the basis of improper placement of silicone or blockage of lymphatics. Chronic irritation and changes in sensation have been reported (33). There is general agreement that migration, ulceration, and many of the horrific sequela of the improper use of adulterated silicone do not occur following the use of small volumes of pure liquid silicone in properly selected patients.

Overcorrection

There are two types of overcorrection. (i) Those which are of esthetic or cosmetic importance only, e.g., overly large lips, which often represent a combination of poor esthetic judgment on the part of the doctor and the patient. (ii) Those which represent specific technique errors (wrong volume, wrong location, and wrong lesion). When relatively small volumes of liquid silicone are employed, most overcorrections are asymptomatic and barely noticeable, often taking the form of poorly defined linear, papular, or circular projections. "Beading," the occurrence of small papules, which may result from too superficial an injection of silicone, is also common when injecting horizontal creases of the face, such as the creases on the forehead, the mental line, and the fine horizontal crease that traverses the philtrum. Injection of shallow V-shaped rhytides of the upper lip can also lead to overcorrection, possibly because silicone may be displaced to the border of these wrinkles while being injected. Greenberg notes overcorrection to occur most commonly in the chin or glabella, where the patient responds by "laying down too much collagen" (65). Dermal nodules, which are asymptomatic, but firm to the touch, can also occur.

Histologically, these are often noninflammatory granulomas (unpublished personal observations). This complication, which has been attributed to the too superficial deposition of silicone in the papillary dermis rather than in the deep reticular dermis, causing excessive fibrohistiocytic proliferation (67), has also been implicated in the development of granulomatous nodules following implantation of Gortex (expanded polytetrafluoroethylene) (126). Noninflammatory nodules are most common in the lips (Fig. 14) and oral commissures, and adjacent to the alae nasi in the proximal nasolabial crease. They may also occur where the skin is very thin or stretched tightly, i.e., periorbital creases (crow's feet, eyelid skin). Bound-down "ice pick scars" can develop a "doughnut-like" elevated collarette where silicone, which cannot elevate the deepest portion of the bound-down scar, elevates its periphery. Pliable atrophic scars, which require mid-dermal implantation, can look well initially, but over a period of time, undergo excessive fibroplasia that resembles hypertrophic scarring. This immunologic process does not appear to be related to technique deficiencies. It may result from abnormal collagen synthesis, which may involve a **cytokine**

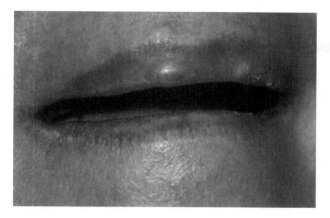

Figure 14
Patient E (12/28/88): These nodules resulted from liquid silicone and partially responded to intralesional steroids.

imbalance modulating overproduction of IL-4, a T_H2 cytokine and decreased levels of interferon gamma, a T_H1 cytokine, a process that is implicated in scleroderma (127–129). Cytokine regulation of angiogenesis may also be involved in the production of telangiectasia which have been noted following silicone injections (27).

Delayed Reactions/Rosacea and Rosacea-like Syndromes—Have Some "Silicone Reactions" Been Misdiagnosed?

A number of syndromes, which clinically and histologically resemble other disease entities, have been reported following use of liquid silicone. Rosacea-like reactions have been reported (65).

Fisher (130) reported the appearance of pruritic nodules in the face at the exact site of previous silicone injections in two patients, who developed complications following breast implantation. Biopsies of these nodules revealed nonspecific inflammation. Periocular nodules have been described, using the ominous term "metastatic silicone granuloma" in association with asymptomatic eyelid edema and erythema of the face and arms, associated with Sjögren syndrome–like annular erythema of the arms, and sicca complex (dry mouth and dry eyes) (131). These bear a striking resemblance to atypical specific presentations of sarcoidosis, which include rosacea-like syndromes and Sjögren's syndrome. Clinical and histological similarities between cutaneous sarcoidosis and complications following liquid silicone implantation are extensive. The differential diagnosis of these lesions includes silicone-induced granulomata, but should also include papular or granulomatous acne rosacea (also referred to as rosacea-like tuberculid or lupus miliaris disseminatus facii). Osofsky (92) also notes that papular or granulomatous acne rosacea may arise as a foreign body reaction from disrupted hair follicles, and that these granulomas are histologically indistinguishable from sarcoidosis. "A biopsy specimen to establish the diagnosis of sarcoidosis should be interpreted with caution if taken from the face." Rapaport's photograph of a widespread facial eruption, which had been triggered by Etanercept in areas treated with liquid silicone about 36 years back, was highly suggestive of granulomatous acne rosacea (61). When one of my patients (KC) developed what appeared to be granulomatous lesions in areas that had never been injected with silicone, biopsy revealed a pattern consistent with granulomatous acne rosacea (unpublished personal observation). Another 40-year-old woman had, one year before, received injections of silicone gel extracted from a breast prosthesis. She developed submandibular lymphadenopathy. Biopsy revealed "silicone granulomas" (88).

Statistics: Past and Present

Almost nothing has been published regarding the frequency of silicone use or of benefits. A survey carried out by the American Academy of Cosmetic Surgery noted that 59,285 injections were carried out in 1990 alone, making it the ninth most popular cosmetic procedure, cited by respondents to a physician questionnaire (65). In addition, a literature review of treatment using the microdroplet technique carried out several years ago indicates that well over 130,000 patients have been treated in America alone. If one includes 10,000 patients treated in Japan using adulterated silicone (33), and the estimate that between 20,000 to 40,000 patients received silicone during the 1960s in Las Vegas, much of which were unquestionably adulterated, it seems reasonable to assume that at least 200,000 patients have been treated with silicone worldwide; the true figure is probably closer to twice that number. Assuming that only 200,000 patients have been treated, and serious complications have occurred or will occur in 0.2 (2/10 of 1%) (55), then at least 400 patients should have been expected to develop serious complications during the last 40 years of silicone use. Nothing in the world literature suggests that this number of complications have occurred, even with egregious misuse of all kinds of injectable agents. The only serious problems reported involved the use of large volumes of silicone. Inflammatory complications following the injection of small volumes of pure liquid silicone are rare, and usually (but not always) small and easily treatable. Estimates of "serious complications" vary from 1 in 10,000 (2) to 1 in 1000 (65). Conversely, extensive granulomas and nongranulomatous inflammatory processes are much more common following the use of large volumes of silicone, particularly those which contain adulterants (55,132). In addition, at the histologic level, more severe inflammatory reactions have been noted when ruptured silicone breast implants spill large volumes of liquid silicone gel into surrounding tissues (19,133).

Facial Site Specificity/Relationship to Complications

Various facial regions exhibit specific patterns of response to implantable agents. For liquid silicone, a permanent implant, an understanding of these differences will lead to uniformly better results.

Four areas merit specific attention. (i) The glabella, because of its proximity to underlying sinuses, is susceptible to colonization by pathogenic bacteria when infectious processes occur. The glabella is also a danger zone for arterial compromise and deep injections in this area may be followed by ulcerations, although to date, I have not had this experience with liquid silicone. (ii) The nasolabial folds are rigid and relatively inelastic at their proximal end near the alae nasi, but they become much more flexible as they extend distally toward the oral commissures. Certain types of nasolabial folds are not suitable for silicone injections. These are very broad, are very deep, or exist adjacent to a fold of redundant skin, a situation often encountered in patients who have either lost a great deal of weight or have developed atrophic changes owing to age and genetic predispositions. Very shallow crease-like nasolabial folds can be easily overcorrected. (iii) The lips may be particularly susceptible to inflammatory and granulomatous reactions following the use of injectable materials for a number of reasons, including their proximity to the oral cavity (the lips are only 2 mm away from a vast reservoir of potentially pathogenic bacteria), which make the lips a common target for a number of other types of granulomatous reactions (22,134–138). In addition, exposure to ultraviolet light can trigger herpetic infections, and traumatically induced bacterial contamination is a common event following both dental procedures and the wear and tear of everyday life. Complications including intermittent or persistent erythema, swelling, and nodularity have been reported following implantation of many types of materials (139–141), including Artecoll [polymethylmethacrylate microspheres (Plexiglas)], suspended in bovine collagen, Bioplastique (polymerized silicone particles in a gel carrier), Gortex (expanded polytetrafluoroethylene threads or patches), and hyaluronic acid (106,126,140,142–144). Silicone injections have also resulted in similar problems (20,52,61,113).

Macrocheilia is fashionable now, resulting in enormous patient interest in fuller, more youthful lips. Accordingly, a great deal of pressure is brought upon practitioners to create permanently larger lips. It is always tempting to provide patients with a permanent solution to their dissatisfaction with what they view as hypoplastic lips. However, in the long term, results are not always optimal (see contraindications in Complications Personal Evaluation), suggesting that permanent implants are not the best initial approach, and should be avoided in certain types of patients. Injections of permanent fillers should be aimed at modest improvements in lip volume. (iv) Oral commissures and melolabial folds (marionette lines) look deceptively easy to treat, but in fact, following injection, there may be protrusion of the implanted material into the oral cavity, resulting in a puffy appearance, and a feeling of nodularity inside the mouth. One needs to understand that elevation of the corners of the mouth does not occur in some individuals, unless enormous volumes of material are used, a process that is contraindicated for permanent fillers. Injections of BOTOX to disable the depressor angularis oris muscles may be an effective and safer method for accomplishing this purpose. (v) Jowliness: the aging process often produces a sagging at the angle of the jaw (jowl). This sagginess can be minimized with small volumes of silicone used between the chin and the jowl area, to produce a more natural and linear definition of the jaw line.

GRANULOMAS AND SILICONE

The carefully researched observation that "Tissue reaction to silicone implants appears to be one of granulomatous inflammation, with a general histologic appearance determined by the type of silicone employed," coupled with the fact that "Migrating silicone can produce granulomas on the surface of organs" (38, pg. 191), should lay to rest the notion that "pure" silicone is unique in evading immune surveillance. It also suggests proof of the principle that an understanding of granulomatous processes and their relationship to a multiplicity of factors, including abnormalities of foreign body processing (145–150), neoplasia (151), trauma (152), collagen vascular disease (153,154), medications (155), relationships between different kinds of granulomas (156) and disease processes activated by infections (154,157–159), is a key element in addressing complications, which occur following the use of liquid silicone, or any type of implant. Many factors can have a profound effect upon the frequency and types of granulomatous complications, and of the specific types of immunologic processing that occur. These include portal of entry, i.e., tissues or organs involved, site of implantation (lips, hands) volume, the presence of particulate matter, adulterants, cellular location of antigen, and the presence or absence of a variety of disease states or drugs, which can interact synergistically with immune processes responsible for granulomata development.

IF IT LOOKS LIKE A DUCK

Some observers are certain that silicone-induced granulomatous complications represent a unique pathological entity. Mastruserio's astute observation (125) that the clinical appearance of a particular case "Exemplifies many of the typical features of silicone induced granulomatous disease" did not spur the realization that silicone granulomata and Weber–Christian disease do not only look alike but share immunopathogenetic mechanisms. Had Mastruserio's intellectual pseudopodia extended just a little farther, (or had knowledge of immunologic processes been more advanced) he might have realized that Weber–Christian disease and silicone granulomata might very well represent different facets of the same disease process, and respond to similarly therapeutic approaches for pathological conditions, which histologically and/or immunophenotypically resemble each other (160–166).

Systemic Complications

Although systemic complications have never been reported following the proper use of pure liquid silicone for soft tissue augmentation, catastrophic complications have occurred following technique failures at the hands of untrained and careless personnel. Pneumonitis, acute respiratory distress syndromes, and sudden death have followed intravascular injections of silicone (31,167). Injection of large volumes of intentionally adulterated or contaminated silicone into the breast has led to necrosis and ulcerations, possibly due to infection and vascular or lymphatic compromise. Large volumes, particularly of low-viscosity silicones, have also led to migration of silicone fluids to distant sites (2,9,26). Erysipelas-like reactions have been reported, and blindness, loss of neurologic function, and death have occurred when liquid silicone entered ophthalmic and meningeal vessels (27).

Autoimmunity/Adjuvant Disease

Although recent studies appear to exonerate all forms of silicone from any causal association with connective tissue disease (38), reports have appeared in the literature since 1964, discussing more than 100 cases of connective tissue disease–like illness occurring in patients who have undergone various forms of breast augmentation (38,98,168–171). Injected materials included paraffin, processed petrolatum jelly, and silicone of unknown purity (2,172–175). Miyoshi introduced the term "adjuvant disease" to describe two patients who developed an arthritic condition, that mimicked "Adjuvant arthritis" in rodents, which had been induced experimentally using mixtures of mineral oil, lanolin and killed tuberculosis bacilli (101,169,176). It was postulated that these "Adjuvants" were directly involved in the pathogenesis of this disorder when the signs and symptoms of their disease were relieved by mastectomy.

Since 1982, periodic anecdotal reports describing connective tissue disease following mammary augmentation with silicone gel–filled elastomer envelope type prostheses (169) have appeared in the world literature, culminating in the temporary prohibition of silicone gel implants for cosmetic mammary augmentation and what may be the most expensive legal battle in American history. Scleroderma has been reported most often, but diseases resembling rheumatoid arthritis (RA), systemic lupus erythematosus (SLE), scleroderma (PSS) or mixed connective tissue disease (MCTD) have also been reported. Polymyositis and dermatomyositis have also been described (172).

INJECTION SITE COMPLICATIONS

Clinical Presentation

Cutaneous complications, which may occur within months to years after injection of both pure and adulterated silicones and other substances, can be manifested in a variety of ways, including severe or moderate persistent or intermittent swelling, sometimes but not always associated with erythema, rock hard induration, or purple discoloration. Winer et al. (28) was the first to term silicone-induced granulomas as "Siliconomas" noting their occurrence following the use of intentionally adulterated silicone and there is general agreement that contaminants in any amount can produce catastrophes (2,9,17,95). The notion that "impurities" can have disastrous implications for permanent implants was used to explain foreign body reactions following the use of Artecoll (177), which were considered to be caused by PMMA (polymethylmethacrylate) impurities, that were attached to the surface of the microspheres. In 1994, the microspheres were changed to "ones with absolutely smooth surfaces" with a substantial reduction in the occurrence of granulomas. Inflammatory and noninflammatory complications, both granulomatous and nongranulomatous, can occur without provocation, following any type of foreign body implantation, or may be precipitated by multiple factors including trauma, vasodilatory conditions (exercise, alcohol, allergies), as well as systemic or localized bacterial or viral infections (178). Certain drugs and allergies have been anecdotally implicated as clinical cofactors for silicone complications (33), including, paradoxically, drugs which might be expected to block the type of immune activation responsible for silicone granulomas (60).

Rapid/Delayed—Granulomas and the Role of Adulterants

Apparently, the concept that implantation of any foreign body without considering the purity or lack thereof, including dextran beads, Plexiglas, silicone and Gortex (106,114,126), tattoos (141,179), and bovine collagen (Fig. 15) (178,180–184), can be followed by granulomas or inflammation at any time has never occurred to observers who speculate that reactions to "Medical-grade silicone occur later than those following the injection of silicone of unknown purity." "From our experience adulterants have not been used for 35 years" (59,95). I see, on a regular basis, patients with severe complications following treatment, in Mexico, within the last three years, using what appears to be large volumes of unquestionably adulter-

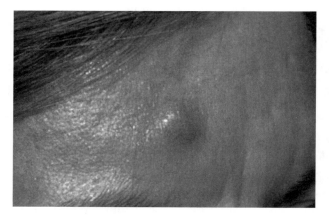

Figure 15
Patient D (8/25/81): Cystic reactions occasionally occur following Zyderm® collagen. This cyst appeared three weeks after treatment of a small scar in this area. Incision and drainage were effective in treating it.

ated silicone. One such patient, who developed massive facial swelling (which revealed granulomas on biopsy), brought with her a small bottle of milky fluid with which she had been injected. This patient, who had the advantage of speaking excellent Spanish, persuaded the physician who treated her to give her a small sample of the material he had used. Her complications began about five years after her first treatment, confirming the fact that although some patients who have received adulterated silicone can develop complications quickly, these complications can also develop many years after treatment. There is no credible support for the idea that the use of adulterants has dropped off, or that adulterants cannot produce late onset complications. A number of well-documented studies describe the occurrence of granulomas at different times following a variety of adulterants (2,9,185). Paraffins (mineral oil) were first employed cosmetically in 1899, and by 1906, disfiguring subcutaneous nodules had been observed in two patients who had received this agent for facial wrinkles. Subcutaneous nodules have been reported to occur more than 30 years after the injection of paraffins (186). In another case, a severe granulomatous reaction occurred 42 years after the injection of paraffin (185). Zyderm® collagen has produced inflammatory nodules, which appeared two years after injection and persisted for four more years (61). Granulomas have followed the use of hyaluronic acid (144), and late-onset granulomatous reactions to Artecoll have been described (177), which mimic delayed reactions to liquid silicone. Delays noted in the occurrence of complications are probably related to infectious processes, which may occur more quickly when a larger antigenic burden is presented in the form of adulterants (19).

Analyzing Granulomata

The analysis of granulomata is best divided into three components: clinical, histologic, and immunological. Several features make this analysis both interesting and complex. (i) "An identical histologic pattern may be produced by multiple causes. Conversely, a single disease process may produce multiple histologic and immunohistochemical patterns" (92). (ii) The clinical appearance of inflammatory granulomatous and nongranulomatous complications provides no clue to the specific immunologic or infectious process underlying them.[h] (iii) Granulomas can evolve through multiple phases over time, which can be distinguished histologically by light microscopy, and are in fact, immunologically heterogenous. This will certainly affect their response to different therapeutic strategies employed at different stages in the disease process (187). New reports of granulomas occurring from a wide variety of causes appear regularly in the world literature. Recently, granulomas have been reported following the injection of sesame

---

[h] Although silicone induced granulomatous inflammation is sometimes much firmer to palpation (perhaps reflecting increased fibrosis) than nongranulomatous inflammatory processes (unpublished personal observations).

seed oil (188), and after the use of acupuncture needles [presumably as a consequence of their coating with liquid silicone; (189)]. It is interesting to note that despite worldwide use of siliconized needles for over 50 years, and in literally billions of injections, granulomas have never been reported.

Etiology/Relationships to Multiple Disease Processes

Originally thought to represent neoplastic growth of granulation tissue, the term "granuloma" now implies a reactive non-neoplastic inflammatory reaction forming as a response to insoluble, nondegradable, or slowly released antigens. Granulomas occur characteristically as a response to persistent microbes (i.e., tuberculosis, or fungi), (117, pg. 302), or in response to particular antigens, which are not readily phagocytized (117, pg. 449). During this process, tissue macrophages (histiocytes) are transformed into activated macrophages, epithelioid cells, and multinucleate giant cells. Clusters of macrophages surround antigen sources (including particulate sources), producing granulomatous inflammation. Histopathologically, granulomas are categorized by the presence or absence of necrosis, necrobiosis, and vasculitis, and the nature of the inflammatory cell infiltrate. Granulomas are associated with a wide variety of etiologic agents including foreign bodies, drugs, genetic syndromes, infectious processes, and neoplastic conditions with a granulomatous component (151), from tattoos (141,179,190,191) to intralesional corticosteroids (192). Although granulomas can occur in otherwise healthy individuals, they are commonly associated with immune-modulated disorders (117, pg. 452,136,144,145,147,155,193–198).

Granulomas and Inflammation Following Implants/Histologic Distinctions

Although liquid silicone and bovine collagen (178,180–184), can induce necrobiotic granulomas associated with focally altered or degenerated collagen, characteristically, silicone granulomas, and indeed granulomata, which follow other types of permanent implants (106,126), are often non-necrobiotic foreign body granulomas with sarcoidal features, i.e., "naked granulomas" with an abundance of epithelioid histiocytes, absence of necrobiotic collagen, and giant cells, either of the foreign body or of the Langerhans type. This pattern is common in a variety of systemic and cutaneous diseases, some of which may have relevance in understanding silicone granulomata (92, pg. 594). Clinically, herpes simplex virus infections mimicking foreign body reactions have been reported after the use of Gortex. Biopsies in these cases revealed inflammatory reactions. Polymerase chain reaction (PCR) suggested herpetic infections (126,142). PCR techniques will unquestionably be useful for evaluating inflammatory complications following liquid silicone, as well as for determining the choice of antimicrobial agents to be employed. As in sarcoidosis, in which conventional bacteriologic and viral cultures are routinely negative, infectious inflammation of implants may be sequestered in such a way as to render the infectious organisms undetectable by conventional culture techniques. Inflammation and granulomas are a generic possibility following any type of implant, permanent or impermanent, including hyaluronic acid (144). For liquid silicone, the "rare inflammatory reactions" reported by advocates (12), may be precursors for the development of end-stage fibrotic granulomas. The distinction between inflammatory and granulomatous reactions to foreign bodies such as silicone may be nothing more than a distinction between acute and chronic inflammatory processes related to the relative balance between exudation and cellular recruitment (199), "Which depending on the nature of the irritant, different profiles of inflammatory mediators and growth factors (collectively referred to as cytokines), are generated locally giving rise to different morphological patterns of chronic inflammation" (199, pg. 1). Different patterns of cytokine secretion may occur for the morphologically distinct giant cells of foreign body and immunologically driven granulomas (199, pg. 4).

IMMUNOPATHOLOGY/SILICONE COMPLICATIONS REDEFINED—NEW NAMES, NEW CONCEPTS, AND NEW LISTS TO MEMORIZE

Although pathologists in years past were familiar with the histologic appearance of granulomas, they could not, as modern immunologists do now, at the molecular level, define granulomas as clusters of activated macrophages and T lymphocytes, which are viewed as forms of **DTH**, the hallmark of which is excessive fibrosis. In the past, tissue fibrosis was viewed as a "passive" response to tissue injury. Fibrosis is in fact a potentially reversible dynamic product of immunomodulatory activity of previously unimagined complexity (127–129). And although pathologists in years past would have recognized fibroblasts and epithelioid cells, they could not have known that these noninflammatory "Bystander" cells might play an important role in producing granulomatous inflammation (200).

Immunologically, epithelioid cells represent activated macrophages, which have developed increased cytoplasm and cytoplasmic organelles that histologically resemble epithelial cells. Driving this transformation is a complex series of immunologic processes, which result in the replacement of phagocytic activity with secretory function and the ability to recruit additional macrophages that mediate fibroplasia and collagen deposition (92,117). Granulomas are commonly triggered by intracellular bacteria, which can survive and duplicate within host cells, including phagocytes. Immunity against these microbes is principally **CMI** involving activated macrophages, **CD4+** T cells, and **CD8+** cytotoxic T cells **(CTLs)** lysing infected cells (117, pg. 363). Distinctions among T cell populations may provide a biologic rationale for the diagnosis and treatment of granulomatous complications. In conditions such as sarcoidosis, which have been carefully studied, the formation of granulomas occurs in steps, beginning with immune activation and T cell activation, followed by inflammatory reactions involving lymphocytes, macrophages, **TNF-α**, **IL-1**, and **Interferon-γ**, and finally, granuloma formation. This is followed by a repair phase when chronic inflammation progresses, resulting in the promotion of fibrosis. In sarcoidosis, a functional predomination of **Th1** cells can be demonstrated, although the capacity for producing **Th2** cytokines seems to be maintained (201). There has been no systematic attempt to apply modern immunologic analytic techniques to determine the molecular nature of complications following permanent implants, despite the fact that such techniques, which are now available in many medical centers, will allow clinicians to diagnose and treat complications "With a level of sensitivity that exceeds that of either clinical examination or routine histopathology" (202). Basic research involving molecular biology and immunology, which has been directed at malignancies and other serious systemic conditions, will provide powerful new tools for precisely identifying immunologic mechanisms responsible for complications following permanent implants (203–205). The potential of these new techniques has been largely ignored, with only a few studies being published (20,109,206–209), which describe the immunophenotypic characteristics of silicone/tissue interactions. Fortunately, immunohistochemical analysis can be performed on paraffin-embedded tissue sections, which may provide scientific clarity to issues that have been dominated by magical thinking, speculations, and less sophisticated diagnostic technologies.

To Learn from a Worm—The Immunologic Basis of Fibrosis

Fibrosis is characterized by the uncontrolled accumulation of collagen in tissues, which depends mainly on increased collagen synthesis by fibroblasts (127). A variety of pathological conditions characterized by increased fibrosis, including hypertrophic scarring, keloids, end-stage granulomatous fibrosis, diffuse cutaneous systemic sclerosis (SSc), bleomycin-induced pulmonary fibrosis, hepatic fibrosis induced by Schistosomes, and scleroderma have been studied at the molecular level (127,128,209–211). In scleroderma, at least five cytokines have been shown to stimulate collagen synthesis (127), in particular, IL-4 produced by T lymphocytes of the Th2 subset is noted during the early stages. The traditional concept of tissue fibrosis as a static pathological endpoint has been replaced by the modern perspective of a potentially reversible process in which cytokines control a sequence of discrete biological events. New cytokines are constantly being discovered. In the case of schistosome-induced fibrosis, a novel lymphokine, mitogenic for fibroblasts produced by CD4+ lymphocytes in the granuloma, has been found in infected livers (209). In addition, yet another step has been discovered in the production of Schistosome granulomas involving specialized receptors, which respond directly to the components of schistosome eggs. IL-4 produced by Th2 cells is a potent activator of collagen synthesis. Interferon-γ, a Th1 cytokine, inhibits fibrosis (129) and may have potential for the treatment of fibrotic conditions including the fibrosis, that accompanies granulomata following permanent implants.

MECHANISM OF COMPLICATIONS

Implant Tissue Interactions—Bacterial Adaptability

Tissue cells have not been programmed by evolution for attachment to implanted biomaterials. Bacteria, on the other hand, have developed adaptive survival strategies for colonizing inanimate substrata and cell surfaces. The fate of any implanted biomaterial has been conceptualized as a "race for the surface" between macromolecules, bacteria, and tissue cells (212,213). Current research also suggests that, for permanently implanted materials to remain undisturbed, they must also elude a broad variety of immune surveillance mechanisms designed to eliminate them.

Implant Scenarios: Bacterial Adhesion, Macrophage Function

Gristina et al. who believed that the proliferation of bacteria that were resistant to antibiotic therapy was the root cause of failure of permanent implants, outlined a stepwise scenario; although it does not take into account bacterially mediated aberrations in immune function, at the very least, it explains quite elegantly the difficulty in treating infectious processes involving permanently implanted silicone elastomers (212–221). Further insights into mechanisms limiting the accessibility of antibiotics to implant-centered infections may be derived from a study, which used the scanning electron microscope to reveal intracellular biofilms resulting from bacterial invasion into superficial bladder cells. Pods of bacteria encased in a polysaccharide-rich matrix were noted "Resting in a matrix, like eggs in a carton" (222). The existence of a similar process following liquid silicone implantation would very neatly explain the difficulty in eradicating these infections and the frequency of recurrent inflammatory episodes. In addition, the intracellular location of these biofilms has important implications for the activation of particular T cell subtypes and therapies directed towards them.

Foreign Materials and Biofilms: The Plot Thickens

In the process of enveloping inanimate surfaces, commensal organisms can express new genes, which transform them from their free-living, or planktonic state, into phenotypically distinct, slime producing, structurally elaborate biofilms bound together by polysaccharides in association with nonbiofilm producers. Under these circumstances, biofilm colonies develop complex architectural features and can act as a unicellular organism complete with signaling systems. Although the existence of biofilms or their equivalents occurring as a consequence of bacterial interaction with liquid silicone has only been postulated (69), the common occurrence of biofilms following the implantation of solid implants is well-documented and similar bacterial adaptations may very well occur involving liquid silicone.

Genetic mutations induced in microbes that are in contact with foreign materials may result in differences in cell wall proteins and decreases in metabolic rate, which make them resistant to antibiotics that target dividing cells, as well as producing enzymes, which break down antibiotics and decrease oxygen tension. Collectively, these bacterial adaptive responses decrease the effect of certain classes of antibiotics on bacterial proliferation. In addition, biofilm bacteria are often undetectable by traditional culture techniques, and can only be found using more elaborate laboratory techniques such as PCR technology. It has been estimated that biofilms are involved in 65% of human bacterial infections. Surface bacteria, and those buried in the depths of the colony, may be both phenotypically and physiologically different from free-floating (planktonic) organisms (219,221,223–227). The slow development of bacterial biofilms or similar adaptive changes in bacteria associated with a concomitant increase in the level of bacterial LPS, which activate multiple components of the immune system, may provide another explanation for the delayed development of granulomatous complications following the use of liquid silicone (69), as well as the failure to culture microorganisms from granulomatous tissue.

Particulates

As bacterial virulence increases, host defenses may be further impaired by the presence of particulates both phagocytosable (approximately one micron in diameter) and nonphagocytosable (25–100 μ in diameter). Particulate matter exhausts the ability of macrophages to produce oxygen radicals necessary for bacterial killing (218). Artecoll, which consists of Plexiglas PMMA microspheres suspended in a solution of partially denatured collagen, attempts to eliminate particulate phagocytosis by creating spheres of nonphagocytosable uniform size (32–40 μm) with a smooth surface (229). Despite these precautions, Artecoll, as with all implants, may be associated with granuloma formation (106,126,143,177). The net result of these factors acting in the long term on the surface of solid silicone implants (elastomers) process may produce an immunoincompetent fibroinflammatory zone in which chronic inflammation persists, macrophage function and killing potential is exhausted, and bacteria proliferate. This sometimes results in the displacement of adjacent healthy tissue cells, which are unable to adapt and integrate with the biomaterial surface. This explanation has been used to explain the failure of tissue implant integration and the presence of inflammatory granulomas around hip joint replacement prostheses. It may also be involved in the formation of extensive granulomas following the injection of adulterated liquid silicone, which routinely contains particulate matter. Moreover, the mechanisms described in the scientific analysis of host implant interactions would explain the occurrence of small granulomas following the use of small volumes of silicone, and larger granulomas when larger implants or adulterated implants were employed (19).

IMMUNE COMPONENTS WHICH PLAY AN IMPORTANT ROLE IN THE SUCCESS OR FAILURE OF CUTANEOUS IMPLANT INTEGRATION

Silicone Granulomas and T Cells

"Skin is the primary interface between the body and the environment ... It is susceptible to a spectrum of insults, including chemical and microbial agents, thermal and molecular, magnetic radiation, and mechanical trauma ... Protection against these challenges has been a fundamental force behind the evolution of the immune system" (158, pg. 1817). Most immune responses depend on the activation of T cells (154), a class of lymphocytes consisting of functionally and phenotypically distinct populations, which are recognized by molecules on their cell surface (**CD nomenclature**) and further divided into subtypes based upon the cytokines that they synthesize. This distinction is important in understanding the immunopathogenesis of pathological entities to which silicone granulomas belong, as well as in understanding the mechanisms underlying the success or failure for a variety of therapies, which interact with various steps in immunologic signaling and processing (230).

Cytokines

Cytokines, the hormones of the immune system, mediate inflammation and play important roles in the development of granulomatous processes. Produced by inflammatory cells (activated T cells and macrophages), two main groups of cytokines are recognized, proinflammatory and anti-inflammatory. Proinflammatory cytokines are produced predominantly by activated macrophages and Th1 cells. They modulate the upregulation of inflammatory reactions. Anti-inflammatory cytokines are secreted by Th2 cells and are involved in the downregulation of inflammatory reactions, as well as humoral immunity. The coordinated synthesis of cytokines is an important feature in the development of the granulomatous response. **DTH reactions** involve multiple cytokines with effects on immune and nonimmune cells, producing inflammatory processes (92,117, pg. 299, 123,231,232). Granulomas occur when activated macrophages fail to eradicate an infection, and continue to produce cytokines and growth factors. Several well-characterized cytokines that are involved in granulomatous processes, including TNF-α, IL-1. IL-4, a Th2 cytokine, may play a critical role in the development of fibrosis as an end-stage product of granulomatous activity (127). The use of immune modulators for diseases such as psoriasis, RA, and Crohn's disease has become a billion dollar business and their application for rare pathological entities may create a niche market for these drugs. The past two decades have witnessed an explosion in the use of biologic therapeutics, which target cytokines and profoundly expand therapeutic options for patients with chronic diseases, for which there have been no new therapies for many years. If TNF-α, a cytokine, which "connects the dots" in multiple inflammatory realms from female hormones (233) to virus infections (234,235) is found to play an important role in the development of silicone granulomata, an incredible variety of therapeutic strategies targeting this cytokine may initiate new treatment possibilities for intractable silicone granulomata (21,232,236–293). As might be noted from reading the references, anti-TNF therapies are not an unmixed blessing. Serious complications can and will occur.

T Cell Types

The best-characterized T cell types are helper T cells and cytotoxic T cells. Distinctive molecules on their surfaces provide markers of these populations, CD4+ for helper T cells and CD8+ for cytotoxic T cells. Naïve CD4+ helper T cells (Th cells, which are also called TH_0 cells) differentiate into one of two specific branches of the immune cell armamentarium, type I helper T cells (TH1) and type II helper T cells (TH2) based upon the cytokines they secrete. Type I helper T cells are proinflammatory, are involved in CMI, and are important for clearing infections caused by intracellular bacteria. They synthesize interferon-γ, and IL-2, and under certain circumstances, TNF-α (249). Type II helper T cells are anti-inflammatory, provide downregulation for Th1 cells, and are critical for fighting extracellular parasitic pathogens and helminthic infections. They principally secrete IL-4, IL-5, IL-6, IL-9, IL-10 and IL-13, which provide downregulation for Th1 cells. Th2 cells also influence B cell development and favor a humoral response (294). Both types are influenced by a variety of factors. Intracellular viral antigens favor Th1, extracellular bacterial antigens favor Th2. Low concentrations of antigens favor Th1, high concentrations favors Th2. Th1 cytokines activate macrophages and natural killer cells, Th2 cytokines suppress macrophage activation. There is a spectrum of immune responses involving Th1 and Th2 cells. At one end, characterized by overstimulation of type I helper T cells (Th1), are diseases, which result from pronounced CMI associated with granuloma formation and/or destructive inflammation, including autoimmune disease. This process involves costimulatory or "second signal" mechanisms (286,294–296), which may induce or sustain the generation of pathogenic type I helper T cells (154). At the other end of the spectrum are a variety of infectious diseases characterized by reduced ratios of type I to type II helper T cells, with impairment of cellular immunity and anergy. The effect of costimulatory function has not been well-established for these conditions. The pathogenesis of certain diseases (and parenthetically the effect of various treatments) appears to be strongly influenced by the type of helper T cells involved (154,297–299).

Naïve and Memory T Lymphocytes/Cutaneous Immune Function

Naïve T lymphocytes (CD45RA, cells in which an immune response has not yet been activated) become memory T cells (CD45RO), with the ability to circulate preferentially into the skin. These cells, which are identified by a marker known as cutaneous lymphocyte antigen (CLA), are generated in lymph nodes draining the skin and are recruited back to the skin during inflammation. CLA+ T cells are implicated in the pathogenesis of multiple pathological processes, including sarcoidosis, trauma, and T cell lymphomas. They also mediate other common skin diseases, including allergic contact dermatitis, psoriasis, atopic dermatitis, alopecia areata, vitiligo, drug-related eruptions, and lichen planus (152,158,300–302). CLA is more than a marker that identifies skin-specific T cells. It is an adhesion molecule, which mediates slowing down and tethering of T cells against forces exerted by blood flow, and permits these specialized T cells to extravasate to targeted areas (158, pg. 1819). The migration of T cells involves specific combinations of adhesion molecules and chemokines as well as a complicated process of activation, which involves T cell antigen receptors and costimulatory signals delivered by antigen presenting cells (APCs). In addition, cytokines, such as TNF-α, IL-1 and Toll-like receptors (TLRs) (and presumably TREMs) activate multiple cellular signaling pathways, including nuclear factor κB (NF-κB) to initiate cutaneous inflammation. These also include the genes for E-selectin, chemokines, cytokines, and defensins (antibacterial peptides), intracellular adhesion molecule I, and vascular cell adhesion molecule I (158, pg. 1819). Each step in the process represents a potential therapeutic target.

T Cells and Granulomas/Laboratory Evaluation

A variety of molecular immunohistological and immunocytochemical analyses are now available to determine the activation of specific components of the immune system, to detect specific cytokines, or to unearth the presence of infectious agents, which are difficult to culture (205). PCR analysis can amplify and identify novel, or unculturable infectious entities (203). Histological similarities between silicone granulomata and various T cell–mediated diseases suggest that an evaluation of T cell populations may be of value. In addition, determining a granulomatous pattern of cytokine gene expression, i.e., a predominance of Th1 or Th2 subtypes could direct specific therapies to restore cytokine balance (204). To date, no one has looked for angiotensin converting enzyme (ACE; 303) elevations in patients with silicone granulomata. ACE is normally produced by endothelial cells in the kidney, and in sarcoidosis by T cell–stimulated epithelioid cells at the periphery of the granuloma. ACE is not specific for sarcoidosis, and is elevated in a variety of diseases, including alpha I antitrypsin deficiency, Melkerson–Rosenthal syndrome, and silicoses hypersensitivity pneumonitis.

ANALYZING AND TREATING GRANULOMAS: IMMUNOLOGICAL AND THERAPEUTIC PARADOXES AND THE POTENTIAL FOR DISASTERS

When analyzing immunologically driven phenomena, one is faced with a puzzling array of conflictual and paradoxical information. For diseases like

psoriasis, the Th1 paradigm fits well, and therapies that block Th1 cytokines, and the T cells that produce them are being developed exponentially.

Granulomatous processes can be driven by either Th1, Th2 or some
combination of the two, leading to therapeutic confusion. Sometimes, a
positive response to therapeutic intervention tells clinicians that they
have used the right drug. In other cases, such as the experimental treatment of toxic epidermal necrolysis with thalidomide (21), fatal results
occur when drugs, which should work, don't. There is general agreement
that sarcoidosis and many other types of granulomas represent Th1-
mediated DTH reactions, in which reducing the production of TNF-α,
Interferon-γ and IL-2 would be beneficial. For example, Thalidomide,
which inhibits Interferon-γ and TNF-α, is regularly used to treat sarcoidosis (304). However, other types of granulomas (granuloma annulare)
have been treated effectively using Interferon-γ (160), a cytokine that theoretically should worsen the condition! In addition, Interferon-γ has been
shown to inhibit DTHs. Interferon-γ has been used effectively for the
treatment of chronic granulomatous disease (136). Blocking TNF-α
and other Th1 cytokines is a fundamental rationale underlying an enormous proliferation of drugs for the treatment of both psoriasis and
sarcoidosis (250,271,277,305–307). And yet, psoriasis has responded to
treatment with TNF itself (241). Indeed, adverse reactions to biological
immune response modifiers may provide immunological clues to
the mechanism underlying the production of implant granulomas
(228,273,274,308). A clearer picture begins to develop when one analyzes
the literature dealing with cutaneous granulomata. Conditions such as
Churg–Strauss syndrome (309) are considered to be Th2-mediated diseases, and have been treated with both Interferon-γ which, among other
things, inhibits Th2 cells and Interferon-α which stimulates Th1 cells. If
silicone granulomas are Th1 driven, their apparently successful treatment
(121), using imiquimod, would be another example of a paradox. Imiquimod (Aldara®) increases the synthesis and release of TNF-α, and *stimulates* the production of Th1 cytokines, while inhibiting the production of
Th2 cytokines (310–318). To make it more confusing, Imiquimod's beneficial effects may be related to the induction of CMI, a category of
immune reactions to which silicone granulomas belong (121). Some of
these paradoxical effects could be explained on the basis of a shift from
Th1 to Th2 cytokine profiles as granulomas become more fibrotic. Imiquimod has also proved to be of value when used with tretinoin for nonsurgical removal of tattoos (122). However, in this report, imiquimod is
associated with fibrosis, which is itself a component of end-stage granulomata. The patient treated by Baumann, most likely had received adulterated silicone, and this reaction probably belonged in the Th2 category
of immune responses. In this respect it is similar to sarcoidosis, in which
early activity (depending on the organ systems involved) may be Th1 driven, followed by a shift to Th2 during chronic phases. Treatment of
other diseases with immunomodulators may also produce paradoxical
results. Rapaport's serendipitous observation (60), of Etanercept®-
induced facial granulomas at the site of silicone injection given 36 years

back, is an even more paradoxical event. Etanercept, a TNF-α blocker, might theoretically be used to treat DTHs, such as silicone granulomata (273,308). This complication may be associated with the presence of CD8 cells, which have "recently been recognized as playing an important role in the mediation of allergic contact hypersensitivity, an activity that "For a long time was attributed to Th1 cells" (319). In this setting, Etanercept may have acted as a hapten, possibly on the basis of memory T cell activation. Paradoxic responses have followed treatment with other types of drugs, including Thalidomide (264), which although approved for the treatment of erythema nodosum, has produced erythema nodosum. Pulsed-dye laser treatments, which successfully treated granuloma annulare (320), have induced ulcerative cutaneous sarcoidosis (321). Topical retinoids, which have been used to treat DTH reactions following tattoos, have caused pyogenic granulomas (322). Infectious granulomata have been reported following antiTNF therapy, possibly on the basis of reduced resistance to infection (287). Allopurinol (323), which has been used effectively to treat subcutaneous sarcoidosis, has induced generalized granuloma annulare (324).

VAN LEEUWENHOEK STARTED IT: THE EVOLUTION OF EVER-LARGER MAGNIFYING GLASSES

Modern immunologists regard light microscopes, with which van Leeuwenhoek "discovered many secrets of nature, now famous throughout the philosophical world" (325), as nothing more than magnifying glasses strong enough to perceive the capital letters in a message left by immunological processes, but too weak to read the fine print. Just as van Leeuwenhoek revolutionized our perception of the physical world by magnifying processes which could not be seen with the naked eye, molecular biologists and immunologists have discovered an even tinier microcosmos which redefines the rules governing biological processes. By illuminating immunopathogenetic mechanisms at the molecular level, relationships are established among disease states, which clinically do not appear to have anything in common. In doing so, they have established a new imperative for understanding, treating, and categorizing old diseases.

No one ever said it better than Gary S. Wood (204) who asks, "What does all this mean to the general dermatologist? ... First, it means we've been able to use modern immunologic methods to redefine the wide array of long recognized but poorly understood skin diseases. ... By putting these disorders in their true biologic context, we have laid the foundation for their eventual cure. ... Second, it means that we have sensitive new tools available that allow us to make diagnoses earlier and with greater confidence, determine the disease state of patients more accurately, and monitor patient response to therapy more precisely. ... No longer must we rely solely on the venerable but dated technology of light microscopy to accomplish these tasks."

Unifying Concepts: Inflammation/Infection

Even in their wildest dreams, the clinicians who pioneered the use of liquid silicone and other implants, viewing inflammation like a Latin catechism of rubor, dolor, calor, and tumor, could have never imagined the complexity and multiplicity of steps involving an octopus-like immune system, whose arms (innate and acquired) are coordinated by signaling systems of enough importance to warrant the devotion of multiple issues of prestigious journals which describe them (302,326–335)[i]. Indeed the same clinicians could have never foreseen the heterogenous identification of look-alike cells (histologically similar white cells) at the molecular level, using CD nomenclature. This, among other things, identifies their lineage, and the role of specific white cells in activation and suppression of genes and enzymes involved in a variety of diseases. For that matter, the notion that human **TLRs**, the equivalent of a protein first identified in fruit flies (*Drosophila* toll receptors), might be the first line of defense in the infectious exacerbation of human diseases such as psoriasis, or connected in any way with the infectious activation of inflammatory events following injections of liquid silicone, or could become therapeutic targets, would have seemed science fiction when liquid silicone was first used for soft tissue augmentation (158,327,331,336–343). The discovery of a multiplicity of steps, signals, and genes, as well as intricate feedback mechanisms involving inflammatory processes, have led to an explosion of novel immunomodulatory therapeutic strategies, which have "shifted the tectonic plates of research (311) and created whole new categories of therapeutic opportunities." No one could have imagined the scope, complexity, and inter-reactivity of inflammatory mechanisms. These cut across seemingly unrelated fields of medicine, and unify disease processes ranging from acne (339,341), atherogenesis (337), strokes and dental disease (344), cancer (345), Parkinson's disease (120,346,347), sarcoidosis (150,249,260,323), pyoderma gangrenosum (269), psoriasis and psoriatic arthritis (244,271,272,347,348), lymphomas (298,349), Crohn's disease (286), and Weber–Christian disease (165,350–353). Who could have dreamed that one type of white cell (T cell) could be the object of so many kinds of treatments for involvement in so many kinds of diseases (152,158,300,298,349,351,352,354–363). Analysis of inflammatory events in the past years was largely limited by the ability to visualize cellular morphology, an investigation which did not yield fundamental insights into molecular processes underlying these events. Advances in cell culture techniques, monoclonal antibody production, immunohistochemistry, recombinant DNA methodology, X-ray crystallography, and the creation of genetically altered animals (especially transgenic and knockout mice), have enabled researchers to identify, synthesize, and assay the effect of immunomodulatory compounds, resulting in a dramatically reconfigured understanding of inflammatory processes and the mechanisms underlying

---

[i] Possibly by increasing potential antigenic burden.

both successful and unsuccessful treatment strategies (203,204,326,277). Although nothing in the practice of everyday medicine prepares clinicians to understand disorders rooted in behavior driven by compounds such as **cytokines**, which exert biological effects in nanograms (billionths) and picograms (trillionths), an understanding of the therapeutic implications of these compounds, and other facets of the immune system, may be a necessity for clinicians in this century, and also provides a driving force for advances in every field of medicine.[j]

PERSONAL EXPERIENCE WITH INJECTABLE SILICONE

My experience using liquid silicone has been overwhelmingly positive, producing results that have generated enormous patient and personal satisfaction. Silicone is truly permanent and for many patients, particularly those of limited means, has provided a welcome and cost-effective relief from endless rounds of painful and expensive injections using temporary tissue fillers. Between 1982 and 2002, I treated over 2200 patients, carefully observing the criteria outlined by established authorities. Most of my patients were treated for depressed scars, rhytides, and atrophic contour defects involving the face and lips. Treatment of facial asymmetry (particularly posttraumatic or congenital) has produced almost miraculous changes in patient appearance and self-confidence. Contour defects involving the nose, whether posttraumatic or following rhinoplasty or Mohs surgery, improved dramatically. Groove-like scars from animal bites (many incurred years back when the patients were small children) have responded beautifully. Silicone is ideal for the treatment of central facial atrophy, which can occur as a consequence of aging, wasting illnesses, or precipitous weight loss, or can occur congenitally. The nasolabial folds, pliable acne scars, perioral rhytides, and atrophy of the lobules of the ears can be treated with results equalled by no other filling agent. Although large volumes of liquid silicone might logically seem most likely to cause serious complications, I have under observation at the time of writing, three patients who were treated for extensive facial atrophy, using relatively large (15–30 cc) volumes of silicone. They have had no problems 15 to 20 years after treatment.

UNPLEASANT REALITIES

I use liquid silicone for a number of reasons. It is permanent, inexpensive, no more antigenic, and less technically difficult to use than agents such as

---

[j] Indeed the popular press has been awakened to the scope and implications of the inflammatory process (353,364).

Bioplastique, Artecoll, and Gortex. It does not carry with it the risk of infectious disease transmission associated with cadaver-derived tissue fillers. From a financial standpoint, there is absolutely no incentive for a reputable physician to use a permanent implant, when the use of a temporary filler would provide a continuing source of income and freedom from covert, overt, blatant, or subtle character assassination by colleagues who have observed complications following the gross misuse of liquid silicone, and other agents masquerading as liquid silicone. Lay publications further fuel patient and physician fears by publishing sensational reports of complications, which have nothing to do with the proper use of liquid silicone. What then is the advantage to legitimate doctors who use silicone? The answer is simple. It appears to be extremely safe when used properly, does not drain the financial resources of patients, or subject them to endless rounds of painful injections. It has, particularly in patients with certain kinds of scarring and posttraumatic contour defects, produced results that have positively transfigured patients' lives, and has been a source of enormous personal gratification as well. I have never employed a modality which was so clearly more advantageous to my patients than it was for my reputation. The specter of scientifically baseless lawsuits adjudicated on the basis of emotional appeal and ignorance has led to the creation of informed consent publications that look as though they have been written in a defensive crouch. For patients who are interested in the use of a permanent implant (those who have often received multiple injections of disappointingly temporary augmenting agents), I routinely provide informed consent material, which includes the most unflattering commentaries I can find (60,61,75,79–81), as well as articles that describe current trends in permanent implantation (33,69,365–367). The stresses inherent in the use of liquid silicone have been anecdotally implicated in the suicide of a physician in New York City who could not face the emotional travail of multiple lawsuits filed in the wake of a searing national television "exposé" of liquid silicone use (56). Another colleague (unpublished personal communication) faced a lawsuit filed by a patient who was completely asymptomatic. Her lawsuit (which was later dismissed) was spurred by another physician, who commented (when he found that she had received liquid silicone) that "The doctor that used it should be in jail." In reality, all permanent implants, indeed all types of implants, can cause foreign body reactions, including granulomas, as well as other inflammatory complications, which can be difficult to treat and which may turn out to be associated with infectious agents when proper diagnostic tools are employed. Silicone, the "S" word, has been singled out as "the great evil," and accordingly, those who use it may be subjected to capricious and prejudicial treatment, both in the legal system and in the court of public opinion. The use of permanent implants represents a triumph of altruism over financial and medico-legal considerations. Those who choose to use liquid silicone or other permanent implants should carefully consider that the Hippocratic admonition: "Above all do no harm," should apply to *both* the patient and themselves.

COMPLICATIONS—PERSONAL EVALUATION AND TREATMENT

In contrast to the horrific and difficult-to-treat complications that I see on a regular basis following the use of adulterated silicone (commonly used in Mexico), my experience following the use of small volumes of pure liquid silicone suggests that serious complications are extraordinarily rare. Most problems which do occur, are small, easily concealed, or respond to treatment.

I have observed both small, localized, noninflammatory complications, and more widespread inflammation associated with edema and erythema, following the use of pure liquid silicone. The results of biopsies, both for histology and immunopathology, are presented at the end of this chapter. Inflammatory complications have often, but not always, occurred in conjunction with an infectious process or allergy. Sinus and dental infections were a common precipitating event. One patient developed transient facial nodules at silicone injection sites, following competition in a marathon, about two years after treatment. These nodules, which were not biopsied, resolved spontaneously. Another patient developed an inflammatory glabellar nodule following silicone injections, associated with a photosensitive reaction. I have not observed ulceration, tissue necrosis, or migration in any patient who has received small volumes of pure liquid silicone.

Lips: Potential Problems

I routinely see swelling, induration, and nodules involving the lips of patients who have also developed inflammatory processes in other areas of the face, following treatment with "Silicone" in Mexico. Two patients gradually developed firm, esthetically unattractive increases in lip volume and asymmetry, following dental work performed 5 to 15 years after receiving small amounts of pure liquid silicone (112). This process may be analogous to keloidal-like fibrogenesis, which occurs occasionally in silicone-augmented scars following trauma (61). Five patients developed intermittent swelling in the lips, six months to four years after injection of small amounts of pure liquid silicone. Two patients reported the swelling to have occurred in conjunction with chronic herpes simplex virus infections (126,142). Prophylactic Valtrex® 500 mg qid has proven effective in preventing swelling in these patients. In the three remaining patients, careful dental evaluation revealed cavities in one, and no dental infection in the other two. In the patient who had dental caries, spontaneous resolution of the swelling was noted after extraction of an infected tooth. Of the two patients with no dental infections, swelling subsided without treatment in one, and in the other, intralesional steroids and oral antibiotics were effective. Many patients prefer what I consider to be an overly large appearance of their lips to the possibility of pseudoatrophy, which may occur following intralesional steroid treatment. Another patient who received multiple injections of small volumes of pure liquid silicone developed massive facial edema each time she ingested alcohol. Her symptoms began following reconstructive surgery for ruptured breast implants, about ten years after her last silicone treatment. In addition, this patient was being treated with medications, which have been associated with rare forms of granulomatous disease (368). (This swelling responded temporarily to oral corticosteroids but recurred when treatment was stopped.) Minocycline, 200 mg daily, has proved effective for the last six months. I recently examined a 49-year-old white female, who developed a severe swelling involving the nasal bridge and glabella, following injections of BOTOX, in the same area where twenty years back she had been treated with silicone of unknown volume and purity. Several months later, when BOTOX injections were carried out again, more severe swelling occurred, this time in association with nontender nodules. Over a six-month period, glabellar swelling has completely subsided; however, the nodules persist, albeit smaller. Cutaneous complications following the use of botulinum toxin is very rare, although one case of a fixed drug eruption has been reported to a constituent (lactose) of a specific form of botulinum toxin (Dysport®, Speywood Pharmaceuticals, Wrentham, U.K.) (369). This case may represent the first reported episode of a BOTOX/silicone interaction. It may have occurred on the basis of traumatic (pathergic) activation of an inflammatory process.

Treatment of Complications

Small noninflammatory fibrotic papular granulomata have generally responded well to a variety of procedures, including injectable corticosteroids, dermabrasion, and CO_2 laser resurfacing. A long-pulse 1064 nd YAG laser was partially effective in reducing the size of a larger granuloma, involving the lower lip (personal experience, unpublished data) Several other publications have described the successful use of lasers for other granulomatous conditions, including sarcoidosis, granuloma faciale, and necrobiosis lipoidica (370), although flare-ups of generalized ulcerative sarcoidosis have been induced by laser treatments (321). In one patient whose hypertrophic scar-like lesions did not respond to dermabrasion, the 532 nm long-pulse laser (VersaPulse, Coherent Corp.) using 55 J effectively flattened these lesions without textural or pigmentary abnormalities (personal experience, unpublished data). In another case, a scar, which became elevated several years after the injection of small amounts of pure liquid silicone, did not respond to dermabrasion or intralesional triamcinolone acetonide (Kenalog 5–80 mg/cc). In this case, biweekly injections of two parts 10 mg/cc Kenalog solution, and eight parts 5% Efudex solution produced satisfactory results (371,372).

In contrast to reports which cite complete success in treating large granulomata, my experience has been less satisfactory. Intermittent severe localized edema and induration, the hallmarks of inflammatory granuloma, often require long-term interventions, with remissions and exacerbations being common. Patients with localized or extensive inflammatory granulomata are often treated with combinations of oral corticosteroids (prednisone 20–40 mg daily in tapering doses), and oral minocycline in doses of 100 to 200 mg daily (373). On the basis of a number of recent clinical articles, I have initiated other treatment protocols for patients who have developed massive granulomas following injection of adulterated silicones in Mexico. These have included allopurinol (323), imiquimod (121), and phonophoresis using topical steroids (374), in an attempt to reduce patient dependence on oral corticosteroids. None of these prove uniformly effective. To date, intermittent intralesional and oral corticosteroids, coupled with minocycline, have been the only effective method for controlling these complications.

CONDITIONS WHICH HAVE RELEVANCE FOR SILICONE COMPLICATIONS

Winkleman et al. (164,375) suggest that a disease entity "starts as a hypothesis based on clinical observations and laboratory data, including pathologic findings." Comparing poorly understood pathological conditions with well-characterized disease entities may produce a rationale for the use of therapies, which have worked for similar diseases. A clear understanding of the mechanisms underlying specific disease processes would eliminate ineffective or potentially dangerous therapies (187). Silicone complications, which appear to embody features of multiple disease processes, are most aptly described by a recent description of sarcoidosis, which notes that sarcoidosis suffers from "a paucity of systematic epidemiologic investigations of cause, diagnostic access, bias, and misclassification of the disease because of insensitive and non-diagnostic testing " and "this disease diagnosis is one of exclusion" (123). For liquid silicone, it might be added that the controversy surrounding its use has introduced a whole new level of contentious bias. Perhaps no condition so closely resembles silicone granuloma clinically, histologically, and, presumably, immunophenotypically as cutaneous sarcoidosis (123,297,376–379), and it is safe to assume that at some point both conditions will be considered to be subtypes of the same pathogenetic processes. Theories advanced regarding the immunopathogenesis of sarcoidosis could easily be applied to silicone granulomata. These include the abnormal processing of particulates and foreign bodies, a prominent feature in sarcoidosis, suggesting yet another connection between sarcoidosis and silicone (17,145–149,262,377,378,380–382). Inoculation of foreign matter from a previous inapparent minor trauma may induce granuloma formation in individuals with sarcoidosis (148). Granuloma annulare, which may evolve into sarcoidosis (157), has been observed with both traumatic and atraumatic presentation as a manifestation of immune restoration syndromes occurring in HIV positive patients whose low CD4+ counts have risen to normal levels following antiviral therapy (159,383). No one is certain whether the etiology of sarcoid/silicone granulomas is multifactorial, or owing to a single antigen driven process. In addition, a variety of immunologic mechanisms, including T cell aberrations, genetic susceptibility, and infectious and environmental agents, which have been implicated as possible causative factors for sarcoidosis, may play a role in the development of silicone granulomata. A recent article (305) details genetic variations in TNF-α genes and HLA-DR loci in determining the clinical spectrum of sarcoidosis, noting that several genes in a particular region may act in concert to define sarcoidal disease susceptibility and prognosis. The same genetic substrate may be operant for silicone granulomata as well. Although familial clusters have been reported in sarcoidosis (378), they have never been looked for or even suspected as a causative agent for silicone complications. An infectious pathogenesis has been suggested for sarcoidosis when PCR studies found mycobacterial DNA sequences in sarcoidal lesions. PCR has also implicated herpes virus (173) in complications of another type of permanent implant. To date, PCR investigations to determine the role of infectious processes in silicone granulomata have not been published.

INFECTIOUS PROCESSES, TRAUMA, AND T CELL ACTIVATION

The mechanism by which silicone complications may be triggered by some uncharacterized or occult bacterial or viral antigenic activation is shared with a variety of conditions characterized by T cell activation. These include psoriasis, sarcoidosis, Weber–Christian disease (panniculitis), and certain types of lymphomas (21,119,150,162,164,262,384–394). Formal studies have linked Weber–Christian disease with silicone granulomas. Therapeutically, minocycline (373), which has been effective for the treatment of silicone granulomas, appears to exert positive therapeutic benefits on certain panniculitides as well (395). This success may be due to the immunosuppressive properties of minocycline, which may resemble the mechanisms using immunosuppressants such as cyclosporine, mycophenolate (Mofetil®), and thalidomide, which have proved effective for Weber–Christian disease (161,165,166,396). Diseases such as chronic granulomatous disease (95,117,124,136) have also been shown to result from T cell–mediated macrophage activation, resulting in the formation of granulomas (117, pg. 453). Infections are commonly associated with granulomatous processes including granuloma annulare (134,159,383). T cell abnormalities underlying neoplastic processes such as Sézary syndrome (151,397) can produce granulomas, which are histologically similar to silicone granulomas. Trauma has been associated with fatal T cell lymphomas (152).

Psoriasis

This condition, which affects some 2.6% of the U.S. population (277), shares no clinical or histological similarities with silicone complications. However, both psoriasis and silicone complications have been traditionally misdiagnosed, and both exhibit similar immunologic features. Psoriasis was once considered incurable (as are to this day some types of silicone complications) and like silicone complications, which are fundamentally viewed as indecipherable, psoriasis was once, mistakenly, viewed as an abnormality of keratinocyte hyperproliferation and abnormal epidermal differentiation. Psoriasis is now recognized to be the most prevalent T cell–mediated inflammatory disease in humans (398). The ability of immunosuppressants, such as methotrexate and T cell toxins (denileukin Diftitox®), to alleviate psoriasis demonstrated that activated T cells were pivotal in the development of this disease. Recent studies (275,399) have clarified the immunologic processes involved. Both silicone complications and psoriasis have been theorized as being driven by some unknown bacterial antigen (357). In the case of psoriasis, it has been postulated that T cells may interact with streptoccocal antigens to produce guttate psoriasis (157,277). Both established psoriasis and guttate psoriasis can be exacerbated by cutaneous infections (158).

Antibiotics/Immunosuppressive Agents

The fact that antibiotics exert both antimicrobial and immunosuppressive effects may also explain their success in treating multiple types of granulomas (114,115,119,373). Indeed, newer antibiotics may be developed with more specificity for the treatment of granulomas. For clinicians who are faced with "intractable" silicone granulomata, immunosuppressive agents developed for conditions which share immunological similarities may provide useful alternatives (21,22,119,121,138,160,165,168,201,232,238,242–244,246–249,252,254–256,258–262,265,266,296,305,320,323,373,374,392,395,399–413).

COMMENTARY: HENNY PENNY VS. PANGLOSS—"A PLAGUE O'BOTH YOUR HOUSES"

Arguments concerning the use of liquid silicone for soft tissue augmentation have become so emotional and corrosive that advocates and critics have abandoned even the thinnest pretense of impartiality. Clinicians who have *personally* observed the immense psychosocial benefits of this highly effective permanent and inexpensive implant, coupled with what appears to be an extraordinarily low incidence of serious complications following its proper use, are convinced that the benefits of this modality far outweigh the risks. There is a perceptual chasm between those who think liquid silicone is too dangerous to use, and those who believe that the utility value of this modality is so great and the risks are so low that they pale in comparison to fatalities that occur following bee stings, or allergies to peanuts, which result in approximately 200 deaths per year (414–417). Indeed, silicone advocates suggest that the energies of those who histrionically attack rare and nonfatal complications, which follow permanent implants, might be better directed to a crusade against bees and peanut butter, whose elimination from our environment would actually save lives. On the other hand, the unwillingness of the passionate advocates to admit the possibility of serious complications following silicone use is just as implausible and antithetical to a proper assessment of risks and benefits, as are the protestations of those who believe silicone is intrinsically evil. In summary, no one has suggested a crusade against bees and peanut butter, and no reasonable person would launch a crusade against a therapy, which produces serious complications in approximately 1 out of every 2000 people treated. Problems, which occur in association with entities of proven utility value, are best approached scientifically with a view toward identifying risk factors and developing methods of treatment.

Those who criticize the use of liquid silicone also note that complications are "Unpredictable and their incidence has not been substantiated." Implicit in this statement is the refusal of those opposed to its use to accept published data regarding the number of patients treated. Those who view the use of liquid silicone as **Henny Penny** did the sky, appear to have given up all hope of either understanding the generic possibility of all types of implant complications or any kind of optimism with respect to evolution of new therapies. In all fairness, there are valid arguments on both sides. Nobody knows what complications may occur from untried or novel procedures and medications, which may interact with permanent implants. The concept that therapies, which utilize thermal energy in a variety of cutaneous applications, could negatively interact with silicone implants (23) had never occurred either to the advocates or to the critics of silicone soft tissue augmentation. Moreover, nobody really needs "to use liquid silicone." Deaths do not occur from scars, facial atrophy, or any kind of cosmetic defects. However, philosophical concerns regarding the merits, or lack thereof, of exposure to any kind of risk for purely "cosmetic benefits" could be applied to the use of Accutane for acne, plastic surgery for correcting protruding ears, or for that matter, any "minor surgery" or pharmacologic treatments for non life–threatening conditions, which can be followed by serious complications. Such concerns do, however, provide a basis for valid arguments (418–421). As with Newcombs' paradox (422–424), which presents the philosophical argument that diametrically opposite opinions can be equally valid, all opinions pertaining to liquid silicone have become matters of faith. Opponents and advocates will not change their opinions, but will voice them more slowly or more loudly. What is obvious to anyone who attempts to interpret data regarding efficacy and risks of liquid silicone impartially is that no one knows with any certainty what the real risks and benefits are. The "magnifying glass" of current immunologic sophistication has not been focused upon the possibilities and drawbacks of this modality. What have become increasingly obvious in evaluating the status of liquid silicone are the forces that shape the opinions and postures of the press, legal, and medical communities, and the laity. The public at large wants a quick fix without any complications, and when complications occur, juries want to punish the villains responsible for them. The media wants something scary to talk about. Trial lawyers smell potential profits, and various physicians, for reasons both venial and noble, have entered the fray. "The gap between the clinician and the basic scientist has increased not diminished in the last quarter century" (425). A gulf between the clinicians' viewpoint of permanent implants, and the evolution of scientific data, which have accrued in the hands of molecular biologists, represent separate noncommunicative entities. While clinicians talk of a "nidus of infection," molecular biologists publish reams of information regarding specific molecular steps and the precise genetic substrata involved in such interactions. Meanwhile, in the "worst case scenario," malpractice suits against physicians who use liquid silicone may, be adjudicated by jurors, who are systematically selected by the plaintiffs, attorneys on the basis of demographic bias, intellectual or educational shortcomings, and gross ignorance of scientific issues. Time and science will inevitably decode the eccentricities of soft tissue implants, and may, hopefully, lead to some improvement in the quality of the jury pool.

Problems and Axioms—The Mathematician's Approach

A clear understanding of the risks and benefits inherent in the use of liquid silicone and other permanent implants resembles the quandary faced by the nineteenth-century mathematicians, who came to the realization that many seemingly intuitive concepts were problematic. David Hilbert, a pre-eminent mathematician, proposed two approaches (426). (i) He suggested that by focusing on hard unsolved problems, which reveal gaps in our knowledge, powerful theories could be developed, which would explain or solve these problems and direct the future course of mathematics. In a similar fashion, our ability to put silicone complications in their true biological and statistical context may predict and perhaps direct the future use of all permanent implants. (ii) Just as clinicians recognized the biases and guesswork, which permeate liquid silicone publications, Hilbert and others attempted to avoid "Misleading dependency on unreliable assumptions and intuitions" by emphasizing the Axiomatic method employed by the ancient Greeks (427).

The Axiomatic Method

In this system, a set of self-evident assumptions (axioms) are presented, which capture the essence of the subject. From these axioms, the truth about a concept or system can be derived by means of logical deduction. Although Gödell (426) demonstrated the limitations to the provability of axiomatic logic, analysis of the mechanics underlying silicone complications using newly developed molecular and immunological tools permit the formulation of fundamental axioms, which explain the behavior of liquid silicone. (i) Liquid silicone is the least immunogenic and permanently implantable material available. It is cost-effective, technique sensitive, and clearly superior to any other available injectable tissue augmentation modality available for certain types of defects. (ii) Used properly, serious complications following the use of small volumes of pure liquid silicone are extremely rare and compare favorably with other elective procedures, which are carried out without fanfare; the triggering of autoimmune systemic problems has not been reported. (iii) Severe local complications (ulceration, necrosis, and edema) may occur following large volumes of pure liquid silicone especially when it is employed in patients with certain types of systemic diseases, particularly those in which inflammatory cytokines play a predominant role. Conversely, large volumes of adulterated liquid silicone will produce these problems in large numbers of patients. (iv) Liquid silicone is a hapten (incomplete antigen). Its ability to generate a localized immune response may be triggered by infectious processes, trauma, and, theoretically, certain classes of drugs (368), and types of immune dysfunction. Such reactions, which involve specific types of inflammatory processing, are a generic possibility following the use of liquid silicone or other implanted substances. The occasional reports of granulomas occurring after both permanent and impermanent implants are a clear warning of this possibility. (v) Clinically, histologically, and immunophenotypically, silicone complications resemble other pathologic entities that have been extensively studied. (vi) Pathogenic mechanisms implicated in related disorders are operant in silicone granulomas. (vii) Knowledge gained by studying the conditions, which resemble silicone complications at multiple levels (histologically, clinically, or immunopathologically), has relevance for the diagnosis and treatment of silicone complications. (viii) Activation of the proinflammatory cascade, including activation of both the innate and the adaptive systems, with associated activation of T cells and cytokine imbalances, plays a dominant role in the production of silicone complications. (ix) Laboratory analysis of the specific steps and components modulating complications may help identify therapeutic targets and patients who are at risk for complications following permanent implants. (x) A wide variety of immunosuppressive drugs, which have proved effective for the treatment of diseases that resemble silicone complications, particularly, biologic therapies resulting from recombinant DNA techniques, can be designed specifically to alter physiologic responses. This will provide a rational and effective treatment for resistant silicone complications.

QUESTIONS AND ANSWERS ABOUT LIQUID SILICONE

1. *Why is it important to discuss liquid silicone now?*
    The availability of FDA approved silicone oils, particularly for AIDS associated facial wasting, in addition to the availability of permanent fillers such as Artecoll, which are on the verge of FDA approval (13,365,366,428–430).

2. *How do silicone and other biologically "inert" materials evade immune surveillance?*
    Epitopes, the specific portion of a macromolecular antigen to which antibody binds (which are produced by antigen processing), are not necessarily presented to or recognized by T lymphocytes (431). Epitopes, which are normally hidden from T cell recognition, are termed "cryptic." Crypticity may involve multiple mechanisms, one of which is anatomical sequestration of antigen, i.e., antigens are located in tissues, which are relatively inaccessible to immune cells, such as the central nervous system. Some epitopes may be cryptic because they are normally destroyed during antigen processing or have

lower affinity for binding MHC molecules. One of the circumstances which can lead to the unmasking of cryptic epitopes includes increasing the concentrations of antigen in APCs. Cryptic T cell epitopes have been demonstrated in microbial antigens as well. In addition, alterations of protease activity can also increase display of cryptic cell epitopes. All these factors provide a rationale for increasing concentrations of liquid silicone–protein complexes to precipitate T cell activation and would neatly explain the development of granulomas in AIDS patients who develop immune restoration syndromes associated with increasing CD4+ cell counts. Epitopes are also involved in autoimmune phenomena (432).

3. *Silicones used for tissue augmentation in the past were considerably less viscous than the newer silicone oils. Should different patterns of response and complications be expected?*
   Probably. Reactions to implants can be implant specific and site specific, i.e., granulomas have never been reported, following the injection of the feet. More viscous silicones require larger needles and deeper injection placement, which may make this procedure more technique dependent. Thin-walled needles, which provide larger inner bore diameters without a concomitant increase in external dimensions, have partially circumvented this problem (433).

4. *Are the more viscous oils a good substitute for 350-centistoke silicone?*
   They are, in every detail, more difficult to use. The use of larger needles necessitated by viscosity often requires a local anesthetic (EMLA™ or nerve blocks). Moreover, it is more difficult to assess the plane of infiltration accurately, and silicone leakage is common through needle tracks. Most importantly, the viscosity of these oils may limit their usefulness for treating bound-down scars or more superficial cutaneous defects. In a few cases I have employed a vacuum device (Mighty VAC®, Prism Enterprises, Inc., Texas, U.S.A.) (434), sometimes in conjunction with subcision (435) to render fibrotic scars more pliable or create a predictable plane of injection.

5. *Have you seen granulomas following the use of FDA approved silicone oils?*
   Yes. I do not know if these complications are related to increased technique sensitivity or the possibility that more viscous silicone oils provide a more favorable substrate for inflammatory granulomas. To date I have not personally encountered any granulomatous complications following the "new silicones," which have not responded to treatment. This does not mean they will not occur.

6. *Can granulomatous reactions be predicted or avoided?*
   There is no foolproof method of doing this.

7. *Will HIV patients treated for facial atrophy be more susceptible to the development of silicone-induced granulomata?*
   Possibly, particularly when immune restoration occurs. In addition, the etiology and increased frequency of localized and generalized granuloma annulare occurring in HIV positive patients has recently been described and discussed (134,159,383). Nevertheless, there is no reasonable alternative to the use of silicone to treat the devastating psychosocial effects associated with this disfiguring form of facial lipoatrophy.

8. *Are future studies planned?*
   Studies are underway to evaluate the usefulness of liquid silicone for the treatment of facial wrinkles, HIV wasting, and podiatric disorder (personal communication; Diane Richard from Richard James, Inc.). Silskin™ (a proprietary name for liquid silicone) is currently undergoing phase one studies involving 150 patients at several treatment sites (75).

9. *If infections are involved, why is it that bacterial cultures taken from affected sites are uniformly negative?*
   Bacteria exist in two forms: planktonic, or free-living, and in the form of structurally complex colonies (biofilm). These are sometimes undetectable by traditional culture techniques, but can be detected using PCR technology. In addition, the ability to quantify cell surface receptors such as TLRs (158,315–317,336,340) and TREM (436) may help distinguish between infectious and noninfectious activation of silicone complications.

10. *Over what time frame have you noted granulomata occurring following the use of pure liquid silicone in small volumes?*
    Several weeks to 15 years.

11. *What does the future hold for reducing the possibility of bacterial infections occurring in permanent implants?*
    Bacterial colonization represents a major obstacle to the usefulness of all types of permanent implants, particularly those which serve critical or life preserving functions, such as catheters, artificial limbs, joints, and arterial stents. Materials are being developed, which employ different stratagems to resist bacterial adhesion. Antimicrobial agents and polyclonal antibodies have been integrated into a variety of implants, which work by releasing active agents at the implant sites. These include nitrous oxide (437), linked to silicone polymers or incorporated in certain implants in the form of sensor activated polymeric films. Biomaterials have been developed which release entrapped drugs when exposed to ultrasound pulses (224,226,438,439). Lactoferrin® (440) chelates iron and alters bacterial surface motility, preventing bacterial adhesion. Intracellular signaling molecules involved in the development of biofilms may be susceptible to genetic manipulation (227). Compounds such as furanones, produced by marine algae, maybe modified to block biofilm formation in humans.

Sirolimus, a macrolide antibiotic with immunosuppressive properties, has been incorporated into coronary artery stents to inhibit smooth muscle cell proliferation following angioplasty (441,442).

12. *Is permanence a virtue?*
     Permanence is intuitively appealing from the standpoint of cost-effectiveness, patient comfort, and convenience. However, no one can predict exactly what undesirable interactions may occur between permanent implants of any sort, not only to infectious agents and other disease processes, but also to the vast assortment of drugs and other treatment modalities (some not yet discovered) to which a person may be exposed in a lifetime. Magro (155) presented 20 patients in whom drug therapy was associated with interstitial histiocytic infiltrates, which mimic early lesions of granuloma annulare. The most frequent clinical differential diagnosis includes cutaneous T cell lymphoma, erythema annulare centrifugum (EAC, GA), and lupus erythematosus. A drug reaction was suspected in only three cases. Drugs implicated included calcium channel blockers, ACE, beta-blockers, lipid lowering agents, antihistamines, anticonvulsants, and antidepressants. In the 15 patients who discontinued the implicated drug, lesional resolution occurred. Over one-third of the patients with drug-related eruptions had other medical illnesses associated with cutaneous granulomatous inflammation, including RA, Crohn's disease, hepatitis C, diabetes mellitus, and thyroiditis. A microbial trigger was implicated in 12 patients, including herpetic or streptococcal infections, Epstein–Barr virus, tuberculosis, leprosy, fungi, and spirochetes. Several other diseases were implicated, including cutaneous T cell lymphomas (CTCL) and idiopathic lichenoid eruptions (443, pg. 126–133). I tell patients that the real virtue and problem with liquid silicone is its permanence. When complications occur, they may be extraordinarily difficult to treat. In my view, the ideal filler would probably last about two years. This would provide a cost-effective incentive for patients without the problems, however rare, which may be associated with permanent implants. Fillers such as hydroxylapatite (Radiance[TM], Bioform Inc., Wisconsin, U.S.) (444), which may act as a matrix for the ingrowth of host tissue and persist for several years, may provide a cost-effective and less controversial alternative to truly permanent (i.e., silicone) implants used for cosmetic purposes.

13. *How will the cause and treatment of complications following permanent implants finally be resolved?*
     A better understanding of the molecular pathology underlying complications following liquid silicone and other types of permanent implants suggest their inclusion in categories of pathological conditions characterized by four processes: (i) delayed hypersensitivity to cutaneous antigens, (ii) T cell and

cytokine regulatory abnormalities, (iii) infectious activation, and (iv) abnormal processing of foreign bodies. The inclusion of silicone complications in these broad and well-characterized categories of pathological processes, whose pathogenesis is slowly being unraveled at the molecular level, will provide both mechanistic insights into how silicone granulomas occur and a rationale for their treatment, using therapies for diseases with similar immunopathogenetic mechanisms (20,285, pg. 47).

14.   *How should resistant granulomata be evaluated and treated?*
      Initially, one should look for a source of occult infection. This includes a careful evaluation of possible sinus, and dental infections, as well as a search for systemic infectious processes, drug therapies, or mechanical thermal procedures carried out in the skin, which could conceivably trigger granulomatous processes. A careful history must be taken to determine, as much as possible, whether the material injected was really silicone, and whether there is a good likelihood that the silicone was adulterated. Routine culture is usually nonproductive. However, if the biopsy reveals only inflammatory cells, PCR analysis can be used to amplify and identify novel or unculturable disease entities (203,204). Immunologic similarities between silicone granulomata and various T cell–mediated diseases (445) suggest that an immunologic evaluation of T cell populations should be carried out. Also an attempt to determine the cytokines modulating this process, i.e., looking for a predominance of Th1 or Th2 subtypes (261), which could direct specific therapies to restore cytokine balance, should be carried out. Intralesional corticosteroids and minocycline have been the mainstay of treatment in this practice, with oral corticosteroids reserved for patients with severe and more widespread inflammatory processes. No one has looked for ACE elevations in patients' silicone granuloma. Cutaneous sarcoidosis can also, in every detail, mimic silicone granulomata. After careful phenotyping, if inflammatory processes are not well controlled, use of biological immune modifiers such as Thalidomide or agents used for T cell mediated pathological entities such as psoriasis should be carefully discussed with clinicians experienced in their use.

15.   *What will happen when immunopathogeneses of silicone granulomata are better understood?*
      As immunologists begin to understand the signaling pathways and the molecular processes involved in the interaction of foreign bodies, infectious organisms, and tissue cells, an orderly and logical understanding of the scientific basis for disorders of tissue–implant integration, as well as methods for diagnosing and treating them, will invariably ensue. As an example, Blau syndrome, which has symptoms that overlap with sarcoidosis and RA, has its "own molecular vocabulary." When

discussing it the authors note that if we could "Define and characterize a cytokine profile in relation to pathology, initiation, and maintenance of granulomas, we may gain insight into the pathogenesis of the disease and consequently develop the means to intercept the progression or even reverse the disease process" (350,354,445–448). Fischer's report of pruritic nodules occurring on the face at the exact site of previous silicone injections, in two patients who later developed complications following breast implants, suggest the presence of specific T cells (CD45RO memory T cells), which "remember" the anatomical site where they first encountered the antigen (117, pg. 506, 158,206). If this is the case, the recombinant protein Alefacept®, which is used to treat psoriatic plaques that are infiltrated with the same type of cell, might provide effective therapy (449). At the same time, other mechanisms underlying effective therapies will also become apparent, e.g., the ability of certain antibiotics to suppress granuloma formation appears to be directly related to their ability to suppress **protein kinase C**, a signaling enzyme for the functional activation of T Cells (114,115,450). Immunohistochemical staining (205), molecular methods of diagnosing skin associated infectious agents (203), and the ability to recognize unique antigen receptors on T and B cell surfaces, as well as the ability to determine and quantify specific types of cytokines and inflammatory cells, will facilitate the use of oral, parenteral, and topical agents that precisely target specific components of the inflammatory cascade (21,129,160,237,249,262,278). These modalities may initiate dramatic advances in the treatment of complications following implants. The notion that silicone granulomata are "untreatable" when conventional therapies such as corticosteroids and antibiotics fail is reminiscent of the therapeutic pessimism that pervaded the medical community in years past regarding diseases such as psoriasis, diabetes, cancer, and infectious processes. This is an attitude that will surely be challenged by emerging therapeutic technologies (20).

16. *What is pathergy?*
    Pathergy (269) is defined as an exaggerated, altered, uncontrolled response to nonspecific stimuli, a process that probably involves memory T cell activation and is operant in the multiplicity of pathologic processes (152,206,278,288,300,377,446,449).

17. *What are adjuvants and molecular mimicry, and what is their relationship to infections and T cell activation, and silicone granulomata?*
    Adjuvants are substances, which, when administered with protein antigens, elicit maximal T cell dependent immune responses. Most adjuvants are microbial products such as LPS, which promote CMI and T cell dependent antibody

production (acquired immunity) while converting an inert nonmicrobial antigen into the equivalent of a microbial antigen (117, pg. 290). It is this ability of microbial products to convert a haptenic compound such as silicone into a "microbial mimic" that would best explain the conversion of this non-antigenic substance into a stimulant for immune reactivity, as well as the putative association between microbes, which contain antigens that cross-react with self-antigens and autoimmune responses against self-tissues (117, pg. 487).

18. *Have you ever carried out CO_2 laser resurfacing and hair removal procedures on areas that have undergone previous silicone augmentation?*

I have routinely carried out CO_2 laser resurfacing and hair removal procedures on areas, which have undergone previous silicone augmentation, without problems. One patient (unpublished personal observation) developed ulcerations following treatment for silicone granulomata involving the lips using a long-pulsed 1064 laser in which stacked pulses were employed. *Sarcoidal* dermal nodules,[k] which anecdotally have been attributed to silicone–heat interactions following radiofrequency (RF) treatments, have been observed on a temporary basis following RF treatment in patients who have never received liquid silicone. This phenomenon has been attributed to the coagulation of dermal proteins (451). Nevertheless, the ability of silicone to retain heat is one of the properties that make it most useful as an insulator in a variety of electrical applications. Heat retention by dermal implanted silicone following procedures which generate high temperatures in the skin may pose a theoretical problem following the use of any heat generating modalities such as CO_2 and hair removal lasers, nonablative resurfacing, and long–wave length lasers for the treatment of vascular anomalies. A small test area carried out before extensive procedures may be of value when treating patients who have received silicone injections. This may be particularly important in areas such as the suborbital grooves where the skin is very thin and silicone is deposited close to the surface.

PERSONAL AND ANECDOTAL OBSERVATIONS

Periodically I have occasion to discuss, observe, and treat complications following the use of adulterated and pure liquid silicone by other practitioners.

---

[k] As have sarcoidal nodules following pulsed-dye laser treatments (321), in patients who have never received silicone. This probably represents traumatic activation of latent cutaneous sarcoidosis.

Case #1. A patient with an allergic diathesis received liquid silicone on two occasions, five years before the development of a firm nodule at the injection site. This followed an episode of erythema nodosum associated with streptococcal infection. This nodule softened after intralesional steroids, but did not completely disappear.

Case #2. In this patient, who was allergic to penicillin, a generalized morbilliform eruption occurred after treatment with Keflex. During this period, a nodule appeared where silicone had been injected several years back. Oral prednisone effected a complete resolution.

Case #3. A patient with a history of ulcerative colitis developed facial nodules at a silicone injection site following the ingestion of seafood. This nodule was successfully treated with intralesional steroids.

Case #4. A 35-year-old white male, who had received liquid silicone injections in the nasolabial folds about five years earlier, developed linear elevations in the treated area following the use of anabolic steroids for weight training. These did not respond to intralesional corticosteroid injections.

Case #5. A 60-year-old white female had received liquid silicone injections in the glabella about twenty years back. She developed nodules at the injection site, following the purchase of a house, which was shown to be contaminated with a mold to which she was allergic. Subsequent repairs to the house resulted in resolution of these nodules, without further intervention.

Case #6. In 1992, a 46-year-old white female was treated in Mexico with 70 cc of some injected substance in each thigh. Two years later, she began to suffer from an episodic, recurrent, flu-like syndrome with fever, chills, and painful, hard swelling of the inner thighs, making it difficult for her to walk. Each attack lasted several days. Treatment with oral and intralesional steroids was only partially effective. Exercise and ambulation precipitated her symptoms. Laboratory analyses indicated a negative autoantibody panel, a significant increase in CD4+ cells, 1800 (normal is 430–1675), and a CD4 to CD8 ratio of 2.07. Venous doppler studies revealed vascular rigidity in the lower extremities. Biopsy noted probable "silicone granuloma."

Case #7. A 77-year-old white female received facial injections in Mexico 12 years before she developed massive facial edema (Figs. 16,17). Biopsy evaluation revealed: "Scattered foci of fat necrosis, characterized by foreign body type giant cells and epithelioid histiocytes, with lipophages and evidence of degenerating fat cells extending into the subcutaneous adipose tissue adjacent to skeletal muscle fibers. No vasculitis, malignancy, or significant cytologic atypia was noted. Polarization was negative for refractile particles. Rare asteroid bodies are noted within the giant cells." This patient's history is noteworthy because she had been treated with methotrexate for several years, for severe RA. Methotrexate is a known immunosuppressant, which has been (paradoxically) associated with granulomatous complications and accelerated rheumatoid nodulosis (452). Immunological evaluation revealed a mixed T and B cell infiltrate with T cell predominance, CD4+ T helper cells predominance, and rare intraepidermal T lymphocytes. Comment: "The immunohistochemical staining pattern favors a reactive process. Result of immunostain: strong staining of lymphocytes with antibodies to pan T cell markers."

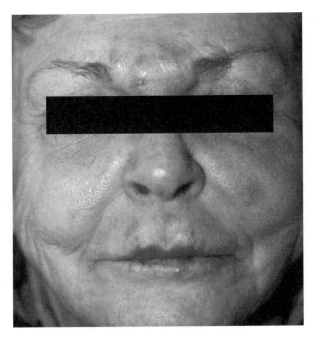

Figure 16
Patient H: This patient presented to our office with massive swelling in the
areas that were injected some 11 years prior in Mexico of an agent, which probably contained silicone along with other adulterants.

Case #8. A 32-year-old female who received large volumes of silicone (of questionable quality and purity) in breast, hips, and buttocks
developed woody induration and severe edema following exercise or after
minor colds or sore throats. Oral prednisone shortened these attacks, but
did not prevent future episodes.

Case #9. A 55-year-old white male and his 51-year-old wife were
treated for facial atrophy with injections of some unknown substance
represented as silicone in Mexico. Two years later, both developed
intermittent, massive, rock-hard facial edema and erythema, which
responded only partially to multiple courses of oral prednisone and
antibiotics.

Case #10. This 68-year-old white female received large volumes of
Sakurai formula from a well-known plastic surgeon in an attempt to
elevate extensive depressed scarring on the right leg, which had resulted
from a crush injury sustained when she was five years old (she was run
over by a truck). The treated area was asymptomatic until she re-trauma-
tized it as a consequence of a fall down the stairs (traumatic activation).
Severe swelling which required systemic corticosteroids and surgical
removal, resulted in a satisfactory response.

Case #11. KC received injections of liquid silicone for facial scarring in 1987. Over a 15-year period, he developed small, nodular swellings

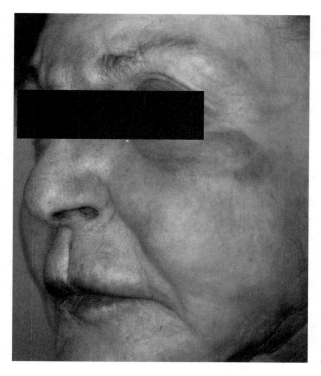

Figure 17
Patient H: What's interesting is that this patient is taking methotrexate, an immunosuppressive drug, which might be expected to ameliorate the effect of this problem but certainly has not. She also has rheumatoid arthritis.

which were initially considered to be silicone granulomatas, but nodules appeared in areas where silicone had never been injected. Biopsy revealed foreign body granulomas consistent with granulomatous rosacea. Treatment with a 532 laser was effective.

Case #12. SG, a 32-year-old white female, developed nodules in the lips following liquid silicone, in conjunction with active herpes simplex lesions involving the areas that were injected. Valtrex and intralesional steroids have effected a resolution in the last two years.

Case #13. A female patient received silicone injections of unknown purity and volume. She developed dermal nodules following RF ablation for facial rhytides. Histologically these were "sarcoidal granulomata." No immunophenotypical data were presented. This may be an example of a pathergic reaction representing an abnormality in foreign body processing, stimulated presumably by the heat released in RF treatments, or it may represent simple thermal coagulation of dermal proteins (451).

Case #14. A 47-year-old female was treated with small volumes of pure liquid silicone suborbitally to elevate groove-like depressions, which she found cosmetically unacceptable. She underwent a lower lid blepharoplasty about five years after silicone treatment. Shortly after surgery, she developed multiple nodules at the silicone injection sites, in association with a sinus infection. These nodules gradually resolved without treatment.

ACKNOWLEDGMENTS

I would like to give great thanks to the courageous Altounian family whose accomplishments have been a continuous source of inspiration. Thanks again to Dr. Jay Barnett for his skill and generosity in teaching me the art and technique of silicone injections and to Dr. Murray Zimmerman, whose intellectual brilliance and keen editorial eye, undimmed by the passage of his 84 years, has directed and molded this publication. Thanks also to Arnie Klein for the honor of being invited to write this chapter. Peggy Goodwin's help was invaluable, and Lisa Elia provided many useful suggestions. Additional thanks to Stephanie Duffy who spent laborious hours sorting out references, and Drs. Scott Binder and Christine Ko, for what may be the first modern day immunologic evaluation of liquid silicone granulomata. Recognition is also owed to the editors of the Archives of Dermatology and the *Journal of the American Academy of Dermatology* for the quality of their publications, which I have used so extensively, and for the unfailing encouragement and support afforded me by Dr. Ronald Reisner, and the late, greatly missed Dr. Arnold Gurevitch.

GLOSSARY—USEFUL TERMS AND CONCEPTS

"*A Plague O'Both Your Houses.*" Shakespeare, Romeo and Juliet (453). This curse was uttered against two parties whose senseless feud produced fatal results. Misunderstandings about liquid silicone unquestionably contributed to the death of an innocent physician, just as the feud between the Capuletes and Montagues destroyed the lives of innocent people.

Accessory Cell. Cell required for, but not actually mediating, a specific immune response. Often used to describe antigen-presenting cells (117, pg. 529).

Adhesion Molecules. Adhesion molecules confer mechanical stability on interactions between cells and the environment. They also act as sensors and signaling molecules, which are essential for cell migration, growth, and survival. It is now well established that the recruitment of leukocytes from the blood to virtually every tissue is regulated by sequential engagement of adhesion molecules on lymphocytes and endothelial cells. Leukocytes make an initial adhesive contact, which allows them to slow down and roll along the vascular wall. This step can be mediated by multiple adhesion molecules including selectins,and integrins. In order for the rolling leukocyte to stop, it must receive an activating signal such as a signal from a chemokine that switches integrins into a highp affinity state and allows the cell to arrest itself. Leukocytes are recruited into a tissue only if they are successful in undergoing each step. Drugs like natalizumab, a recombinant monoclonal antibody against integrins, have been used for multiple sclerosis and Crohn's disease. This drug presumably blocks the binding of specific integrins to a vascular cell adhesion molecule (154).

Affinity. A measure of the binding constant of a single antigen combining site with a monovalent antigenic determinant (117, pg. 469).

Allelic. Relating to one of a series of two or more alternate forms of a gene that occupy the same position or locus on a specific chromosome (117, pg. 499).

Antigen. Any foreign material that is specifically bound to antibody or lymphocytes; also used loosely to describe materials used for immunization. Antigens may also be immunogens if they are able to trigger an immune response, or haptens if not (117, pg. 470).

Antigen Processing. T cells recognize antigens only after considerable processing and gene activation. Antigen processing includes the introduction of protein antigens to APCs, their degradation into peptide fragments by proteases, and the binding of these peptides to MHC molecules which display peptide–MHC complexes on the APC surface for T cell recognition. The type of processing that occurs. i.e., intra or extra cellular, which determines the operant class of MHC molecules, is important for understanding the immunopathogenesis of postimplant granulomata as well as for determining appropriate therapies (285,446,454).

Antigen-Presenting Cells (APC). When faced with microbial invasion, the immune system must decide whether or not to respond, and then if a response occurs, it must be tailored to cope with a specific microbe. Although B and T lymphocytes can respond to antigens, the decision making process is shaped by the nature of the antigen, its concentration, and portal of entry as well as by dendritic cells (DCs) which are scattered throughout the body (326,327,455). DCs can be viewed as immunological sensors, which can decode and integrate signaling systems and transfer information to naïve T cells. DCs can fine tune the immune response by modulating the amplitude or class of the response. Langerhans cells (LCs) and their precursors reside in the skin and mucus membranes. When a microbe infects tissue, DCs sense its presence via surface receptors such as TLRs. DCs can be divided into several subsets. In the skin two subsets can be found, LCs in the epidermis and interstitial DCs in the dermis. Although LCs are the professional antigen presenting cells of the skin, other dendritic cells and dermal macrophages may also present antigen. In addition, LCs promote T cell differentiation on expressed surface receptors, which regulate a large number of immune functions. These include surface receptors for IL-6, IL-1, TNF-α, as well as integrins and adhesion molecules. LCs also secrete cytokines (proteins which mediate communication between cells of the immune system), such as IL-1b, IL-6, IL-12, IL-15, IL-18, and MIP (macrophage inflammatory proteins). The pharmacological manipulation of cytokines and adhesion molecules and the gene activation of cytokine imbalances, (285) is rapidly becoming a billion dollar business (117, pg. 490, 542).

B Lymphocyte (B Cell). The precursors of antibody-forming plasma cells; these cells carry immunoglobulin and class II MHC antigens on their surfaces (117, pg. 532).

CD Nomenclature. Various subsets of T cells are distinguished based upon the types of proteins expressed on their cell membranes. These are referred to as cell-surface molecules, which are recognized by monoclonal antibodies and are also called antigens because antibodies can be raised against them, creating markers that identify or discriminate different cell populations. Each cell-surface molecule has been assigned a number—prefaced by the letters "CD," standing for the cluster of differentiation, which specifies the type of T cell upon which that molecule can be found. Additional letters and symbols appearing after the CD number represent the life cycle stage (isoform) of the molecule (456). Their value in classifying lymphocytes is enormous. This system allows immunologists to identify cells participating in different immune responses as well as isolate or analyze their specificities in the monitoring of disease states (117, pg. 533–534).

Cell-Mediated Immunity (CMI). This form of adaptive immunity, mediated by T cells, is especially important for destroying intracellular viruses and bacteria, which survive within phagocytes or infect nonphagocytic cells. It is also important for the destruction of tumor cells. CMI responses include CD4+ T cell (helper T cell) –mediated activation of macrophages that have phagocytosed microbes as well as CD8+ cytolytic T lymphocyte (CTL) killing of infected cells. These responses are especially important for destroying intracellular pathogens, eliminating viral infections, and destroying tumor cells (117, pg. 534).

Chemotaxis. Migration of cells along a concentration gradient of an attractant (117, pg. 473).

Cytokines. Cytokines play an important regulatory role in a variety of basic physiologic functions such as cellular/humoral immunity, fever, inflammation, chemotaxis, tumor regression, hematopoiesis, and wound repair. Cytokines are the "hormones" of the immune system and mediate a variety of responses by acting in an endocrine, paracrine, or autocrine fashion on target cells. As a result of advances in recombinant DNA technology, the genes that encode these proteins have been cloned, allowing the investigators to use unlimited quantities of these cytokines to treat disease. When administered at super physiologic doses, recombinant cytokines produce pharmacologic effects different from their physiologic functions. These biologic properties may render them particularly useful to treat cutaneous disease, i.e., IL-10 produced by TH2 cytokines inhibits TH1 proliferation and function, which may be useful for the treatment of allergic contact dermatitis and psoriasis. IL-12 produced by APCs promotes TH1 immune responses that inhibit TH2 F1 mediated immunity. A cytokine like IL-12 would be useful for the treatment of TH2 F1 mediated diseases such as atopic dermatitis or cutaneous T cell lymphomas. Cytokines (117, pg. 536, 249,274,326,457–459) have been named on the basis of their origin, i.e., lymphokines are cytokines secreted mainly by activated Th1 lymphocytes. Monokines are immunoregulators produced by activated macrophages and monocytes. Cytokines are also named according to their functions (interferons, growth and differentiation factors and colony stimulating factors). Unlike classic hormones, cytokines are usually inactive in serum or plasma. They can be synthesized by many cell types. They are heterogenous in their effect and possess redundancy or overlap of their effects. Individual cytokines can have pleiotropic (multiple, overlapping, and sometimes contradictory) functions, depending on their concentration, the cell type they are acting on, and the presence of other cytokines and mediators. Thus, the information which an individual cytokine conveys, depends on the pattern of regulators to which a cell is exposed and not on only one cytokine. It is postulated that all cytokines form a specific system or network of communicating signals between cells and the immune system, and between the immune system and other organs. Because of their potent and profound biological effects, it is not surprising that their activities are tightly regulated, most notably at the levels of secretion and receptor expression. Cytokines can display redundancy (the ability of different cytokines to induce the same response), synergy (cooperative induction of cell responses), and antagonism (in addition to cytokine activation). Many cytokines stimulate or inhibit other cytokines and the action of a specific cytokine can be influenced by the microenvironment of the cell depending on, for example, the growth state of the cell, the type of neighboring cells, cytokine concentrations, the combination of other cytokines present at the same time, and even the temporal sequence of several cytokines acting on the same cell. The biological activity of cytokines is mediated by specific membrane receptors, which can be expressed on virtually every cell type known. Cytokines interact first with high-affinity cell surface receptors (distinct for each type or even subtype) and then regulate the transcription of cellular genes, which can enhance or inhibit changes in cell behavior. The production of cytokines is not constitutive, but is inducible and transient. Additional regulatory mechanisms are provided by the concomitant action of different cytokines and the presence of specific inhibitory proteins, cytokine binding factors, and specific autoantibodies in biological fluids. When cytokine production is sustained or systemic, cytokines contribute to the signs, symptoms, and pathology of inflammatory, infectious, autoimmune, and malignant diseases. TNF-α is an excellent example of such dual action. Locally, it has important regulatory and antitumor activities, but when TNF-α circulates in concentrations higher than that produced by the organ of origin, it may be involved in the pathogenesis of endotoxic shock, cachexia, and other serious diseases.

From the inflammation point of view, there are two main groups of cytokines, proinflammatory and anti-inflammatory. Proinflammatory cytokines are produced predominantly by activated macrophages and activated CD4+ T cells, which are involved in the upregulation of inflammatory reactions. Anti-inflammatory cytokines predominantly belong to the Th2 class of T cell–derived cytokines, and act to downregulate inflammatory reactions by suppressing Th1 cytokines (459). "The past two decades have witnessed an explosion in the use of biologic therapeutics which target cytokines and cells involved in chronic inflammatory and auto-immune diseases." (237). These agents profoundly expand the therapeutic options for patients with chronic diseases for which there have been no new therapies for many years. The new biologic immunomodulators include interferons, TNF-α inhibitors, interleukin-1 receptor antagonist, monoclo-nal antibodies that interfere with B and T cell activation (antiCD20, antiCD40 and antiCD25), complement protein inhibitors, and numerous other important immune modifying agents (409,460).

Cytolytic or Cytotoxic T Lymphocytes (CTL). Also known as "killer T cells." These lymphocytes are effector cells, which recognize and kill host cells infected with viruses or other intracellular microbes. CTLs usually express CD8+ and recognize microbial peptides displayed by class I MHC molecules (117, pg. 536).

Delayed-Type Hypersensitivity (DTH). An immune reaction in which T Cell–dependent macrophage activation and inflammation cause tissue injury. A DTH reaction to the subcutaneous injection of antigen is often used as an assay for CMI, e.g., the purified protein derivative skin test for immunity to mycobacterium tuberculosis. DTH is a frequent accompaniment of protective CMI against microbes (117, pg. 536).

Dendritic Cells. Immune cells with tentacle-like branches. Among dendritic cells are the cutaneous LCs and follicular dendritic cells of the lymph nodes. Most dendritic cells function as APCs, although follicu-lar dendritic cells do not (117, pg. 536).

Epitope. An epitope is a portion of a molecule capable of binding to the combining site of an antibody. For every given antigenic determinant, the body can construct a variety of antibody-combining sites, some of which fit almost perfectly and others barely fit at all. In the case of a pro-tein antigen recognized by a T cell, an epitope is a peptide portion that binds to an MHC molecule for recognition by T cell receptors (TCRs). In contradistinction to B cell function, T cells only recognize peptide frag-ments bound to MHC molecules expressed on the surface of another cell (117, pg. 475).

Freund's Complete Adjuvant. A water-in-oil emulsion that con-tains an immunogen, an emulsifying agent, and killed mycobacteria, and which enhances the immune response to the immunogen; termed "incomplete" Freund's adjuvant if mycobacteria are not included (117, pg. 530).

Hapten. A compound, usually of low molecular weight, that is not by itself immunogenic, but after conjugation to a carrier protein or cells, becomes immunogenic and induces antibody, which can bind the hapten alone in the absence of a carrier.

Henny Penny—An Old English Fable. Those who irrationally describe complications following liquid silicone as indecipherable or untreatable, can be accurately compared to Henny Penny, who inter-preted a blow to the head as a sign of cosmic collapse (461).

Innate and Adaptive Immunity. "The rapid translation of insults into cutaneous inflammation (innate immunity), and the recruitment of memory T lymphocytes that have clonally expanded in response to antigens encountered at the cutaneous interface with the environment (acquired immunity) are both required for successful cutaneous immune surveillance" (158, pg. 1817). Innate immune responses are mediated largely by white cells (neutrophils and macrophages), which phagocytize and kill pathogens, and concurrently coordinate additional host responses by synthesizing inflammatory mediators and cytokines. Molecules produced during innate immune responses stimulate adaptive immunity and shape the nature of adaptive immune responses. In addition, recently discovered receptors (TLRs), (337,340,342,343) and TREM-1 receptors (436) also play key roles in tying the innate and adaptive immune systems together.

Interferons. A group of proteins having antiviral activity and capable of enhancing and modifying the immune response (117, pg. 541).

Lipopolysaccharides (Also known as endotoxins). This component of the cell wall of gram-negative bacteria is released from dying bacteria and stimulates many innate immune responses. The immune system of higher organisms probably evolved in the veritable sea of endotoxin, and so it is not surprising that this substance evokes a powerful response. In addition, endotoxins can elicit T cell proliferation and have been described as a superantigen for T cells (117, pg. 476, 459).

Macrophage. A large phagocytic cell of the mononuclear series found within tissues. Properties include phagocytosis, and antigen presentation to T cells.

Major Histocompatibility Complex (MHC). MHC molecules are membrane proteins whose only known function is to bind and transport peptides for presentation to T lymphocytes. After antigen processing, a fundamental step is the introduction of immunity to foreign antigens (230,462). Initially named MHC molecules because they were the principle targets of rejection in grafts, these molecules control the immune response to recognition of self and nonself, and consequently serve as targets in transplantation rejection. MHC restriction refers to a characteristic of T lymphocytes, which recognizes a foreign peptide antigen only when it is bound to a particular allelic form of an MHC molecule following antigen processing. Different classes of MHC molecules are involved in processing antigens from different cellular compartments, resulting in the activation of specific types of lymphocytes. Protein antigens synthesized by intracellular cytosolic microbes generate peptides bound to class I MHC molecules for recognition by CD8+ CTLs, which eradicate cells harboring intracellular infections. Conversely, proteins from extracellular microbes generate peptides bound to class II MHC molecules for recognition by CD4+ helper T cells (117, pg. 544, 230,462,463).

Class I MHC Molecules. These proteins are associated with cell-mediated responses and are present on the surface of virtually all nucleated cells in the body with the exception of human red blood cells (117, pg. 486).

Class II MHC Molecules. These proteins, associated with antibody responses, are present on the surface of a limited number of cells including macrophages, dendritic cells, LCs, veiled cells, and B cells (117, pg. 487).

Natural Killer Cells (NK Cells). NK cells are part of a group known as the "large granular lymphocytes." These cells are generally nonspecific, MHC-unrestricted cells involved primarily in the elimination of neoplastic or tumor cells. The precise mechanism by which they recognize their target cells is not clear. Probably, there is some type of NK-determinant expressed by the target cells that is recognized by an NK-receptor on the NK cell surface. Once the target cell is recognized, killing occurs in a manner similar to that produced by the CTL (117, pg. 546).

Nuclear Factor-κ. Sometimes called the master switch of the immune system, it is a cellular signaling pathway which regulates many genes central to the initiation of cutaneous inflammation, and appears to be a final common pathway "For the translation of environmental insults into inflammation, and is a crucial element of innate immunity" (158, pg. 1819). IL-1, and TNF-α (primary cytokines), which can be activated by ultraviolet radiation from sunlight, activate several mechanisms that can in turn activate NF-κB. Corticosteroid effects are related to activation of NF-κB (285,117, pg. 489).

Pangloss. Voltaire's Pangloss, whose absurdly illogical philosophy of optimism ignored the grim realities of his own life can accurately be compared to the equally absurd aura of perfection, which permeates the writings of those with the magical belief that liquid silicone is flawless (464).

Protein Kinase C and Protein Tyrosine Kinase (PTKs). Both protein kinase C and protein tyrosine kinases are enzymes involved in numerous signal transduction pathways in cells of the immune system. Protein kinase C has been found to be the target of antibiotics such as tetracycline. It activates pathways leading to transcription activation for T and B lymphocytes (285,329,330,335,465).

TH1 and TH2 Cells. Two different T helper cell populations have recently been discovered in mice based on their ability to secrete different cytokines. The cytokines that a cell secretes reflects the different biological functions of that cell. Multiple disease states can be accurately defined and treated on the basis of distinctions in Th1 and Th2 cells populations (350,354,355,445–448,455,466–473).

Relevance for Clinicians. Therapies can be designed to direct the differentiation of T_H0 cells and specific TH cell subtypes (T_H1 or T_H2), and patients suffering from TH-mediated diseases may derive some benefit by redirection of T_H0 cell maturation into the appropriate T_H subtypes.

It is always tempting to try to distinguish various disease entities on the basis of Th1 or Th2 activation and phenotypes. However, most diseases involve a balance of these cytokines or changes in cytokine profiles as the disease progresses (355,465–470).

TH1 and TH2 Cell Functions. TH1 cells are responsible for classical cell-mediated functions, for example, for DTH and activation of T cells; TH2 cells function primarily as helpers for B cell and macrophage activation. Th2 cells provide help for IgE production and antibody formation (117, pg. 550).

Toll-Like Receptors (TLRs). These cell surface protein receptors "the eyes of the innate immune system" were named because of their similarities to the Toll family of receptors discovered in fruit flies (Drosophila). TLRs, which are present on many cell types including lipocytes, serve an important function by offering dendritic cells a means of discriminating between various stimuli (319). They do this by recognizing common bacterial and viral motifs (PAMPs), (474) and transmitting or transducing a signal to APCs that a foreign object has been encountered. TLRs are linked to a variety of diseases including lung damage following ozone exposure and premature birth, and acne (331,341,475). They may also be involved in defense against virus infections (336). TLR recognition of microbial motifs is followed by cell activation and represents a crucial link between innate and adaptive immunity. TLRs probably represent mammalian homologs of proteins present on plants and invertebrates millions of years ago. The human genome contains at least 10 genes encoding TLRs. TLR-4 is crucial in mediating effects of LPS immune stimulation. Genetic variants in TLRs may be related to the development of atherosclerosis (337). TLR-7 is a ligand for imiquimod.

Tumor Necrosis Factor-α (TNF-α). TNF-α, the first identified member of a large family of proinflammatory cytokines, plays a major role in host immune responses to infection, tumors, foreign proteins, and apoptotic processes. Produced mainly by mononuclear phagocytes and in certain pathological states by Th1 cells, TNF-α is extremely pleiotrophic, exerting its effects on inflammatory processes in a multiplicity of ways. ·This includes overexpression of adhesion molecules (246) and promotion of maturation of LCs, which increases their capacity to activate T cells. In addition, TNF-α produced by dermal dendrocytes exerts a spatially coordinated increase in the expression of other immunomodulatory cytokines such as IL-8, and tumor growth factor-α. TNF elevations are noted in psoriasis, erythema nodosum leprosum, contact dermatitis, and cutaneous lupus. In sarcoidosis, TNF-α promotes granulomatous inflammation. TNF-α levels are also elevated in aphthous ulcers, graft versus host disease, and toxic epidermal necrolysis. TNF-α, which has receptors on almost every cell, is involved in an enormous diversity of inflammatory processes in almost every tissue of the body. The role of TNF-α and ultraviolet-induced apoptosis and immunosuppression has been studied. UV radiation (UVR) is absorbed by the epidermis resulting in "sunburned" keratinocytes, which have undergone apoptosis (476). UVB radiation has been shown to stimulate TNF production, as well as NF-κB activation. Paradoxically, TNF-α may inhibit LC migration and its activity as APCs (477). TNF-α is also involved in cutaneous wound healing and plays a principal role in the acute inflammatory response to LPS by stimulating the activation of neutrophils and monocytes and their recruitment to the sites of infection. By increasing the expression of adhesion molecules by endothelial cells, TNF-α facilitates margination of leukocytes, and promotes leukocyte chemotaxis to the sites of infection. In times of severe infection, TNF-α levels rise and circulate to cause a variety of systemic abnormalities, acting as a pyrogen to induce fever, cachexia, life threatening hypoglycemia, and cardiovascular collapse. TNF plays a particularly important role in Crohn's disease and rheumatoid arthritis. TNF plays a prominent role in HIV AIDS (251). It can be detected in the skin using a variety of different antibodies (240) and is associated with a variety of genetic syndromes and inflammatory diseases of muscles (239). TNF-α is a key cytokine in innate immune responses (237). It also increases NF-κB production and this increases TNF-α levels (285). The effect of TNF-α may vary from one tissue to the next. For example in rheumatoid arthritis, TNF-α does not induce apoptosis in rheumatoid synovial fibroblasts, but stimulates them to proliferate. Again, paradoxically, fibroblasts do undergo apoptosis if NF-κB is inhibited when they are treated with TNF-α. There is an association between TNF and subcorneal pustular dermatosis (SPD; 247), which is in itself associated with pyoderma gangrenosum, rheumatoid arthritis, and inflammatory bowel disease, all of which are united by TNF-α. TNF-α also plays a role in the pathogenesis of ankylosing spondylitis (242). Modulating TNF-α activity in the skin has become the rationale for dozens of new therapies, for both cutaneous and disease processes (21,237,478).

   Vascular Endothelial Growth Factor (VEGF). VEGF and TNF-α share a complex and highly pleiotropic relationship. TNF directly induces the expression of VEGF messenger RNA, which in turn produces the stepwise process of new vessel growth (angiogenesis) in several ways (479), including direct mitogenic effects on endothelial cells, the promotion of endothelial cell migration, and inhibition of apoptosis. Estrogens are known to influence VEGFs (480) perhaps by regulating TNF-α (233). Drugs such as minocycline directly inhibit endothelial cell proliferation while Thalidomide inhibits angiogenesis by inhibiting the biosynthesis of TNF-α (439).

REFERENCES

1. Rubin L, ed. Biomaterials in Reconstructive Surgery. St. Louis: C.V. Mosby Co., 1983.
2. Orentreich DS, Orentreich NO. Injectable Fluid Silicone: Principles of Dermatologic Surgery. New York: Marcel Dekker, Inc., 1989:1349–1395.
3. Latish E. From Eric Latish, Chief Dental, ENT, and Ophthalmic Devices Branch, Division of Enforcement II, Office of Compliance, Center of Radiologic Health, U.S. Food and Drug Administration [letter]. Int J Cosmet Surg 1999; 7.
4. Personal communication from a colleague December 2003.
5. Tolbolsky AV. Properties and Structure of Polymers. New York: John Wiley & Sons, 1960.
6. Council on Scientific Affairs, American Medical Association. Silicone Gel Breast Implants. JAMA 1993; 270:2602–2606.
7. Baier RE. Adhesion in Biological Systems. New York: Academic Press, 1970.
8. Yasuda H. The Polymer Handbook. 2d ed. New York: John Wiley & Sons, 1975.
9. Orentreich NO. Soft tissue augmentation with medical-grade fluid silicone. In: M Biomaterials in Reconstructive Surgery. St. Louis: C.V. Mosby Co., 1983:859–881.
10. Frisch EE. Technology of silicones in biomedical applications. In: Rubin L, ed. Biomaterials in Reconstructive Surgery. St. Louis: C.V. Mosby Co., 1983:73–90.
11. Carine HM, et al. Efficacy of injected liquid silicone in the diabetic foot to reduce risk factors for ulceration. Diabetes Care 2002; 23(5):634–638.
12. Orentreich D. Liquid injectable silicone. Clin Plast Surg 2000; 27(4).
13. Jones DH. Injectable silicone for facial lipoatrophy. Cosmet Dermatol 2002; 15(6):13–15.
14. Carruthers J, Carruthers A. An AIDS patient's experience with injectables. CST Sep 2003; 12.
15. Wallace WD. The histological host response of liquid silicone injections for prevention of pressure-related ulcers of the foot: A 38 year study. Presented at The Los Angeles Society of Pathology, May 13, 2003.
16. Palmer A. Hands across the table. Am J Cosmet Surg 1990; 7(1):15–17.
17. Blocksma R, Braley S. Implantation materials. In: Grabb WC, Smith JW, eds. Plastic Surgery. 2d ed. Boston: Little, Brown, 1973:131–156.
18. Ashley FL, Braley S, McNall EG. The current status of silicone injection therapy. Surg Clin North Am 1971; 51:501.
19. Sanger JR, Komorowski RA, Larson DL, Gingrass RP, Yousif JN, Matloub HS. Tissue humoral response to intact and ruptured silicone gel prosthesis. Plast Reconstr Surg 1995; 95:1033.
20. Duffy D. Silicone granulomata management. Dermatol Times 2003; 75–76.
21. La Duca J, Gaspari A. Targeting tumor necrosis factor alpha: new drugs used to modulate inflammatory diseases. Dermatol Clin 19(4);617–635.
22. Thomas P, Walchner M, Ghoreschi K, Rocken M. Successful treatment of granulomatous cheilitis with Thalidomide. Arch Dermatol 2003; 139:136–138.
23. Zager W, Huang J, McCue P, Reiter D. Laser resurfacing of silicone-injected skin. Arch Otolaryngol Head Neck Surg 2001; 127:418–421.
24. Selmanowitz VJ, Orentreich NO. Medical-grade fluid silicone: a monographic review. J Dermatol Surg Oncol 1977; 3:597–611.
25. Webster RC, Fuleihan NS, Gaunt JM, Haindan US, Smith RC. Injectable silicone for small augmentations: twenty year experience in humans. Am J Cosmet Surg 1984; 1(4):1–10.
26. Kopf EH, Vinnik CA, Bongiovi JJ, et al. Complications of silicone injections. Rocky Mountain Med J 1976; 73:77–80.
27. Ellenbogen R, Rubin L. Injectable fluid silicone therapy, human morbidity and mortality. JAMA 1975; 234:308–309.
28. Winer LH, Sternberg TH, Herman R, et al. Tissue reactions to injected silicone liquids. Arch Dermatol 1964; 90:588–593.

29. Duffy, DM. Silicone: a critical review. Adv Dermatol 1990; 5:93–110.

30. Leong ASY. Silicone: a possible iatrogenic cause of hepatic dysfunction in hemodialysis patients. Pathology 1983; 15:193–195.

31. Bommer J. Silicone storage disease in long-term hemodialysis patients. Contrib Nephrol 1983; 36:115–126.

32. Leong ASY, et al. Spallation and migration of silicone from blood-pump tubing in patients on hemodialysis. N Eng J Med 1982; 306:135–140.

33. Duffy DM. Tissue injectable liquid silicone: New perspectives. In: Klein A, ed. Augmentation in Clinical Practice: Procedures and Techniques. New York: Marcel Dekker, 1998:237–263.

34. Blumenthal R. New York Dermatologist is fighting with FDA over silicone injections. The New York Times, July 19, 1984.

35. Adatosil package insert.

36. Kagan HD. Sakurai injectable silicone formula: a preliminary report. Arch Otolaryngol 1963; 78:663–668.

37. http://www.caringmedical.com/therapies/mesotherapy.asp/ Uses for mesotherapy.

38. Safety of silicone Breast implants, Bondurant S, Ernster V, Herdman R. eds. Institute of Medicine. Copyright 2000 National Academy of Sciences; National Academy Press. 22, 146, 241, 247, 112, 169, 182, 183, 186, 191.

39. Rathjen. The dermabrasion, chemical peel, silicone and collagen symposium. American Society for Dermatologic Surgery, Tulane University Medical School, July 4–8, 1984.

40. Ortho Pharmaceutical Corporation. Investigational new device clinical protocol. Protocol #H87–046. Silicone Investigation Meeting, New York City, NY, June 10, 1987.

41. Leif WE. Product Manager, New Products, Ortho Pharmaceutical Corporation. Jan 8, 1988. Personal Communication.

42. Webster RC, Fuleihan NS, Hamdan US. Injectable silicone: report of 17,000 facial treatments since 1962. Am J Cosmet Surg 1986; 3:41–48.

43. Webster RCP, Hamdan VS, Gaunt JM, et al. Rhinoplastic revisions with injectable silicone. Arch Otolaryngol Head Neck Surg 1986; 112:269–296.

44. Balkin SW. Plantar keratoses: Treatment by injectable liquid silicone. Clin Orthop 1972; 87:235–247.

45. Balkin SW. Treatment of painful scars on soles and digits with injection of fluid silicone. J Dermatol Surg Oncol 1977; 3:612–614.

46. Balkin SW. Fluid silicone augmentation in the diabetic foot: A fifteen year study (scientific exhibit). Presented at the 1979 annual meeting of the American Diabetes Association, Los Angeles, CA June 9–12, 1979.

47. Balkin SW. The fluid silicone prosthesis. Clin Podiatry 1984; 1:145–164.

48. Balkin SW. Treatment of corns by injectable silicone. Arch Dermatol 1975; 3:1143–1145.

49. Balkin SW, Kaplan L. Injectable silicone and the diabetic foot: a 25-year report. Foot 1991; 2:83.

50. Balkin SW. Fluid silicone implantation of the foot. In: Lorimer D, ed. 5th ed. Neale's Common Foot Disorders: Diagnosis and Management. 5th ed. Edinburgh: Churchill Livingstone, 1997:387–400.

51. Carine HM, et al. Efficacy of injected liquid silicone in the diabetic foot to reduce risk factors for ulceration. Diabetes Care May 2002; 23(5):634–638.

52. Duffy D. Liquid silicone for soft tissue augmentation, J Dermatol Surg 2005:31. In press.

53. Duffy DM. Liquid silicone for soft tissue augmentation. In: Lask G, Moy R, eds. The principles and techniques of cutaneous surgery. New York: McGraw-Hill, 1996:403–417.

54. Stegman SJ. What's new in dermatology? Soft tissue implants. Lecture presented before American Academy of Dermatology, 45th Annual Meeting, New Orleans, LA, 1986.

55. Clark DP, Hanke CW, Swanson NA. Dermal implants; safety of products injected for soft tissue augmentation. J Am Acad Derm 1989; 21(5):997.

56. 60 Minutes, CBS. Aug 2, 1992.
57. Hilts PJ. "Doctors Continue to Inject Silicone Despite F.D.A. Warnings, Agency Says," NY Times, Feb 1, 1992.
58. American Academy of Dermatology. Soft tissue augmentation task force on liquid injectable silicone. Dec 1993.
59. Rapaport MJ, et al. Injectable silicone: cause of facial nodules, cellulitis, ulcerations and migration. Aesth Plast Surg 1996; 20:267–276.
60. Rapaport M. Silicone injections revisited. J Dermatol Surg 2002; 28(7):594–595.
61. AAD 61st Annual Meeting, San Francisco; Course 102, Fri., Mar 21, 2003. Silicone Redux: Caution, Dr. Rapaport.
62. Aronsohn RB. A 22 year experience with the use of silicone injection. Am J Cosmet Surg 1984; 1:21–28.
63. Webster RC, Gaunt JM, Hamdan VA, et al. Injectable silicone for facial soft-tissue augmentation. Arch Otolaryngol Head Neck Surg 1986; 112:290–296.
64. Webster RC, Hamdan US, Fuleihan NS, Gaunt JM, Smith RC. Injectable silicone: it's history and it's current status. Am J Cosmet Surg 1986; 3(2):31–39.
65. Greenberg JH: Information postal survey of selected physicians in dermatology. Presented to American Academy of Dermatology, Dallas, TX, Dec, 1991.
66. Auerbach R. Subdermal silicone injections fill in acne, other scars. Dermatol Times 1986:4–6.
67. Yarborough JM. The Dermabrasion, Chemical Peel, Silicone and Collagen Symposium. Lecture presented before American Society for Dermatologic Surgery. Tulane University Medical School, New Orleans, LA, July 4–8, 1984.
68. Waxman J. Silicone fears—How real are they? In: Mutaz B. Habel et al., eds. Advances in Plastic and Reconstructive Surgery. Vol 12. Saint Louis: Mosby Year Book Inc., 1996:1–8.
69. Duffy D. Silicone conundrum: a battle of anecdotes. Dermatol Surg 2002; 28(7):590–594.
70. Wilke TF. Late development of granuloma after liquid silicone injections. Plast Reconstr Surg 1977; 60:179–188.
71. New reports relating to silicone, collagen implants. FDA truth and information report, No. 16974, 16875.
72. Angell M. Science on Trial: The clash of medical evidence and the law in the breast implant case. New York: W.W. Norton & Company, 1996.
73. Erderly SR. Pretty at a price. Self Magazine, Nov 2003, 168.
74. Shearer L. Have doctors found the fountain of youth? Parade, Feb 16, 1964, 6–7.
75. Kron J. Inject at your own risk. Allure Magazine, Sep 2002, 146–152.
76. "Silicone Kills Eight Transvestites". San Francisco Chronicle, Feb 4, 1983.
77. http://msnbc.msn.com/id/4610301/ 3/26/04. Man charged with murder for silicone injection death. (Pumping Parties).
78. Silicone could be deterrent for breast cancer. San Francisco Examiner, Aug 5, 1994.
79. Diaz J, Smith S Miami Herald FL, April 29, 2001.
80. www.ABCnews.com. Black market beauty. Jan 28, 2002.
81. Singer S. Sun-Sentinel. June 19, 2001.
82. www.MSNBC.com/Health. Dangerous beauty julia sommerfeld. June 4, 2001.
83. Field LM. A new adulterated silicone epidemic: Java, Indonesia. Dermatol Surg 2002; 28(3):301–302.
84. Huffman T. Court allows class action against doctor. Toronto Star, Dec 12, 2003.
85. Rees TD, Platt J, Ballantyne DL. An investigation of cutaneous response to dimethyl-polysiloxane (silicone liquid) in animals and humans: a preliminary report. Plast Reconstr Surg 1965; 35:131–139.
86. Otero J. Silicone issues and controversies. Presented at Valley Medical Center Hospital Bulletin, Vol. 16, No.7 Fullerton, CA, July 15, 1991, 5–6.

87. Ruffenach G. Study links silicone gel to cancer. Wall Street Journal, Nov 10, 1988, B-1.
88. Mustafa D, et al. Diagnosis of silicone lymphadenopathy. Gazi Medical Journal-Turkey 1997; 8:93–95.
89. Zirkin H, Avinoach I, Edelwitz P. A tattoo and localized lymphadenopathy: a case report. Cutis 2001; 67:471–472.
90. Eller AW, et al. Migration of silicone oil into the brain: a complication of intraocular silicone oil for retinal tamponade. Am J Ophthal 2000; 129:685–688.
91. Garrido L, et al. Detection of silicone migration and biodegradation with NMR; NMR Center, Dept of Radiology, Massachusetts General Hospital and Harvard Medical School, Charlestown, MA, 1993.
92. Osofsky L, Zaim T. A clinicopathologic approach to granulomatous dermatoses. J Am Acad Dermatol 1996; 35(4):588–600.
93. Plediderer B, Ackerman JL, Garrido L. Migration and biodegradation of free silicone from silicone gel-filled implants after long-term implantation. Dept of Radiology, NMR Center, Massachusetts General Hospital and Harvard Medical School, Charlestown, MA, 1993.
94. Haycox CL, et al. Quantitative detection of silicone in skin by means of spectroscopy for chemical analysis (ESCA). J Am Acad Dermatol 1999; 40:719–725.
95. Pearl RM, Laub DR, Kaplan EN. Complications following silicone injections for augmentation of the contours of the face. Plast Reconstr Surg 1978; 61:888–891.
96. Immunology Tests. F.D.A. Consumer, Nov 1995, 13.
97. Taubes G. Silicone in the system. Discover Magazine 1995; 65–75.
98. Dow-Corning Position Statement. Reported immunologic reactions to silicone fluid and devices. Dec 30, 1987.
99. Nosanchuk JS. Injected dimethylpolysiloxane fluid: a study of antibody and histologic response. Plast Reconstr Surg 1968; 42(6):562–566.
100. Kossovsky N, Heggers JP, Robson MC. Experimental demonstration of the immunogenicity of silicone-protein complexes. J Biomed Mater Res 1987; 21:1125–1133.
101. Kossovsky N, Heggers JP, Robson MC. The bioreactivity of silicone. Critical reviews in biocompatibility 1987; 21:1125–1133.
102. Kossovsky N, et al. Ventricular shunt failure: evidence of immunologic sensitization. Surgical Forum 1983; 34:527.
103. Heggers JP, et al. Immunologic responses to silicone implants; Fact or fiction? Plast Surg Res Forum 1990; 13:13–18.
104. Reilly DA, Heggers JP, Goldblum RM, Pelley RP. Immuno-globulins binding to polydimethylsiloxane "Silastic" tubing in the serum of women with "Silicone Bag and Gel" mammary prostheses: Relationship of serology to clinical parameters and histopathology. Submitted to the Conference on Silicone in Med. Devices 12–7-90.
105. Application to AMGEN Corporation for study of granuloma histology and phenotyping Nov 2003.
106. Reisberger, Eva-Maria, Landthaler M, Wiest L, et al. Foreign body granulomas caused by polymethylmethacrylate microspheres. Arch Dermatol 2003; 139:17–20.
107. Kossovsky N, Heggers JP, et al. Acceleration of capsule formation around silicone implants by infection in a guinea pig model. Plast Reconstr Surg 1984; 73(1):91–96.
108. Virden CP, Dopke MK, Stein B, et al. Subclinical infection of the silicone breast implant surface as a possible cause of capsular contracture. Aesth Plast Surg 1992; 16:173–179.
109. Wells AF, Daniels S, Gunasekaran S, et al. Local increase in hyaluronic acid and Il-2 in the capsules surrounding silicone breast implants. Ann Plast Surg 1994; 33:1-5.
110. Wells AF, Daniels S, Wells KE, et al. Il-6 and multi-nucleated giant cells in capsular biopsies from patients with silicone breast implants [abstr]. Arthritis Rheum 1994; 37(suppl 9):S422.
111. FDA Medical Bulletin, Vol. 22, No. 2, Sept 1992, 3.

112. Duffy D. Presentation #AS 352. Silicone granulomas: causation and treatment. ASDS, New Orleans, October 11, 2003.
113. Duffy D. Complications of Fillers: An overview. J Derm Surg 2005:31. In press.
114. Webster GF, Toso SM, Hegemann L. Inhibition of a model of in vitro granuloma formation by tetracyclines and ciprofloxacin. Involvement of protein kinase C. Arch Dermatol 1994; 130(6):748–752.
115. Webster GF, Layden, Mussen, Douglas. Resistant Propioni Bacterium Acnes. Acne Pathogenesis Update on Therapy. Yale University/Fujisawa Healthcare Inc., Lectureship series in dermatology, 2002.
116. Webster G. Acne pathogenesis and update on therapy. Yale University/Fujisawa Healthcare, Inc. Lectureship series in dermatology 2002; Lecture 3.
117. Abbas A, Lichtman A, Pober J. Cellular and Molecular Immunology. 4th ed. W.B. Saunders Co., 2000.
118. Duffy D. Silicone granulomata management. Dermatol Times May 2003, 75–76.
119. Bachelez H, Senet P, Cadranel J, Kaoukhov A, Dubertret L. Observation: The use of Tetracyclines for the treatment of sarcoidosis. Arch Dermatol 2001; 37:69–73.
120. Du Y, Ma Z, Lin S, Dodel RC, Gao F, Bales KR, Triarhou LC, Chernet E, Perry KW, Nelson DLG, Luecke S, Phebus LA, Bymaster FP, Paul SM. Minocycline prevents nigrostriatal dopaminergic neurodegeneration in the MPTP model of Parkinson's disease. PNAS 2001; 98(25):14669–14674.
121. Baumann LS, Halem ML. Lip silicone granulomatous foreign body reaction treated with Aldara (Imiquimod 5%). Dermatol Surg 2003; 29:429–432.
122. Solis R, Diven D, Colome-Grimmer M, Snyder N, Wagner R, Jr. Experimental nonsurgical tattoo removal in a guinea pig model with topical imiquimod and tretinoin. Dermatol Surg 2002; 28:83–87.
123. English J, Patel P, Greer K. Sarcoidosis. J Am Acad Dermatol 44:725–743.
124. Achauer BM. A serious complication following medical grade silicone injection of the face. Plast Reconstr Surg 1983; 71:251–254.
125. Mastruserio DN, Pesqueira MJ, Cobb MW. Severe granulomatous reaction and facial ulceration occurring after subcutaneous silicone injection. J Am Acad Dermatol 1996; 34:849–852.
126. Hoffmann C, Schuller-Petrovic, Soyer HP, Kerl H. Adverse reactions after cosmetic lip augmentation with permanent biologically inert implant materials. J Am Acad Dermatol; 40(1):100–102.
127. Salmon-Her V, Serpier H, Nawrocki B, Gillery P, Clavel C, Kalis B, Birembaut P, Maquart FZ. Expression of Interleukin-4 in scleroderma skin specimens and scleroderma fibroblast cultures. Arch Dermatol 1996; 132:802–806.
128. Sapadin A, Fleischmajer R. Treatment of Scleroderma. Arch Dermatol 138:99–105.
129. Varga J. Recombinant cytokine treatment for scleroderma. Arch Dermatol 1997; 133:637–642.
130. Fisher AA. Reactions at silicone-injected sites on the face associated with silicone breast implant "Inflammation" or "Rejection." Curr Contact News 1990; 45:393–395.
131. Suzuki K, Aoki M, Kawana S, Hyakusoku H, Miyazawa S. Metastatic silicone granuloma: lupus miliaris disseminatus faciei-like facial nodules and sicca complex in a silicone breast implant recipient. Arch Dermatol 2002; 138.
132. Travis WD, Balogh K, Abraham JL. Silicone granulomas: Report of three cases and review of the literature. New England Deaconess Hospital, Path Dept., Boston, MA and Upstate Medical Center, Syracuse, NY, Jan 27, 1984.
133. Rudolph R, et al. Myofibroblasts and free silicone around breast implant. Plast Reconstr Surg 1978;62:195.
134. Cohen PR. Editorial. Granuloma annulare: a mucocutaneous condition in immunodeficiency virus affected patients. Arch Dermatol 135:1404–1407.

135. Urbatsch A, Frieden I, Williams ML, Elewski BE, Mancini AJ, Paller AS. Extrafascial and generalized granulomatous periorificial dermatitis. Arch Dermatol 2002; 138:1354–1358.

136. Dohil M, Prendiville JS, Crawford RI, Cutaneous manifestations of chronic granulomatous disease. J Am Acad Dermatol 36(6):899–907.

137. Rogers R. Granulomatous cheilitis, Melkersson-Rosenthal syndrome and orofacial granulomatosis. Arch Dermatol 2000; 136:1557–1558.

138. Guttman-Yassky E, Weltfiend S, Bergman R. Resolution of orofacial granulomatosis with amalgam removal. J Euro Acad Dermatol Venereol 2003; 17(3):344–347.

139. Andre P. Filler Complications. Dermatol times 2003; 24(10):51.

140. Blanchard M. Filler material may cause nodules, lumps in lips. Cosmet Surg Times 2002; 5:20–21.

141. Duke D, Urioste S, Dover J, Anderson R. A reaction to red lip cosmetic tattoo. J Am Acad Dermatol 1998; 39(3):488–490.

142. Rudolph CM, Mullegger RR, Schuller-Petrovic S, Kerl H, Soyer HP. Unusual herpes simplex virus infection mimicking foreign body reaction after cosmetic lip augmentation with expanded polytetrafluoroethylene threads. Dermatol Surg 2003; 29:195–197.

143. Mang WL, Sawatzki K. Complications after implantation of PMMA (polymethylmethacrylate) for soft tissue augmentation. Zeitschrift Fur Hautkrankheiten 1998; 73:42–44.

144. Fernandez-Acenero MJ, Zamora E, Borbujo J. Granulomatous foreign body reaction against hyaluronic acid: Report of a case after lip augmentation. Dermatol Surg 2003; 29:1225–1225.

145. Callen J. Editorial. The presence of foreign bodies does not exclude the diagnosis of sarcoidosis. Arch Dermatol 2001; 137:485–486.

146. Marcoval J, et al. Foreign bodies in granulomatous cutaneous lesions of patients with systemic sarcoidosis. Arch Derm/2001; 137:427–430.

147. Kim YC, Triffet MK, Gibson LE. Foreign bodies in sarcoidosis. Am J Dermatopath 2000; 22(5):408–412.

148. Marcoval J, Mana J, Moreno A, Gallego I, FortunoY, Peyri J. Foreign bodies in granulomatous cutaneous lesions of patients with sarcoidosis. Arch Dermatol 2001;137:427–430.

149. Zimmerli W, Waldvogel A, Vandaux P, et al. Pathogenesis of foreign body infections: Description and characteristics of an animal model. J Infect Dis 1982; 146:487–497.

150. Katoh N, Mihara H, Yasuno H. Sarcoidosis is a disorder characterized by macrophage and T-cell mediated responses to as yet unidentified infectious antigens or autoantigens. Washington whispers. J Drugs Dermatol 2002; 3:340–351.

151. Gregg P, Kantor GR, Telang GH, LLessin SR, Nowell PC, Vonderheid EC. Sarcoidal tissue reaction in Sézary syndrome. J Am Acad Dermatol 2002; 43(2):372–374.

152. Narasimhan P, Arora A, Hitti I, Glasberg S, Kanzer B. Rapidly progressive fatal cutaneous T-cell lymphoma with a trauma related presentation. Cutis 2000; 66:195–196.

153. Chu P, Connolly MK, LeBoid PE. The histopathologic spectrum of palisaded neutrophilic and granulomatous dermatitis in patients with collagen vascular disease [abstr]. Arch Dermatol 1994; 130(10):1278–1283.

154. Reiser H, Stadecker MJ. Costimulatory B7 Molecules in the pathogenesis of infectious and autoimmune diseases. N Engl J Med 1996; 335(18):1369–1377.

155. Magro CM, Crowson AN, Schapiro BL. The interstitial granulomatous drug reaction: A distinctive clinical and pathological entity. J Cutan Pathol 1998; 25(2):72–78.

156. Lupton JR, et al. Can granuloma annulare evolve into cutaneous sarcoidosis? Cutis 2000; 66:390–392.

157. Herbst R, Hoch O, Kapp A, Weiss J. Guttate psoriasis triggered by perianal streptococcal dermatitis in a four-year-old boy. J Am Acad Dermatol 2000; 42(5):885–887.

158. Robert C, Kupper T. Inflammatory skin diseases, T cells, and immune surveillance. N Eng J Med 1999; 341(24):1817–1828.

159. Toro J, Chu P, Ben Yen TS, LeBoid PE. Granuloma Annulare and Human Immunodeficiency Virus Infection. Arch Dermatol 1999; 135:1341–1346.

160. Weiss J, Muchenberger S, Schopf E, Simon JC. Treatment of granuloma annulare by local injections with low-dose recombinant human interferon gamma. J Am Acad Dermatol 39(1):117–119.

161. Viravan S, Wisnthsarewong W, Manonulcul J. Successful treatment of cytophagic histiocytic panniculitis by cyclosporine A: a case report. Asian Pac J Allergy. Immunol 1997; 15(3):161–166.

162. Phelps RG, Shoji T. Update on panniculitis. Mt Sinai J Med 2001; 68:262–267.

163. Wick MR, Patterson JW. Cytophagic histiocytic panniculitis—a critical reappraisal. Arch Dermatol 2000; 136:922–924.

164. White JW, Winkelmann RK. Weber-Christian panniculitis: a review of 30 cases with this diagnosis. J Am Acad Dermatol 1998; 39:56–62.

165. Enk AH, Knop J. Treatment of relapsing idiopathic nodular panniculitis (Pfeifer-Weber-Christian disease) with mycophenolate mofetil. J Am Acad Dermatol 1998; 39:508–509.

166. Levy ML, Lifshitz O. Weber-Christian Disease. http://www.emedicine.com.

167. Chastre J, et al. Acute pneumonitis after subcutaneous injections of silicone in transsexual men. N Eng J Med 1983; 308:764–767.

168. Gabriel SE, D'Fallon WM, Kurtland LT, et al. Risk of connective tissue diseases and other disorders after breast implantation. N Eng J Med 1994; 330(24):1697–1702.

169. Baldwin CM, Kaplan EN. Silicone-induced human adjuvant disease. Ann Plast Surg 1983; 10:270–273.

170. Okana Y, Nishikai M, Sato A. Scleroderma, primary cirrhosis and Sjögren's syndrome after cosmetic breast augmentation with silicone injection: A case report of possible human adjuvant. Ann Rheum Dis 1984; 43:520–522.

171. Fock FM, Feng PH, Tey BH. Autoimmune disease developing after augmentation mammoplasty: report of three cases. J Rheumatol 1984; 11:98–100.

172. Houpt KR, Sontheimer RD. Autoimmune connection tissue disease and connective tissue disease-like illnesses after silicone gel augmentation mammoplasty. J Am Acad Dermatol 1994; 3(4):626–642.

173. Kumagai Y, Shiokawa Y, Medsger TA Jr, Rodnan GP. Clinical spectrum of connective tissue diseases after cosmetic surgery. Arthritis Rheum 1984; 27:1-12.

174. Sergott TJ, Limoli MD, Baldwin CM, Laub DR. Human adjuvant disease, possible autoimmune disease after silicone implantation: a review of the literature, case studies, and speculation for the future. Plast Reconstr Surg 1986; 78:104–114.

175. Kumagai Y, Abe C, Shiokawa Y. Scleroderma after cosmetic surgery; four cases of human adjuvant disease. Arthritis Rheum 1979; 22:532–537.

176. Miyoshi K, Shiragami H, Yoshida K. Adjuvant disease of man. Clin Immunol 1973; 5:785–794.

177. Alcalay J, Alcalay R, Gat A, Yorav S. Late-onset granulomatous reaction to Artecoll. Dermatol Surg 2003; 29:859–862.

178. Hanke CW. Adverse reactions to bovine collagen. In: Klein A, ed. Augmentation in Clinical Practice: Procedures and Techniques. New York: Marcel Dekker, 1998:147.

179. Schwarze H, Giordano-Labadie F, Loche F, Gorguet B, Bazex J. Delayed-hypersensitivity granulomatous reaction induced by blepharopigmentation with aluminum-silicate. J Am Acad Dermatol 2000; 42(5):888–891.

180. Stegman SJ, et al. Adverse reactions to bovine collagen implant: clinical and histologic features. J Dermatol Surg Oncol 1988; 14(suppl 1):39–48.

181. Ruiz-Esparza J, et al. Necrobiotic granulomas formation at a collagen implant treatment site. Cleve Clin Q 1983; 50:163–165.

182. Barr RJ, et al. Necrobiotic granulomas associated with bovine collagen test site injections. J Am Acad Dermatol 1982; 6:867–869.

183. Barr RJ, Stegman SJ. Delayed skin test reaction to injectable collagen implant (Zyderm). J Am Acad Dermatol 1984; 10:652–658.

184. Brooks NA. Foreign body granuloma produced by an injectable collagen implant at a test site. J Dermatol Surg Oncol 1982; 8:111–114.

185. Feldmann R, Harms M, Chavaz P, Salomon D, Saurat JH. Orbital and palpebral paraffinoma. J Am Acad Dermatol 1992; 26:833–835.

186. Cohen J, et al. Penile paraffinoma: self-injection with mineral oil. J Am Acad Dermatol 2001; 45:S222–224.

187. Sharma O, Maheshwari A. Lung diseases in the tropics. Part 1: Tropical granulomatous disorders of the lung: Diagnosis and management. Tuber Lung Disease: 1993; 74(5):295–304.

188. Darsow U, Bruckbauer H, Worret WI, Hofmann H, Ring J. Subcutaneous oleomas induced by self-injection of sesame seed oil for muscle augmentation. J Am Acad Dermatol 42(2):292–294.

189. Alani R, Busam K. Acupuncture granulomas. J Am Acad Dermatol 2001; 45:S225–226.

190. Jacob CI. Tattoo-associated dermatoses: a case report and review of the literature. Dermatol Surg 2002; 28:962–965.

191. Tope WD, Arbiser JL, Duncan LM. Black tattoo reaction: the peacock's tale. J Am Acad Dermatol 1996; 35(3):477–479.

192. Brancaccio R, Zappi G. Delayed type hypersensitivity to intralesional triamcinolone Acetonide. Cutis 2000; 65:31–33.

193. Tomasini C, Pippione M. Interstitial granulomatous dermatitis with plaques. J Am Acad Dermatol 46(6):892–899.

194. Kanathur N, Byrd RP, Fields CL, Roy TM. Non-caseating granulomatous disease in common variable immunoefficiency Granulomatous disease (CVID). South Med J 1993; 93(6):631–633.

195. Verneuil L, Dompmartin A, Comoz F, Pasquier CJ, Leroy D. Interstitial granulomatous dermatitis with cutaneous cords and arthritis: a disorder associated with autoantibodies. J Am Acad Dermatol 2001; 45:286–291.

196. O'Brien J, Regan W. Actinically degenerate elastic tissue is the likely antigenic basis of actinic granuloma of the skin and of temporal arteritis. J Am Acad Dermatol 1999; 40(2):214–222.

197. Skin granulomas. http://www.thedoctorsdoctor.com/diseases/skin_granuloma.

198. Granel B, Serratrice J, Rey J, Bouvie CR, Weiller-Merli C, Disdier P, Pellissier JF, Weiller PJ. Chronic hepatitis C virus infection associated with a generalized granuloma annulare. J Am Acad Dermatol 2000; 43:918–919.

199. Wakefield D, Kumar RK. Inflammation: Chronic. Encyclopedia of Life Sciences. 2001. Nature publishing Group/www.els.net.

200. Kunkel SL, Chensue SW, Strieter RM, Lynch JP, Remick DG. Cellular and molecular aspects of granulomatous inflammation. Am J Respir Cell Mol Biol 1989; 1(6):439–447.

201. Karrer S, Abels C, Wimmershoff MB, Landthaler M, Szeimies RM. Successful treatment of cutaneous sarcoidosis using topical photodynamic therapy. Arch Dermatol 2002; 138:581–584.

202. Wood GS. Management of cutaneous T-cell lymphoma: the future is here. J Am Acad Dermatol 2001; 45:317.

203. Payne D, Straten MV, Carrasco D, Tyring SK. Molecular diagnosis of skin-associated infectious agents. Arch Dermatol 2001; 137:1497–1502.

204. Wood G. T-cell receptor and immunoglobulin gene rearrangements in diagnosing skin disease. Arch Dermatol 2001; 137:1503–1506.

205. Schach C, Smoller BR, Hudson AR, Horn TD. Immunohistochemical stains in dermatopathology. J Am Acad Dermatol 43(6):1092–1100.

206. Abbodenzo SL, Young VL, Wei MQ, Miller FW. Silicone gel-filled breast and testicular implant capsules: A histologic and immunophenotypic study. Mod Pathol 1999; 22(7):706–713.

207. Wells AF, Daniels S, Wells KE, et al. Il-6 and multi-nucleated giant cells in capsular biopsies from patients with silicone breast implants [abstr]. Arthritis Rheum 1994; 37(suppl 9):S422.

208. Katzin WE, Feng LJ, Abbuhl M, Klein MA. Phenotype of lymphocytes associated with the inflammatory reaction to silicone gel breast implants. Clin Diagn Lab Immunol 1996; 3(2):156–161.

209. Wyler DJ. Schistosomes, fibroblasts, and growth factors: how a worm causes liver scarring. New Biol 1991; 3(8):734–740.

210. Yamamoto T. Animal model of sclerotic skin induced by bleomycin: a clue to the pathogenesis of and therapy for scleroderma. Clin Immunol 2002; 102:209–216.

211. Stege H, Bemeburg M, Humke S, Klammer M, Grewe M, Grether-Beck S, Boedeker R, Diepgen T, Dierks K, Goerz G, Ruzicka T, Krutmann J. High-dose UVA$_1$ radiation therapy for localized scleroderma. J Am Acad Dermatol 36(6):938–944.

212. Gristina AG. Particle-induced in vivo priming of alveolar macrophages for enhance oxidative response: a novel system of cellular immune augmentation. J Leukoc Biol 1993; 54:439–443.

213. Gristina AG. Biomaterial-centered infection: microbial adhesion versus tissue integration. Science 237:1588–1595.

214. Naylor P, Jennings R, Myrvik Q, Webb L, Gristing A. Antibiotic sensitivity of biomaterial-adherent staphylococcus epidermidis. Orthop Trans 1988; 12:524–525.

215. Nichols WW, Evans JJ, Slack MPE, et al. The penetration of antibiotics into aggregates of mucoid and non-mucoid Pseudomona Aeruginosa. J Gen Microbiol 1989; 135:1291–1301.

216. Gristina AG, Jennings RA, Naylor PT, et al. Comparative in vitro antibiotic resistance of surface colonizing coagulase-negative staphylococci. Antimicrob Agents Chemother 1989; 33:813–816.

217. Gristina AG. Implant failure and the immunoincompetent fibro-inflammatory zone. Clin Orthop Relat Res 1994; 298:106–118.

218. Gristina AG. Simple technique for the preparation of silicone gel particles: The effect of silicone gel particles on oxidative responses of macrophages. J Biomed Mater Res 1995; 29:101–105.

219. Gristina AG, Giridhar BL, Naylor PT, Nyrvik, QN. Cell biology and molecular mechanisms in artificial device infections. J Artif Organs 1993; 16:755–764.

220. Gristina AG, Naylor PT, Myrvik QN. Mechanisms of musculoskeletal sepsis. Orthop Clin North Am 1991; 22(3).

221. Gristina AG, Webb LX, Barth E. Microbial adhesion, biomaterials and man. In: Coombs R, Fitzgerald R, eds. Infection in the Orthopaedic Patient. 30. London: Butterworths, 1989.

222. Anderson GG, Palermo JJ, Schilling JD, Roth R, Heuser J, Hultgren SJ. Intracellular bacterial biofilm-like pods in urinary tract infections. Science 2003; 301:105–107.

223. Nichols WW, Dorrington SM, Slack MPE, et al. Inhibition of tobramycin diffusion by binding to alginate. Antimicrob Agents Chemother 1988; 32:518–523.

224. Gorman J. Getting out the thorn: biomaterials become friendlier to the body. Sci News 2002; 161:13–14.

225. Portera C. Forging a link between biofilms and disease. Sci Mag 1999; 283(5409):1837–1839.

226. Netting J. Sticky situations. Sci News 2001; 160(2):28.

227. Davies DG, Parsek MR, Pearson JP, Iglewski BH, Costerton JW, Greenberg EP. The involvement of cell-to-cell signals in the development of a bacterial biofilm. Sci Mag 1998; 280:295–297.

228. Sanders S, Busam K, Tahan ST, Johnson RA, Sachs D. Granulomatous and suppurative dermatitis at interferon alfa injection sites: report of 2 cases. J Am Acad Dermatol 46(4):611–616.

229. Skin Therapy Letter 1999; 4(2).

230. Sauder DN. Br J Dermatol 2003; 149(suppl 66).

231. Skin Granulomas. http://www.thedoctorsdoctor.com/diseases/skin_granuloma.

232. Lee J, Koblenzer P. Disfiguring cutaneous manifestations of sarcoidosis treated with thalidomide: A case report. J Am Acad Dermatol 1998; 39(5):835–838.

233. Zuckerman SH, Ahmari SE, Bryan-Poole N, Evans GF, Short L Glasebrook AL. Estriol: A potent regulator of TNF and IL-6 expression in a murine model of endotoxemia. Inflammation 1996; 20(6):581–597.

234. Benedict CA, Ware CF. Virus targeting of the tumor necrosis factor superfamily. Virology 2001; 298(1):1–5.

235. Cvancara J, Meffert JJ, Elston DM. Estrogen-sensitive cutaneous polyarteritis nodosa: Response to tamoxifen. J Am Acad Dermatol 1998; 39(4):643–646.

236. Weinberg J, Saini R, Tutrone WD. Biologic therapy for psoriasis—the first wave: Infliximab, Etanercept, efalizumab, and alefacept. J Drugs Dermatol 2002; 3:303–310.

237. Wolf R, Matz H, Orion E, Ruocco V. Anti-TNF therapies—The hope of tomorrow. Clin Dermatol 2002; 20:522–530.

238. Wakefield PE, et al. Tumor necrosis factor. J Am Acad Dermatol 1991; 24(5):675–685.

239. Toro JR, Aksentijevich I, Hull K, Dean J, Kastner DL. Tumor necrosis factor receptor-associated periodic syndrome: a novel syndrome with cutaneous manifestations. Arch Dermatol 2000; 136(12):1487–1494.

240. Van der Laan N, de Leij LFMH, Buurman W, Timens W, ten Duis HJ. Tumor necrosis factor alpha (TNF-alpha) in human skin: a comparison of different antibodies for immunohistochemistry. Arch Dermatol Res 2001; 293(5):226–232.

241. Creaven PJ, Stoll HL Jr. Response to tumor necrosis factor in two cases of psoriasis. J Am Acad Dermatol 1991; 24(5):735–737.

242. Dayer JM, Krane S. Anti–TNF-α therapy for ankylosing spondylitis—A specific or nonspecific treatment? N Engl J Med 2002; 346:1399–1400.

243. Gorman J, Sack K, Davis J. Treatment of ankylosing spondylitis by inhibition of tumor necrosis factor α. N Engl J Med 346(18):1349–1356.

244. Mease PJ, Goffe BS, Mets J, Vanderstoep A, Finck B, Burge DJ. Anti-tumor necrosis factor α therapy in psoriatic arthritis and psoriasis. Arch Dermatol 2001; 137:784–785.

245. Muller H. Tumor necrosis factor as an antineoplastic agent: pitfalls and promises. Cell Mol Life Sci 1998; 54(12):1291–1298.

246. Oh C, Das KM, Gottlieb AB. Treatment with anti-tumor necrosis factor alpha (TNF-α) monoclonal antibody dramatically decreases the clinical activity of psoriasis lesions. J Am Acad Dermatol 2000; 42:829–830.

247. Voigtlander C, Lüftl M, Schuler G, Hertl M. Infliximab (Anti-tumor necrosis factor α antibody). Arch Dermatol 2001; 137:1571–1574.

248. Schopf RE, Aust H, Knop J. Treatment of psoriasis with the chimeric monoclonal antibody against tumor necrosis factor alpha, infliximab. J Am Acad Dermatol 2002; 46(6):886–891.

249. Yee A, Pochapin M. Treatment of complicated sarcoidosis with Infliximab anti-tumor necrosis factor-alpha therapy. Ann Intern Med 2001; 135(1):27–31.

250. Gottlieb A, Masud S, Ramamurthi R, Abdulghani A, Romano P, Chaudhari U, Dooley L, Fasanmade A, Wagner C. Pharmacodynamic and pharmacokinetic response to anti-tumor necrosis factor-α monoclonal antibody (infliximab) treatment of moderate to severe psoriasis vulgaris. J Am Acad Dermatol 2003; 48:68–75.

251. Drexler AM. Tumor necrosis factor: Its role in HIV/AIDS. Seattle Treatment Education Project (STEP) Perspective, Vol. 7, No. 1- Spring 1995. www.Aegis.com/pubs/step/1995/STEP7107.html/.

252. O'Quinn RP, Miller JL. The effectiveness of tumor necrosis factor α antibody (Infliximab) in treating recalcitrant psoriasis. Arch Dermatol 2002; 138:644–648.

253. Callen JP. Tumor necrosis factor antagonists associated with heart failure. Journal Watch – Dermatology. Sponsored by Medicis. Published by the Massachusetts Medical Society. July 2003, 56.

254. Hassard PB, Binder SW, Nelson V, Vasiliauskas EA. Anti-tumor necrosis factor monoclonal antibody therapy for gastrointestinal behcet's disease: A case report. Gastroenterology 2001; 120:995–999.

255. Fleisher MR, Fulmer J, Barwick K, Etzkorn K, Turner RJ, Hopkins K. A case report: Infliximab in the treatment of Behcet's syndrome. Am Col of Gastroenterol 66th Annual Scientific Meeting. Poster #P198, Oct 22, 2001.

256. Bertken R. Behcet disease associated with severe gastroparesis: A dramatic response to combination therapy with methotrexate and infliximab. Am Col of Rheum. 65th Annual Scientific meeting, San Francisco, CA, Nov 10–15, 2001.

257. Sfikakis PP, Theodossiadis PG, Katsiari CG, Kaklamanis P, Markomichelakis NN. Effect of infliximab on sight-threatening panuveitis in Behcet's disease. Lancet 2001; 358:295–296.

258. Travis SPL, Czajkowski M, McGovern DPB, Watson RGP, Bell AL. Treatment of intestinal Behcet's syndrome with chimeric tumour necrosis factor α antibody. Gut 2001; 49:725–728.

259. Baughman RP, Lower EE. Infliximab for refractory sarcoidosis. Sarcoidosis Vasc Diffuse Lung Dis 2001; 18:70–74.

260. Oliver SJ, Kikuchi T, Krueger JG. Thalidomide induces granuloma differentiation in sarcoid skin lesions associated with disease improvement. Clin Immunol 2002; 102:225–236.

261. Mavroleon G. Restoration of cytokine imbalance by immunotherapy. Clin Exp Allergy 1998; (28):917–920.

262. Rousseau L, Beylot-Barry M, Doutre MS, Beylot C. Cutaneous sarcoidosis successfully treated with low doses of Thalidomide. Arch Dermatol 1998; 134:1045–1046.

263. Bahl S, Mutasim F. How to use Thalidomide in your practice. Skin and Aging 2000; 41–45.

264. Camisa C, Popovsky JL. Effective treatment of oral erosive lichen planus with Thalidomide. Arch Dermatol 2000; 136:1442–1443.

265. George S, Hsu S. Lichen planopilaris treated with thalidomide. Letters. J Am Acad Dermatol 2001; 965–966.

266. Clinical trial review. Thalidomide and Interferon alpha in treating patients with mycosis fungoides. J Drugs Dermatol 2002; 2:235–245.

267. Hwu WJ, et al. Temozolomide plus thalidomide has antitumor activity in patients with advanced melanoma. J Clin Onc 2002; 20(11):2610–2615.

268. Singhal S, Mehta J, Desikan R, Ayers D, Roberson P, Eddlemon P, Munshi N, Anaissie E, Wilson C, Dhodapkar M, Zeldis J, Barlogie B. Antitumor activity of thalidomide in refractory multiple myeloma. N Engl J Med 341:1565–1571.

269. Tan MH, Gordon M, Lebwohl O, George J, Lebowhl MG. Improvement of pyoderma gangrenosum and psoriasis associated with necrosis factor α monoclonal antibody. Arch Dermatol 2001; 137:930–933.

270. Jo M, et al. Apoptosis induced in normal human hepatocytes by tumor necrosis factor-related apoptosis-inducing ligand. Nat Med 2000; 6(5):564–567.

271. Cruz P. Ed. Biologic agents—new hope for psoriasis. Dermatology Focus 20(4):1–7.

272. Wilson F. Psoriasis Tx quartet—TNF-alpha inhibitors Etanercept, infliximab two of four drugs signaling new era of treatment. Derm Times 2002; 16–18.

273. Werth V, Levinson A. Etanercept-induced injection site reactions—Mechanistic insights from clinical findings and immunohistochemistry. Editorial. Arch Dermatol 2001; 137:953–955.

274. Asnis L, Gaspari AA. Cutaneous reactions to recombinant cytokine therapy. CME. J Am Acad Dermatol 33(3):393–412.

275. Gottlieb A. Psoriasis: Immunopathology and immunomodulation. Derm Clinics 2001; 19(4):649–657.

276. Correia O, Delgado L, Roujeau JC, Le Cleach L, Fleming-Torrinha JA. Soluble Interleukin 2 receptor and Interleukin 1alpha in toxic epidermal necrolysis. Arch Dermatol 2002; 138:29–32.

277. Krueger, J. The immunologic basis for the treatment of psoriasis with new biologic agents. J Am Acad Dermatol; 46(1):1–23.

278. Geyer AS, Anhalt GJ, Nousari HC. Effectiveness of Infliximab in the treatment of refractory perineal cutaneous Crohn's disease. Arch Dermatol 136:459–460.

279. Lorincz A. Dermatology and the evolution of therapies to control inflammatory tissue injury. Arch Dermatol 130:781–782.

280. Miyachi Y. Pharmacologic modulation of neutrophil functions. Clin Dermatol 2000; 18:369–373.

281. Victor F, Gottlieb A. TNF-α and apoptosis: implications for the pathogenesis and treatment of psoriasis. J Drugs Dermatol 2002; 3:264–275.

282. Turtone W, Kagen MH, Barbagallo J, Weinberg JM. Biologic therapy for psoriasis: a brief history, II. Cutis 2001; 68:367–372.

283. Koo J, Khann D, Nguyen K. The new biological fight against psoriasis. Skin and Aging 2001.

284. Lebwohl M. New developments in the treatment of psoriasis. Arch Dermatol 2002; 138:686–688.

285. Greaves MW. The immunopharmacology of skin inflammation: the future is already here! Br J Dermatol 2000; 143:47–52.

286. Najarian DJ, Gottlieb AB. Connections between psoriasis and Crohn's disease. J Am Acad Dermatol 2003; 48:805–821.

287. Walsh N. Granulomatous infection reports were higher for infliximab than Etanercept. Skin and Allergy News 2003; 34(9).

288. Robinson ND, Guitart J. Recalcitrant, recurrent aphthous stomatitis treated with Etanercept. Arch Dermatol 2003; 139:1259–1262.

289. Edwards KR, Mowad CM, Tyler WB. Worsening injection site reactions with continued use of Etanercept. J Drugs Dermatol 2003; 2:184–187.

290. Victor FC, Gottlieb AB, Menter A. Changing paradigms in dermatology: tumor necrosis factor alpha (TNF-α) blockade in psoriasis and psoriatic arthritis. Clin Dermatol 2003; 21:392–397.

291. De Rycke L, Elli Kruithof, Nancy Van Damme, Ilse E.A. Hoffman, Nancy Van den Bossche, Filip Van Den Bosch, Eric M. Veges, Filip De Keyser. Antinuclear antibodies following infliximab treatment in patients with rheumatoid arthritis or spondylarthropathy. 2003; 48:1015–1023.

292. Simpson S, Marshall E. Immune control, memory, and vaccines. Science 2001; 293:233–245.

293. DePrisco G, Bandel C, Cockerell CJ, Ehrig T. Interstitial heparan sulfate in granulomatous inflammatory skin diseases. J Am Acad Dermatol 2004; 50:253–257.

294. www.Biologictherapy.org. Functions of TH1 and TH2 Cytokines, Oct 2002.

295. von Andrian U, Engelhardt B. α₄Integrins as therapeutic targets in autoimmune disease. N Engl J Med 348(1):68–72.

296. Ghosh S, Goldin E, Gordon FH, Malchow HA, Rask-Madsen J, Rutgeerts P, Vyhnalek P, Zadorvoa Z, Palmer T, Donoghue S. Natalizumab for active Crohn's disease. N Engl J Med 348(1):24–32.

297. Shetty A, Gedalia A. Sarcoidosis. eMedicine (www.emedicine.com) Journal Oct 31, 2001, Vol. 2, No. 10.

298. Suchin K, et al. Treatment of cutaneous T-cell lymphoma with combined immunomodulatory therapy. Arch Dermatol 2002; 138;1054–1060.

299. Ellis CN, Krueger GG. Treatment of chronic plaque psoriasis by selective targeting of memory effector T lymphocytes. N Engl J Med 2001; 345:248–255.

300. Guitart J, et al. Long-term remission after allogenic hematopoietic stem cell transplantation for refractory cutaneous T-cell lymphoma. Arch Dermatol Bol 2002; 138:1339–1364.

301. Guitart J, Carnisa C, Ehrlich M, Bergfeld WF. Long-term implications of T-cell receptor gene rearrangement analysis by southern blot in patients with cutaneous T-cell lymphoma. J Am Acad Dermatol 2003; 48:775–779.

302. Sprent J, Tough D. T cell death and memory. Science 2001; 293:245–250.

303. SydPath Internet. St. Vincents. Angiotensin converting enzyme (ACE), May 2002.

304. Nguyen YT, Dupuy A, Cordoliani F, Vignon-Pennamen MD, Lebbe C, Morel P, Rybojad M. Treatment of cutaneous sarcoidosis with thalidomide. J Am Acad Dermatol 2004; 50:235–241.

305. Mallbris L, Ljungberg A, Hedblad MA, Larsson P, Stahle-Backdahl M. Progressive cutaneous sarcoidosis responding to anti-tumor necrosis factor-α therapy. J Am Acad Dermatol 2003; 48:290–293.

306. Lebwohl M, Ali S. Treatment of psoriasis. Part 2. Systemic therapies. J Am Acad Dermatol 2001; 45:649–661.

307. Asadullah K, et al. Interleukin 10 treatment of psoriasis. Arch Dermatol 1999; 135:187–192.

308. Zeltser R, Valle L, Tanck C, Holyst MM, Ritchlin C, Gaspari AA. Clinical, histological, and immunophenotypic characteristics of injection site reactions associated with Entanercept. Arch Dermatol 2001; 137:893–899.

309. Termeer C, et al. Low-dose interferon alpha-2b for the treatment of Churg-Strauss syndrome with prominent skin involvement. Arch Dermatol 2001; 137:136–138.

310. Gupta AK, Browne M, Bluhm R. Imiquimod: a review. J Cutan Med Surg 2002:554–560.

311. Schwarz R. A Molecular star in the wars against cancer. N Engl J Med 347(7):462–463.

312. Skinner RB, Theirs BH. Consulting Ed. Imiquimod. Dermatol Clin 2003; 21:291–300.

313. Lambert WC. Imiquimod and the treatment of cutaneous T-cell proliferative diseases: at the threshold Ph.D. Commentary. SKINmed 2003; 5:273–274.

314. Do JH, McLaughlin S, Gaspari AA. Case studies: Topical imiquimod therapy for cutaneous T-cell lymphoma. SKINmed 2003; 5:316–318.

315. Hurwitz DJ, Pincus L, Kupper TS. Imiquimod: a topically applied link between innate and acquired immunity. Arch Dermatol 2003; 139:1347–1350.

316. Urosevic M, Maier T, Benninghoff B, Slade H, Burg G, Dummer R. Mechanisms underlying Imiquimod-induced regression of basal cell carcinoma in vivo. Arch Dermatol 2003; 139:1325–1332.

317. Sauder DN. Imiquimod: Modes of action. Br J Dermatol 2003; 149(suppl 66):5–8.

318. Sullivan TP, Dearaujo T, Vincek V, Berman B. Evaluation of superficial basal cell carcinomas after treatment with Imiquimod 5% cream or vehicle for apoptosis and lymphocyte phenotyping. Dermatol Surg 2003; 29:1181–1186.

319. Schwarz T. Skin immunity. Br J Dermatol 2003; 149(suppl 66):2–4.

320. Derk M, Elston MC. Tx of granuloma faciale with a pulsed-dye laser. Cutis 2007; 65:97.

321. Green J. Vignettes: generalized ulcerative sarcoidosis induced by therapy with the flashlamp-pumped pulsed dye laser. Arch Dermatol 2001; 137:507–508.

322. Baran R. Pyogenic granuloma-like lesions associated with topical retinoid therapy. J Am Acad Dermatol 2002; 47(6):970.

323. Voelter-Mahlknecht S, Benez A, Metzger S, Fierlbeck G. Treatment of subcutaneous sarcoidosis with Allopurinol. Arch Dermatol 1999; 135:1560–1561.

324. Becker D, Enk A, Bräuninger W, Knop J. Allopurinol-induced generalized granuloma annulare. Der Hautarzt 1994; 46(5):343–345. ISSN:1432–1173 (electronic version).

325. http://www.ucmp.berkeley.edu/history/leeuwenhoek.html Antony van Leeuwenhoek (1632–1723).

326.　Zinkernagel R, Hengartner H. Regulation of the immune response by antigen. Science 2001; 293:251–253.

327.　Pulendran B, et al. Sensing pathogens and tuning immune responses. Science 2001; 293:253–256.

328.　Simpson S, Marshall E. Immune control, memory, and vaccines. Science 2001; 293:233–245.

329.　Ray, LB, Gough N. Orienteering strategies for a signaling maze. Science 296:1632–1633.

330.　Nelson J. A call to arms: The cytokine selection service. Science STKE 17 July, 2001. www.stke.org/cgi/content/full/OC_sigtrans:2001/91/pe2.

331.　Germain R. The art of the probable: system control in the adaptive immune system. Science 293:240–250.

332.　Schwartzberg P. Tampering with the immune system. Science 293:228–229.

333.　Johnson G, Lapadat R. Mitogen-activated protein kinase pathways mediated by ERK, JNK, and p38 protein kinases. Science 2002; 298:1911–1934.

334.　Chin GJ. Remembrance of T-shirts past; Editors' choice. Science Magazine, March 2003, p. 299.

335.　Ray LB, Adler EM, Gough NR. Building a case for signaling. Science 2003; 300:1523.

336.　Travis J. Taking a Toll: antiviral drugs activate immune system. Science News 2002; 161:84–85.

337.　Kiechl, S, Lorenz E, Reindl M, Wiedermann CJ, Oberhollenzer F, Bonora E, Willeit J, Schwartz DA. Toll-like receptor 4 polymorphisms and atherogenesis. N Engl J Med 2002; 347(3):185–192.

338.　Travis, J. Biologists reveal the proteins that first see dangerous microbes. Science News 2001; 160(10).

339.　Guttmann C. TLRs linked to origin of inflammatory acne. Dermatol Times 2002; S13.

340.　Aderem A, Ulevitch RJ. Toll-like receptors in the induction of the innate immune response. Nature 2000; 406:782–787.

341.　Jones DA. Exploring inflammation throughout acne vulgaris. Face to face monograph UCSF 2002.

342.　Meyer T, Nindl I, Schmook T, Ulrich C, Sterry W, Stockfleth E. Induction of apoptosis by Toll-like receptor-7 agonist in tissue cultures. Br J Dermatol 2003; 149(suppl 66):9–13.

343.　Travis J. Immune cells carry concealed weapons. Of Note; biology. Science News 2002; 161:237.

344.　Glurich I, Grossi S, Albini B, Ho A, Shah R, Zeid M, Baumann H, Cenco RJ, De Nardin E. Systemic inflammation in cardiovascular and periodontal disease: comparative study. Clin Diagn Lab Immunol 2002:425–432.

345.　www.intelihealth.com. "Aspirin to be tested in cancer fight". Aug 13, 2003. Associated Press.

346.　http://12.42.224.152/healthNews/reuters/NewsStroy0407200310. Common painkillers may help treat Parkinson's.

347.　Kimball AL, Kawamura T, Tejura K, Boss C, Hancox AR, Vogel JC, Steinberg SM, Turner Ml, Blauvelt A. Clinical and immunologic assessment of patients with psoriasis in a randomized, double-blind, placebo-controlled trial using recombinant human Interleukin 10. Arch Dermatol Bol 138.

348.　Biologic Agents: new hope for psoriasis. Dermatol Focus 2001; 220(4).

349.　Shapiro M, Rook AH, Lehrer MS, Junkins-Hopkins JM, French LE, Vittorio C. Novel multimodality biologic response modifier therapy, including bexarotene and long-wave ultraviolet A for a patient with refractory stage IVa cutaneous T-cell lymphoma. J Am Acad Dermatol 2002; 47:956–961.

350.　Mossmann TR, Coffman R. Th1 and Th2 cells: Different patterns of lymphokine secretion lead to different functional properties. Ann Rev Immunol 1987; 7:145–173.

351. Wood GS. Management of cutaneous T-cell lymphoma: The future is here. J Am Acad Dermatol 2001; 45:317.

352. Burzynski Research Inst. Clinical Trial Review. Phase II study of Roferon (interferon alpha) and Accutane for patients with T-cell malignancies. J Drugs Dermatol 2002; 2:235–245.

353. Stein R. Inflammation may spur diseases. Washington Post, Feb 18, 2003. www.msnbc.com/news/873592.asp?0cl=cR.

354. Morinobu A, Kumagai S. Cytokine measurement at a single-cell level to analyze human Th1 and Th2 cells. Rinsho Byori 1998; 46(9):908–914.

355. Viola JP, Rao A. Molecular regulation of cytokine gene expression during the immune response. J Clin Immunol 1999; 19(2):98–108.

356. Huittinen T, Leinonen M, Tenkanen L, Virkkunen H, Mänttäri M, Palosuo T, Manninen V, Saikku P. Synergistic effect of persistent *Chlamydia pneumoniae* infection, autoimmunity, and inflammation on coronary risk. Circulation 2003; 107:2566–2570.

357. Krueger J. The central role of T-cell adhesion molecules in the immunopathogenesis of psoriasis: Implications for targeted therapy. Clinical Corner 2000; Gardiner-Caldwell SynerMed (00GN221).

358. Sheih, S, Mikkola DL, Wood GS. Differentiation and colonality of lesional lymphocytes in pityriasis lichenoides chronica. Arch Dermatol 2001; 137:305–308.

359. Pielop JA, et al. Transient CD30+ nodal transformation of cutaneous T-cell lymphoma associated with cyclosporine treatment. Int J Dermatol 2001; 40:505–511.

360. Woo E, Cassin M, Lesin SR, Rook AH. Complete molecular remission during biologic response modifier therapy for Sézary syndrome is associated with enhanced helper T type 1 cytokine production natural killer cell activity. J Am Acad Dermatol 2001; 45:208–216.

361. Lord CJM, Lamb JR. Th2 cells in allergic inflammation: a target of immunotherapy. Rev Clin Exp Allergy 1996; 26:756–765.

362. Sallusto F, Lanzavecchia A, Mackay CR. Chemokines and chemokine receptors in T-cell priming and Th1/Th2-mediated responses. Rev Immunol Today 1998; 19:568–574.

363. Martin AG. Bexarotene gel: a new skin-directed treatment option for cutaneous T-cell lymphomas. J Drugs Dermatol 2003; 2:155–167.

364. Gorman C, Park A. The fires within. Time Magazine Feb 23, 2004, 37–46.

365. Allen J. Injecting a look of good health. LA Times, Feb 10, 2003.

366. Vincent R. Times staff writer. FDA panel smoothes way for permanent wrinkle remover. LA Times, Mar 1, 2003.

367. Kemper V. Times staff writer. Panel calls for end to silicone implant curbs. LA Times, Oct 16, 2003.

368. Perrin C, Lacour JP, Castanet J, Michiels JF. Interstitial granulomatous drug reaction with a histological pattern of interstitial granulomatous dermatitis. Am J Dermatopathology 2001; 23(4):295–298.

369. Cox N, Duffey P, Royle J. Fixed drug eruption caused by lactose in an injected botulinum toxin preparation. J Am Acad Dermatol 1999; 40(2):263–264.

370. Lewis AT, Benedetto AV. Lasers in Dermatology: unapproved treatments. Clin Dermatol 2002; 20:700–714.

371. Fitzpatrick R. Intralesional 5-FU for Hypertrophic Scars. Presented at AAD Surgical Pearls, Orlando FLA, July 26, 1996.

372. Blugerman G, Schavelzon D, Dreszman R. Intralesional use of 5-FU in subcutaneous fibrosis. J Drugs Dermatol 2003; 2:169–171.

373. Sente P, Bachelez H, Ollivaud L, Vignon-Pennamen D, Dubertret L. Minocycline for the treatment of cutaneous silicone granulomas. Br J Dermatol 1999; 140:963–991.

374. Gogstetter D, Goldsmith A. Treatment of cutaneous sarcoidosis using phonophoresis. J Am Acad Dermatol 1999; 40:767–769.

375. Forstrom L, Winkelmann RK. Granulomatous panniculitis and erythema nodosum. Arch Dermatol 1975; 111(3):335–340.

376. Robertson S. Sarcoidosis, Jan 9, 1997. http://hsc.virginia.edu/medicine/clinical/internal/conf/chiefs/sarcoidosis.htm.

377. Pinali. ATS/ERS/WASOG Statement on Sarcoidosis. Sarcoidosis, vasculitis and diffuse lung diseases 1999; 16:149–173. www.pinali.unipd.it/sarcoid/clpres.htm.

378. Giuffrida T, Kerdel F. Sarcoidosis. Dermatol Clin 2002; 20:435–447.

379. Kawaguchi H, et al. Second Dept. Internal Med., Nagoya City University, Med. Sch., Nagoya Japan.IL-12 and IL-10 released from peripheral blood mononuclear cells in sarcoidosis is associated with differential modulation of B7-1 (CD80) and B7-2 (CD86) expression on monocytes. www.med.nagoya-cu.ac.jp/NMJ/45-17.html.

380. Personal communication; September 2001. Diane Richard from Richard James, Inc.

381. Vacuum assisted tissue augmentation, presented at American Academy of Dermatology, Association of Surgical Faculty, Feb 24, 2002.

382. Personal Communication with Patient (G.C.), May, 9, 1996.

383. Murray CA, DeKoven J, Spaner DE. Foreign body granuloma: a new manifestation of immune restoration syndrome. J Cutan Med Surg 2003; 38–42.

384. Khan GA, Lewis FA. Recognizing Weber-Christian disease. Tenn Med 1006; 89:447–449.

385. White WL, Wieselthier JS, Hitchcock MG. Panniculitis: recent developments and observations. Semin Cutan Med Surg 1996; 15:278–299.

386. Akama H, Tanaka H, Yoshida T, Kameda H, Kawai S. Glucocorticoid-unresponsive fever in a patient with Weber-Christian disease. Br J Clin Pract 1994; 48:161–162.

387. Miyasaki N. Steroid-resistant Weber-Christian disease. Intern Med 1999; 38:522.

388. Asauliuk IK. Pfeifer-Weber-Christian disease with 20-year course. Lik Sprava 1998; 7:154–159.

389. Hyun SH, Kang SH, Kim CD, Lee Jm, Kim IT, Kim SN. Weber-Christian disease presenting with proptosis: a case report. J Korean Med Sci 2000; 15(2):247–250.

390. www.whonamedit.com. Pfeiffer-Weber-Christian disease.

391. Hurley TH, Sullivan JR, Hurley JV. Reaction to Kveim test material in sarcoidosis and other diseases. Lancet 1975; 1(7905):494–496.

392. Clinical Trial Review. Denileukin Diftitox in treating patients with stage I, stage II, or stage III cutaneous T-cell lymphoma. J Drugs Dermatol 2002; 2:235–245.

393. Wolf R, Matz H, Orion E, Tüzün B, Tüzün Y. Miscellaneous treatments, I: sulfasalazine, pentoxifylline: unapproved uses, dosages, or indications. Clin Dermatol 2002; 20:531–546.

394. Assmann T, Ruzicka T. New immunosuppressive drugs in dermatology (mycophenolate mofetil, tacrolimus): unapproved uses, dosages, or indications. Clin Dermatol 2002; 20:505–514.

395. Ginarte M, et al. Treatment of α_1—Antitrypsin-deficiency panniculitis with minocycline. Cutis 2001; 68:86–88.

396. Iwasaki T, Hamano T, Ogata A, Hashimoto N, Kakeshita E. Successful treatment of a patient with febrile, lobular panniculitis (Weber-Christian disease) with oral cyclosporine A? implications for pathogenesis and therapy. Intern Med 1999; 38:612–614.

397. Clinical trial review. Interleukin-2 in treating patients with mycosis fungoides or Sézary syndrome. J Drugs Dermatol 2002; 2:235–245.

398. Gottlieb A, Krueger JG, Wittkowski K, Dedrick R, Walicke PA, Garovoy M. Psoriasis as a model for T-cell-mediated disease. Arch Dermatol 2002; 138:591–600.

399. Nickoloff BJ. The search for pathogenic T cells and the genetic basis of psoriasis using a severe combined immunodeficient mouse model. Cutis 2000; 65:110–114.

400. Nousari H, et al. Mycophenolate mofetil in autoimmune and inflammatory skin disorders. J Am Acad Dermatol 1999; 40(2):265–268.

401. Boyd A. Use of mycophenolate mofetil in erythema nodosum. Letters; J Am Acad Dermatol 2001; 967.
402. Fivenson D, Breneman DL, Rosen GB, Hersh CS, Cardone S, Mutasim D. Nicotinamide and tetracycline therapy of bullous pemphigoid. Arch Dermatol 1994; 130:753–758.
403. Wolf R, Matz H, Orion E, Tüzün B, Tüzün Y. Miscellaneous treatments, II: Niacin and Heparin: unapproved uses, dosages, or indications. Clin Dermatol 2002; 20:547–557.
404. Orion, E, Matz H, Wolf R. Interferons: unapproved uses, dosages, or indications. Clin Dermatol 2002; 20:493–504.
405. McGinnis KS, et al. Denileukin diftitox for the treatment of panniculitic lymphoma. Arch Dermatol 2002; 138:740–742.
406. Schanz S, Ulmer A, Rassner G, Fierlbeck G. Effects of mycophenolate mofetil (MMF) on treatment of extensive skin lesions secondary to subacute cutaneous LE (SCLE). Br J Dermatol 2002; 147(1):174–178.
407. Ritter MS, George MR, Serwatka LM, Elston DM. Long-term suppression of chronic sweet's syndrome with colchicines. J Am Acad Dermatol 2002; 47:323–324.
408. Termeer C, et al. Low-dose interferon alpha-2b for the treatment of Churg-Strauss syndrome with prominent skin involvement. Arch Dermatol 2001; 137:136–138.
409. Singri P, et al. Biologic therapy for psoriasis. Arch Dermatol 2002; 138:657–663.
410. Nousari H, et al. The effectiveness of mycophenolate mofetil in refractory pyoderma gangrenosum. Arch Dermatol 1998; 134:1509–1511.
411. Plevy S, Valentine J, Fleischer MR, Lichtenstein GR. Successful treatment of IBD-associated pyoderma gangrenosum with infliximab. AAD 60th meeting, Poster #P176, Feb 22–27, 2002.
412. Limova M. Treatment of pyoderma gangrenosum with intravenous Infliximab. AAD 60th Annual meeting, Poster #P150, Feb 22–27, 2002.
413. Sofen H. New therapies for psoriatic diseases presentation, January 8, 2004. Chez Melange, Torrance. Sponsored by Amgen, Inc.
414. McConnaughey J. Experimental drug may help sufferers of peanut allergies. The Daily Breeze Tues. Mar 11, 2003, 1.
415. Lack G, Fox D, Northstone K, Golding J. Factors associated with the development of peanut allergy in childhood. N Engl J Med 2003; 348:977–985.
416. Park R. Bee and hymenoptera stings. eMedicine Journal, April 10 2002, Vol. 3, No. 4; http://www.emedicine.com/emerg/topic55.htm/.
417. Gorman C. Fighting over peanuts. Time Magazine March 24, 2003, 59.
418. Ringel EW. The morality of cosmetic surgery for aging. Arch Dermatol 1998; 134:427–431.
419. Glogau R. Cosmetic dermatology: no apologies, a few regrets. Arch Dermatol 1998; 134.
420. Werth V, et al. Preserving medical dermatology: a colleague lost, a call to arms, and a plan for battle. Derm Clinics 2001; 19(4):583–592.
421. Wolff K. Quo vadis dermatology: a scenario for the future. J Am Acad Dermatol 2003; 48:605–608.
422. Essays in honor of Carl G. Hempel. Published by D. Reidel, 1970.
423. Craig WL. Divine foreknowledge and Newcomb's paradox. www.origins.org source "Divine Foreknowledge and Newcomb's Paradox, Philosophia." 1987; 17:331–350.
424. Piotrowski EW, Stadkowski J. Quantum solution to the Newcomb's paradox. RePEc:-sla:eakjkl:10, Poland, Nov 14, 2002.
425. Rees J. Complex disease and the new clinical sciences. Science 2002; 296.
426. Gouvea FQ. A most influential problem set. Science 2002; 296:853–854.
427. Devlin K. Kurt Gödell—Separating truth from proof in mathematics. Science 2002; 298:1899–1900.
428. Hilton L. Silicone… the next rage in permanent fillers? CST 2002; 5(8):17.
429. Brown L, Frank PJ. The silicone conundrum. Skin and Aging 2002; 15.

430. Tobin HA. Microdroplet silicone injection shows pout possibilities. CST 2003; 13.

431. Warnock M, Goodacre J. Cryptic T-cell epitopes and their role in the pathogenesis of autoimmune diseases. Br J Rheumatol 1997; 36:1144–1150.

432. Weigle WO. Advances in basic concepts of autoimmune disease. Clin Lab Med 1997; 17(3):329–340.

433. Maxflo Needles. Richard James Corp. Peabody, MA.

434. Duffy D. Vacuum assisted tissue augmentation. Presented at American Academy of Dermatology, Association of Surgical Faculty, Feb 24, 2002.

435. Orentreich DS, Orentreich N. Subcutaneous Incisionless (Subcision) surgery for the correction of depressed scars and wrinkles. Dermatol Surg 1995; 21:543–549.

436. Bouchon A, Facchetti F, Weigand MA, Colonna M. TREM-1 amplifies inflammation and is a crucial mediator of septic shock. Letters to Nature Magazine. Nature 2001; 410:1103–1107.

437. Nablo BJ, Chen TY, Schoenfisch MH. Sol-gel derived nitric-oxide releasing materials that reduce bacterial adhesion. J Am Chem Soc 2001; 123:9712–9713.

438. Christensen D. Ultrasound boosts drug delivery to tumors. Science News 2001; 160:391.

439. http://www.sigmaaldrich.com/Area of Interest/Life Science/Cancer Research/ Mechanisms of Action.html/. Anti-tumor agents by mechanisms of action. Mar 18, 2004.

440. Singh PK, Parsek MR, Greenberg EP, Welsh MJ. A component of innate immunity prevents bacterial biofilm development. Nature 2002; 417:552–555.

441. Marie-Claude M, et al. A randomized comparison of a sirolimus-eluting stent with a standard stent for coronary revascularization. N Eng J Med 346:1773–1780.

442. AP. Cardiology advance is hailed. LA Times, Mar 18, 2002.

443. Magro CM, Crowson AN. Lichenoid and granulomatous dermatitis. Int J Dermatol 2000; 39(2):126–133.

444. Misiek D, et al. Soft Tissue Responses to Hydroxylapatite particles of different shapes. J Oral Maxillofac Surg 1984; 42:150–60.

445. Ewida AS, Raphael SA, Abbasi JA, Geslani GP, Bagrasra O. Evaluation of Th-1 and Th-2 immune responses in the skin lesions of patients with Blau syndrome. Appl Immunohistochem Mol Morphol 2002; 10(2):171–177.

446. Murray JS. How the MHC selects Th1/Th2 immunity. Immunol Today 1998; 19:157–163.

447. Cordes H. The Th1/Th2 paradigm: Biological allergy research.

448. Desmedt M. Macrophages induce cellular immunity by activating Th1 cell responses and suppressing Th2 cell responses. J Immunol 1998; 160:5300–5308.

449. Ellis CN, Krueger GG. Treatment of chronic plaque psoriasis by selective targeting of memory effector T lymphocytes. N Engl J Med 2001; 345:248–255.

450. Prose NS. Recent advances in pediatric dermatology. Yale University/Fujisawa Healthcare, Inc. Lectureship series in dermatology 2002; Lecture 4.

451. Syneron Aesthetics Workshop. Westwood, CA, Mar 24, 2004.

452. Goerttler E, Kutzner H, Peter HH, Requena L. Methotrexate-induced papular eruption in patients with rheumatic diseases: a distinctive adverse cutaneous reaction produced by methotrexate in patients with collagen vascular diseases. J Am Acad Dermatol 1999; 40:702–707.

453. http://www.allshakespeare.com/quotes/. "A plague o' both your houses!"

454. Kenneth B, Gordon MD, Thomas S, McCormick. Review: Evolution of biologic therapies for the treatment of psoriasis. SKINmed 2003; 5:286–294.

455. Mullen A, High FA, Hutchins AS, Lee HW, Villarino AV, Livingston DM, Kung AL, Cereb N, Yao TP, Yang SY, Reiner SL. Role of T-beta in commitment of T_H1 cells before IL-12-depenent selection. Science Bol 2001; 292:1907–1910.

456. Updates in Biodermatology - #1. Looking beneath the surface: Identifying the immunologic basis of psoriasis. Biogen, Inc. 2002.

457. Dalong MA. Beijing Medical University http://mededucation.bjmu.edu.cn/ek10.htm/.

458. Immune network. http://webmed.unipv.it/immunology/network.html/.

459. Stvrtinova V, Jakubovsky J, Hulin I. Computing Centre, Slovak Academy of Sciences, Slovakia online. © 1995 ISBN 80-967366-1-2. Cytokines mediating inflammatory and effector functions. http://nic.sav.sk/logos/books/scientific/node32.html/.

460. Heinzerlling L, Dummer R, Kempf W, Hess Schmid M, Burg G. Intralesional therapy with anti-CD20 monoclonal antibody rituximab in primary cutaneous B-cell lymphoma. Arch Dermatol 2000; 136:374–378.

461. Henny Penny. http://www.authorama.com/english-fairy-tales-23.html/.

462. Cohen J. Escape artist par excellence. Science Mag 299:1505–1508.

463. Grafenstein HV. Phar 441 Immunology; Lecture 6—Coordination and organization of a normal immune response. http://www-hsc.usc.edu/~grafen/teaching/lectures/lecture6.htm/.

464. Voltaire. Pangloss. In: Kuklok, Allison. "BookRags Book Notes on Candide." 8 April 2004. http://www.bookrags.com/notes/can/.

465. Manning G, Whyte DB, Martinez R, Sudarsanam S, Sugen Inc., SF, CA, Hunter T, Salk Inst, La Jolla CA. The human kinome: Cell signaling science mag. Pull-out 2002.

466. Katzin WE, Feng LJ, Abbuhl M, Klein MA. Phenotype of lymphocytes associated with the inflammatory reaction to silicone gel breast implants. Clin Diagn Lab Immunol 1996; 3(2):156–161.

467. Hessian PA, Highton J, Kean A, Sun CK, Chin M. Cytokine profile of the rheumatoid nodule suggests that it is a Th1 granuloma. Arthritis Rheum 2003; 48(2):334–338.

468. Torre D, Speranza F, Giola M, Matteelli A, Tambini R, Biondi G. Role of Th1 and Th2 cytokines in immune response to uncomplicated Plasmodium falciparum malaria. Clin Diagn Lab Immunol 2002; 9(2):348–351.

469. Oriss TB, McCarthy SA, Morel BF, Campana MA, Morel PA. Cross regulation between T helper cell (Th) 1 and Th2: Inhibition of Th2 proliferation by IFN-gamma involves interference with IL-1. J Immunol 1997; 158(8):3666–3672.

470. Zingoni A. Cutting edge: The chemokine receptor CCR8 is preferentially expressed in Th2 but not in Th1 cells. J Immunol 1998; 161:547–551.

471. Lo-Man R. A recombinant virus-like particle system derived from parvovirus as an efficient antigen carrier to elicit a polarized Th1 immune response without adjuvant. Euro J Immunol 1998; 28:1401–1407.

472. Walters IB, Ozawa M, Cardinale I, Gilleaudeau P, Trepicchio WL, Bliss J, Krueger JG. Narrowband (312-nm) UV-B suppresses Interferon γ and Interleukin (IL) 12 and increases IL-4 transcripts. Arch Dermatol 2003; 139:155–161.

473. Malissen B. Switching off TCR signaling. Science 2003; 302.

474. Tigelaar RE. T Cells, B Cells & immunoglobulins, and antigen presenting cells. AAD course #110; San Francisco, 2003.

475. Guttmann C. TLRs linked to origin of inflammatory acne. Dermatol Times 2002; S13.

476. Raskin C. Apoptosis and cutaneous biology. J Am Acad Dermatol 1997; 36(6):885–898.

477. Bhushan M, Cumberbatch M, Dearman RJ. TNF-α induced migration of human Langerhans cells: The influence of ageing. Br J Dermatol 2002; 146:32–40.

478. Hossein C, et al. Bullous pemphigoid treated with leflunomide. Arch Dermatol 136:1204–1205.

479. Neufeld G, Cohen T, Gengrinovitch S, Poltorak Z. Vascular endothelial growth factor (VEGF) and its receptors. FASEB J 1999; 13:9–22.

480. www.obgyn.net/newsheadlines/womens_health-Breast_Cancer-20030408-3.asp. Estrogen influences vascular endothelial growth factor in a biphasic manner.

10

Resurfacing Procedures and Topical Therapy

Melvin L. Elson

Cosmeceutical Concepts International, Inc., Nashville, Tennessee, U.S.A.

As soft tissue augmentation products have become more effective, safer, and have increased in number over the years, so too have adjunctive therapies used to treat other aspects of the aging face. Much of the development in both soft tissue products and topical therapies has evolved most recently owing to the demographics of the aging population, particularly the "baby boomers." This is beneficial in that science has attempted to keep up with the demands; however, this has also led to overpromising by manufacturers and greater expectations on the part of the patient than is realistic. This is particularly true in the area of topical therapy and especially of some of the newer noninvasive procedures that have been developed. This chapter will take a close look at products, claims, and the marketing of drugs, cosmetics, and cosmeceuticals. It is, however, important to review the concept of the interacting factors of the aging face to understand the potential for improvement with a filler or neuromuscular blocking agent, as well as understand where noninvasive procedures and topical therapy fit into the armamentarium available to reverse the aging appearance.

The aging face comprises five interacting factors—intrinsic aging, sleep lines, gravity, expression lines, and photoaging (1). The great majority of what is perceived as aging, perhaps as much as 80%, is in actuality sun damage. To demonstrate the degree of damage due to the sun, to the patient (especially those who state "I never get in the sun") one need only compare the backs of the hands with the tops of the feet or the face with the buttocks. Fine lines over the surface, play on color with lentigines and pseudoscars, play on texture with coarse wrinkles, broken vessels, enlarged pores, and a sallowness that the skin acquires—all are due to the sun. It is this particular aspect of the aging face that has been primarily addressed by dermatologists who continue to be the experts in this area, by developing the devices and procedures used to treat other aspects of the aging face.

Using the proper modality to treat each factor of the face results in the desired correction for both patient and physician. One modality should not and indeed cannot be used interchangeably with another to treat other factors or delay treatment, e.g., soft tissue augmentation will not delay the need for a face-lift. Intrinsic aging, where tissue has been lost by true aging, requires replacement of the lost tissue, i.e., the use of solid implants or lipotransfer (2). Sleep lines, which occur unilaterally from sleeping with the face in the same position every night, can be filled for temporary benefit, alleviated by use of a satin pillowcase or by attempts to change the sleep pattern (3). The gravity factor must generally be treated by some significant invasive procedure, such as rhytidectomy, rhinoplasty, blepharoplasty, etc. (4). Photoaging may be treated with a number of different modalities from sunscreens and topical agents, to chemical peels. This chapter will mainly address the issue of treatment of photoaging. Expression lines are best treated by soft tissue augmentation and this is where injectable materials, as well as neuromuscular blocking agents, come into play.

There are some adjunctive procedures, which may be able to both enhance and/or prolong the benefits of soft tissue augmentation. Laser resurfacing and some of the other more invasive type of procedures are covered elsewhere in this text. Chemical peeling, which produces a deep level of injury in the skin (such as Jessner's/35% Trichloroacetic acid (TCA) peel and TCA or variants of phenol), may provide a significant decrease in the appearance of fine lines and wrinkles (5,6). Soft tissue augmentation combined with appropriately timed chemical peeling produces excellent results in softening and smoothing the face. It is important that the peel be separated from the augmentation procedure by at least six weeks to avoid destruction of the augmentation material by collagenase induced by the peel. Dermabrasion (7) can be utilized similarly, again keeping in mind the issue of collagenase production. Liposuction and lipotransfer are frequently used in conjunction with injectable materials, both to fill material in larger defects with other fillers "topping off" and to produce a full rounded appearance to the entire face (8). These types of procedures are described in detail in other portions of the text.

Although surgical intervention is another alternative to aid in the patient's overall appearance following soft tissue augmentation, it is in the realm of topical therapy, both pharmaceutical and cosmetic, that even greater strides have been made. Although it is sometimes difficult to separate fact from fiction and marketing from science, a great deal has been learned through reliable and reproducible scientific investigation about the aging process and how best to treat it.

In the evolution of the available products for the treatment of photoaged skin, the early years were dominated by two types of products—retinoids and alpha hydroxy acids. Unquestionably, the single most important event in the history of treatment of aging skin was the discovery of the benefits of Retin-A for this indication as well as in the treatment of acne. Dr. Albert Kligman of the University of Pennsylvania has been thought to be the leader in this field and is the inventor of Retin-A®.

Retin-A was developed by Dr. Kligman in the 1960s in an attempt to find a nontoxic topical agent that could be used in the treatment of acne, as is oral vitamin A (Retinol). His discovery and clinical studies led to its approval by the U.S. Food and Drug Administration (FDA) for use in the treatment of acne. Shortly after, both Dr. Kligman and his patients noticed that as they used the cream to clear the acne problem, fine lines and wrinkles also improved. Clinical studies confirmed these anecdotal reports and he began publishing information on the use of Retin-A in the treatment of aging skin as early as 1993 (9).

Further studies revealed that patients treated with tretinoin demonstrated improvement in epidermal atrophy, dysplasia, keratosis, and dyspigmentation (all manifestations of photodamage) (10). These studies eventually led to the approval by the FDA, of Renòva®, a formulation of tretinoin, for photoaging.

It is important to understand that all retinoids are vitamin A or its derivatives. The newer materials designated as having retinoid-like activity are not true retinoids (e.g., adapalene), but are chemically derived entities that have certain chemical effects like true retinoids.

Although popular belief is that retinoids work by peeling the skin, in actuality retinoids affect cell growth, differentiation, homeostasis, and apoptosis, by regulating gene transcription at the molecular level. In the 1970s, retinoid-binding proteins were discovered (11) and in 1987, the discovery of retinoic acid receptors led to the designation of tretinoin as a "hormone" (12,13). The effects of retinoic acid and other retinoids are now known to be mediated by a number of receptors, both cellular and nuclear, which interact with receptors in the cell, as well as among one another, in complex manners not yet completely delineated. Retinoids have long been known to be beneficial in the treatment of photoaging, but have now been determined to be of benefit in true intrinsic aging as well. Retinoids have a particularly effective method of blocking the action of collagenase on types I and III collagen and therefore should always be used in conjunction with collagen injections, since these are always types I and III collagen. The beneficial effects of the soft tissue augmentation devices appear to be enhanced with pretreatment and continuous usage of retinoids following injection.

Although retinol (vitamin A) is actually the parent compound of all true retinoids, it is only recently that cosmetic formulations have begun to incorporate this compound. It must be converted to retinal and then retinoic acid by the keratinocyte before it can actually become active (14), but retinol is still considered a cosmetic. One of the problems with the use of retinol in cosmetic formulations is the inherent instability of the molecule. For this reason, many compounds contain an extremely small amount of retinol, present merely for marketing purposes, which is ineffective. There are products that use retinol in a stabilized form, which are effective. Retinoic acid has been shown to be approximately 20 times more potent than retinol (15); thus, a stabilized formulation with

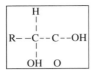

Figure 1
Alpha hydroxy acid structure.

0.25% retinol is probably equivalent to 0.025% retinoic acid. In this form, there is also less irritation with the effect. It is important then to be certain that the formulation has a stabilized form of retinol and in a concentration high enough to be effective. A formula that lists retinol as an ingredient far down the list of ingredients most likely does not have a concentration high enough to have any effect.

The other highly touted products over the last couple of decades are those that contain alpha hydroxy acids. Although some would have us believe that these are new additions in the treatment of aging and other skin disorders, they have actually been used for centuries (16). Ancient Egyptians bathed in sour milk (lactic acid) to moisturize and smooth their skin. After wine was fermented in ancient Greece, the sludge was removed from the bottom of the vat and applied to the face to make it smoother and prettier (tartaric acid).

Glycolic acid has been the ingredient of choice from this group of chemicals, because it is the smallest molecule of the group and somewhat easier to work with and formulate (17). Alpha hydroxy acids are a class of compounds characterized by the presence of a hydroxyl group on the alpha carbon (18; Fig. 1). R is H for glycolic acid. Lactic acid contains two carbons, butyric has four etc.

Table 1 indicates the natural commonly used acids; however, the natural source is rarely used by any manufacturer of cosmetic agents. Almost all products containing alpha hydroxy acids are chemically manufactured and, for compounding, are generally quite pure (19).

Table 1
Common Acids Derived from Foods

Acid	Structure	Natural Source
Glycolic	$CH_2OHCOOH$	Sugar cane
Lactic	$CH_3CH_2OH\ COOH$	Sour milk
∂OH Butyric	$CH_3CH_2\ CHOHCOOH$	Rancid butter
Malic	$HO_2C–CH\ OHCH_2CO_2H$	Apples
Oxalic	$HO_2C–CO_2H$	Sauerkraut
Tartaric	$HO_2C–CH_2(OH)_2CO_2H$	Grapes
Citric	$HO_2C–CH_2COH$ CO_2HCH_2COOH	Lemons

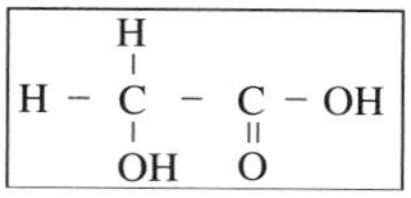

```
        H
        |
  H  -  C  -  C - OH
        |     ||
        OH    O
```

Figure 2
Glycolic acid structure.

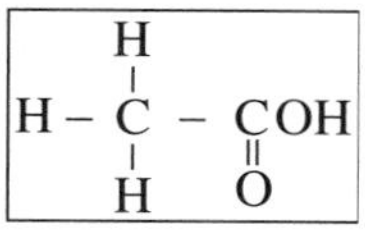

```
        H
        |
  H  -  C  -  COH
        |     ||
        H     O
```

Figure 3
Acetic acid structure.

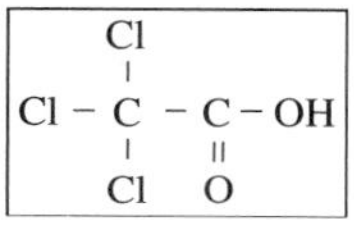

```
        Cl
        |
  Cl -  C  -  C - OH
        |     ||
        Cl    O
```

Figure 4
Trichloroacetic acid structure.

The concept of utilizing glycolic acid in products is an extension of the benefits of chemical peeling of the skin to reverse the manifestations of photoaging. One of the most commonly used substances by dermatologists for chemical peels in office has been trichloroacetic acid (TCA). It is interesting to note the similarity in the structures of glycolic acid in Figure 2, acetic acid (vinegar) in Figure 3, and TCA in Figure 4. The strength of an acid is determined by the ease with which it donates a proton, i.e., its hydrogen ion. Under ordinary circumstances TCA is a stronger acid than acetic acid, because of the attraction of the Cl groups for electrons, pulling negative charges away from the hydrogen and freeing it up. TCA is a much stronger acid than glycolic acid because the hydroxyl group is a relatively weak electron attractor and frees up the hydrogen ion much less readily. It would, therefore, seem that the higher the concentration of the acid, the greater the strength of the acid. The deeper the penetration, the greater the benefit. This is true for TCA, but not necessarily for glycolic acid. For both chemical peels and products derived from glycolic acid, three parameters are necessary to determine the "strength" of the material—concentration, pH, and formulation (20).

Chemical peeling will not be dealt with in depth here, but it is important to have an understanding of the chemistry of glycolic acid, particularly when used in formulations. The natural tendency is to compare each product based merely on concentration and assume that the greater the concentration, the greater the benefit, but this is not necessarily the case. No formulation of any product on the market is pure glycolic acid. These products are combinations of the acid, its salts or its esters, and adjustments are made to the pH and the amount of free acid in the product. It is with the introduction of these products at the time when baby boomers were coming to the age of concern about aging that the great difficulty has arisen separating fact from fiction and science from marketing.

Alpha hydroxy acids, including glycolic acid, despite a great deal of claims and press, remain acids. The effect of an acid on the skin is simple—it wounds the skin and then the skin heals, looking better owing to the processes involved in wound healing. There is also a peeling effect, which will remove debris, make-up, and dead skin to make the skin appear smoother and healthier.

In addition to the effects mentioned above, there is a loosening of the cells of the epidermis by these types of products, leading to increased permeability of other agents. This may play a significant role in the usefulness of these agents in a skincare program to combat aging, allowing penetration of agents, such as tretinoin and other topical vitamins (21).

Ascorbic acid (vitamin C) has been the subject of intense research by a number of centers for years. It is a well-known free-radical scavenger, but studies of topical vitamin C have failed to yield reproducible data in humans that there is a significant difference with its use. Animal experiments have shown that vitamin C blocks the effects of UV-A, that there is a reservoir of vitamin C that can collect in the skin and that there are indications of collagen repair (22). There are a great deal of anecdotal data indicating significant cosmetic improvement in terms of fine lines, dullness to the skin, and discoloration.

One of the major problems in working with vitamin C is formulating the product. It is a very unstable compound and oxidizes very easily once exposed to air after formulation. Also, the skin can only utilize L-ascorbate and no other form. Most of the products sold containing vitamin C are improperly formulated, unstable, and decompose within hours of opening the product. There are some products such as Skinceuticals' vitamin C products that were developed by Darr and Pinnell (23) and have been shown to be stable and effective. Basically, one must be very careful and recommend to patients only those products that are stable and have clinical data to support them.

Although vitamin E has been used topically for years, particularly in treating scars, there are no studies indicating its usefulness in the treatment of aging or any other skin disorder.

Recently, topical vitamin K has been introduced for the treatment and prevention of actinic purpura, bruising associated with procedures such as laser resurfacing and soft tissue augmentation, and more recently in the treatment of ruddiness and telangiectasia (24,25). Probably, the most common cosmetic use at present is in the treatment of dark circles under the eyes (26). Vitamin K was discovered in Germany in 1929; the K stands for "koagulations vitamin" (27). It is necessary for the production of prothrombin, factor VIII and IX, as well as other factors that are manufactured by the liver and control the cascade of blood coagulation (28). Natural sources are green leafy vegetables, especially kale, and normal flora of the gastrointestinal tract. In modernized countries, newborns are given IM vitamin K since they have no natural sources at birth.

I became interested in topical vitamin K while seeking a treatment for actinic purpura. This entity occurs when the support collagen breaks down in the dermis and the interdigitation between the dermis and epidermis comes apart and the protective veil cell is destroyed (29). Clinically, this is manifested by easy bruising and shearing with the least bit of trauma to the skin, such that the arms and hands are constantly purpuric. This is very disconcerting cosmetically, and patients also experience discomfort and these areas serve as a nidus of infection. In a double-blind study of vitamin K_1 (phytonadione) versus its base cream, patients in the active group had faster resolution of the lesions and with continued use, had decreased appearance of the lesions as well. Since then, laser resurfacing, the medication has proved useful for both treating and preventing bruises due to surgery, laser resurfacing, and soft tissue augmentation, decreasing or eliminating downtime from procedures, and allowing faster return to work and social activities (30).

Topical vitamin K also decreases the neovascularization after sclerotherapy and there appears to be some benefit to small telangiectasias due to the application of vitamin K. The most common use of topical vitamin K is currently in the treatment of dark undereye circles. Most of the formulations utilize 0.5% to 1% phytonadione combined with 0.025% retinol. There have been a number of studies published on the benefits of this therapy for dark circles under the eyes (31,32). Figures 5 and 6 are demonstrative of the benefit after use for 16 weeks.

Ongoing research continues to uncover more clinical uses for topical vitamin K as well as to delineate possible mechanisms of action, including the presence of the ubiquinone (Fig. 7) moiety within the molecule, indicating possible antioxidant capabilities, its ability to decrease pigmentation by virtue of the fact that it is a quinone and that recent research has begun to delineate receptors for vitamin K in certain cells (33).

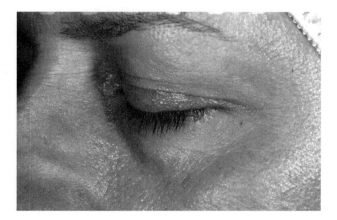

Figure 5
Dark circles (before treatment).

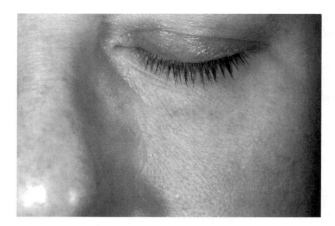

Figure 6
After 16 weeks of treatment with 1% phytonadione and 0.5% retinol in a micro-sponge base.

Recently, there have been appearing on the market, various formu-lations containing growth factors, both as mixtures taken from cellular incubation baths and as individual substances, particularly TGF-beta. There are a number of factors that must be kept in mind with these sub-stances. First of all, all these factors are very large molecules that cannot penetrate the epidermis. It is certainly possible that they may influence activity from the surface, but this has not been shown to be the case. Second, these factors act in very short bursts, beginning a cascade of activity that proceeds very rapidly. It is highly unlikely that these factors

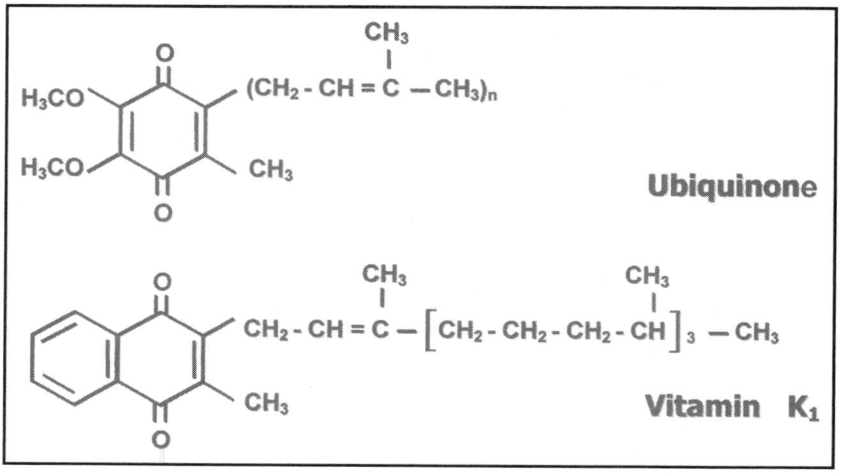

$$H_3CO \quad \overset{O}{\underset{O}{\cdots}} \quad (CH_2\text{-}CH = \overset{\overset{CH_3}{|}}{C} - CH_3)_n$$

$$H_3CO \quad \cdots \quad CH_3$$

Ubiquinone

$$CH_2\text{-}CH = \overset{\overset{CH_3}{|}}{C} - \left[CH_2\text{-}CH_2\text{-}CH_2\text{-}\overset{\overset{CH_3}{|}}{CH} \right]_3 - CH_3$$

$$CH_3$$

Vitamin K$_1$

Figure 7
Structure of phytonadione and ubiquinone.

act in this manner in formulations. Additionally, there is some evidence that the factors are stable in formulations in terms of chemical integrity, but there is no evidence as yet that they retain their physiologic activity. Basically, there are anecdotal data with some before and after photographs that seem to indicate activity, but more research is necessary to make any conclusion regarding this new technology.

Of all the methods available to prevent and treat photoaging and to maintain the youthful glow, the most important is the daily application of sunscreen. Although the dangers of the sun in terms of acute sunburn have been recognized for centuries, as evidenced by the wearing of long robes in areas of intense sun and sitting in the shade of trees, it was only in the 1950s that lotions began to appear on the market to prevent sunburn, and only in the 1970s did the first effective sunscreens (para-amino benzoic acid, PABA) appear. There are basically two types of protection—sunblocks and sunscreens. Sunblocks physically block the ultraviolet radiation and have been in use for many years. Zinc oxide was in frequent use in the past, and a number of years ago colored zinc oxide appeared on the market for a period of time. Most interesting now are the sunblocks that contain micronized zinc (Skinceuticals) and melanin as a sunblock that has been introduced (Integrative Aesthetics) quite recently.

Sunscreens act chemically rather than as physical blocks. As mentioned, the first in use in the United States was PABA, which actually binds to epidermal cells and blocks UVB. This sunscreen had a tendency to stain and there was a significant presence of allergic reactions—both contact and photocontact, hence it has fallen out of favor. There are many other UVB blockers in sunscreens, such as esters of PABA, cinnamates, salicylates, etc. There are also UVA blockers, which are extremely important, since UVA has more influence on inducing pigment problems in the skin as well as a factor in the development of malignant melanoma. Patients should be instructed to pay more attention to the fact that a product should be both a UVA and UVB blocker, rather than a product having a very high sun protection factor (SPF), as these numbers are based on the ability of the product to block UVB only.

Obviously, sunscreen application should be part of an everyday health routine with application every morning.

It is obvious that great strides have been made in the treatment and prevention of photoaging using topical therapy. When used in conjunction with injectable materials for soft tissue augmentation and other modalities, a significant benefit occurs in the patient's appearance and overall self-esteem, sense of health, and well-being.

Since a good portion of this chapter has dealt with substances that do not require a prescription, it is appropriate at this juncture to discuss the concept of cosmeceuticals. The Federal Food, Drug and Cosmetic Act of 1938 defines both drugs and cosmetics. Drug is defined as a substance "intended to affect the structure and function of the body." In this act, cosmetic is defined as "articles intended to be rubbed, poured, sprinkled or sprayed on, introduced into, or otherwise applied to the human body or any part thereof for cleansing, beautifying, promoting attractiveness, or altering the appearance." More than two decades ago, Albert Kligman (34) used the term cosmeceuticals at a meeting of the Society of Cosmetic Chemists. He felt this category should be added, and, although still not officially recognized, the term is frequently used to describe products that are known to have a biologic action but are regulated as cosmetics rather than as drugs.

The conundrum that the cosmetic industry is in at the current time is that they have developed products that have significant benefits on the skin; however, if clinical trials are performed to prove this and the product is marketed as having an effect, they have just proven it is a drug and cannot market the product. It is this catch 22 situation that has led to the games played by companies in labeling their products. A good example of this situation is the claim "reduces wrinkles," which is a drug claim and the claim "reduces the appearance of wrinkles," which is a cosmetic claim. The FDA would not allow a cosmetically marketed product to make a drug claim. It is, however, even a bit more complicated, because if a claim is made or implied by a cosmetic company that a product reduces the appearance of wrinkles, there must be substantiation of the claim or the Federal Trade Commission will see this as false advertising.

This obviously makes for a very complicated and difficult situation. This is one of the major reasons cosmeceuticals have come to the forefront of the cosmetic market. These are products, which have been shown through clinical trials of various sorts to be safe and effective, but the expense and time necessary to take them through the entire FDA process for drug approval have not been fulfilled nor will they be. The companies have "data on file," testimonials, before and after pictures, etc., but are careful as to what they claim and this is the key point.

It is true that companies do not have to prove safety and efficacy for a cosmetic product to enter the market; however, all reputable companies demonstrate the safety of products prior to distribution and most will also be certain of the efficacy. One would be surprised at the amount of research done by cosmetic companies to develop, test, and prove their products.

As seen from this review, a great deal has been accomplished in the area of topical therapy in the treatment of aging and photoaging. As the population continues to age and science attempts to produce more and newer advances, there is no limit as to what will be achieved in this area of dermatologic therapy.

REFERENCES

1. Elson ML. Evaluation and treatment of the aging face. In: Elson M, ed. Evaluation and Treatment of the Aging Face. New York: Springer-Verlag, 1995:1–9.
2. Coleman WP. Lipotransfer. In: Elson M, ed. Evaluation and Treatment of the Aging Face. New York: Springer-Verlag, 1995:101–109.
3. Stegman SJ. Sleep creases. Am J Cosmet Surg 1987; 4:277.
4. Chrisman BB. The facelift. J Dermatol Surg Oncol 1988; 15(8):812–822.
5. Brody HJ. Current advances and trends in chemical peeling. Dermatol Surg 1995; 21(5):385–387.
6. Monheit GD. The Jessner's-trichloroacetic acid peel. A medium depth chemical peel. Dermatol Clin 1995; 13(2):277–283.
7. Yarborough JM Jr. Wherefore dermabrasion. Dermatol Surg 1995; 21(5):381–382.
8. Collins PC, Field LM, Narins RS. Liposuction surgery and cutaneous fat transplantation. Clin Dermatol 1992; 10(3):365–372.
9. Kligman AM, Leyden JJ. Treatment of photoaged skin with topical tretinoin. Skin Pharmaceut 1993; 6(suppl 1):78–82.
10. Kligman L, Kligman AM. Photoaging—Retinoids, alpha hydroxy acids, and antioxidants. In: Gabard B, Elsner P, Surber C, Treffel P, eds. Dermatopharmacology of Topical Preparations. New York: Springer, 2000:383.
11. Chytil F, Ong D. Cellular retinoid-binding proteins. In: Sporn MB, Roberts A, Goodman D, eds. The Retinoids. Vol. 2. Orlando: Academic Press, 1984:89.
12. Giguere V, Ong ES, Segui P, et al. Identification of a receptor for the morphogen retinoic acid. Nature 1987; 330:624.
13. Petkovich M, Brand NJ, Krust A, et al. A human retinoic acid receptor which belongs to the family of nuclear receptors. Nature 1987; 330:440.
14. Kligman L, Kligman AM. Photoaging—Retinoids etc.op.cit.
15. Duell EA, Kang S, Voorhees JJ. Unoccluded retinol penetrates human skin in vivo more effectively than unoccluded retinyl palmitate or retinoic acid. J Invest Dermatol 1997:301.
16. Harris DR. Treatment of the aging skin with glycolic acid. In: Elson M, ed. Evaluation and Treatment of the Aging Face. New York: Springer-Verlag, 1995:22–23.
17. Elson ML. The molcecular structure of glycolic acid and its importance. Cosmet Dermatol 1993; 6(7):31–35.
18. Solomons T. Organic Chemistry. 5th ed. New York: John Wiley and sons, 1995.
19. Glypure Specifications Sheet. E. I. Du Pont de Nemours & Co., Wilmington, DE, 1994.
20. Elson ML. Treatment of photoaging—A personal comment and open study of the use of glycolic acid. J Dermatol Treat (Wales, UK), Dec 1993.
21. Dial WF. Use of AHAs add new dimenstion of chemical peeling. Cosmet Dermatol 1990; 3:32–34.
22. Pinnell S. Topical vitamin C protects porcine skin from ultraviolet radiation-induced damage. Br J Dermatol 1992; 127(3):247–253.
23. Darr D, Pinnell SR. Stable ascorbic acid composition. US Patent #5,140,043, Aug 18, 1992.
24. Elson ML. Topical phytonadione (vitamin K) in the treatment of actinic and traumatic purpura. Cosmet Dermatol 1995; 8(12):25–27.
25. Bernstein LJ, Geronemus R. Poster presentation. Meeting of ASDS, Palm Desert, CA, May 15–17, 1996.
26. Elson ML, Nacht S. Treatment of periorbital hyperpigmentation with topical vitamin K/ vitamin A. Cosmet Dermatol 1999; 10:32–34.
27. The Merck Index. Vitamin K_1 Rahway NJ: Merck and Co, 1989:1580.
28. O'Reilly RA. Vitamin K and the oral anticoagulant drugs. Ann Rev Med 1976; 27:245–261.

29. Ryan TJ. The microcirculation of the skin in old age. Gerontol Clin 1966; 8:327.
30. Elson ML. Method of treating blood vessel disorders of the skin using vitamin K. US Patent #5, 510, 391. Apr 23, 1996.
31. Ghosh D, Elson M, Nacht S. Treating dark under-eye circles with topical vitamins A and K. Cosmet and Toilet 2001; 116(6):51–54.
32. Eury R, Patel R, Longe K, et al. Microsponge Delivery Systems (MDS): A Topical Delivery System with Multiple Mechanism for Triggering the Release of Actives. Cosmetic and Pharmaceutical Applications of Polymers. New York: Plenum Press, 1991:169–179.
33. Posternak ME, Damonte SH, Ferraro, et al. The effects of topical vitamin K_1 on the skin pH and also on the facial erythema. 2002. In Press.
34. Kligman AM. Cosmeceuticals: Do we need a new category? In: Elsner P, Maibach H, eds. Cosmeceuticals. New York: Marcel Dekker, 2001:1.

11

Nonablative Skin Rejuvenation as an Adjunct to Tissue Fillers

Joshua A. Tournas
Irvine Department of Dermatology, University of California, Los Angeles, California, U.S.A.

Teresa T. Soriano and Gary P. Lask
David Geffen School of Medicine, Dermatologic Surgery and Laser Center, University of California, Los Angeles, California, U.S.A.

INTRODUCTION

Various techniques have been used for the improvement of cutaneous changes seen with photoaging to complement the effects of tissue fillers. These include dermabrasion, chemical peels, botulinum toxin, and lasers. They attain varying degrees of clinical improvement of rhytides, dyschromia, and textural irregularities. For optimal results, laser choices for attenuation of rhytides were initially limited to the CO_2 and Er:YAG lasers. These systems ablate the epidermis leading to a protracted recovery period. Prior to re-epithelialization, the initial phase of postoperative healing can be associated with significant morbidity, including serous discharge, erythema, bleeding, pain, and infection. In addition, treatments can result in complications, including hypopigmentation, hyperpigmentation, persistent erythema, and scarring (1–9). However, nonablative laser and light sources have presently gained popularity as another modality for skin rejuvenation.

BACKGROUND

The mechanisms underlying the clinical improvement seen with traditional treatments are not well understood. Photoaging from repeated sun exposure has been characterized by reduced amounts of type I collagen and decorin and by increased amounts of elastin, fibrillin, and versican (10,11). Members of the matrix metalloproteinase family have been suggested to play a role in the degradation of dermal collagen seen in photoaged skin (12). Topical applications of tretinoin and

251

alpha-hydroxy acids lead to increased papillary dermal collagen and diminished rhytides (13). Increased deposition of new collagen have been reported after CO_2 laser resurfacing, dermabrasion, and chemical peels (14–17). It has been suggested that tissue ablation leading to collagen shrinkage and new collagen deposition contribute to the clinical results after traditional laser resurfacing (18–20). In addition, changes in long-term wound healing and associated dermal remodeling likely play a role in sustained improvement. Dermal wounding and new collagen deposition have been shown with the nonablative laser devices. Several nonablative systems have become available. These systems will be discussed in this chapter.

1320 NM LONG-PULSED ND:YAG LASER

The 1320 nm long-pulsed Nd:YAG laser is a nonablative laser used for facial rejuvenation. It has a pulsed waveform composed of three 300 μs duration pulses delivered at 100 Hz pulse repetition frequency; thus, this yields a 20 ms duration macropulse containing three micropulses.

The theory behind the effect of the 1320 nm laser was the introduction of a dermal wound, which would lead to tissue remodeling and collagen deposition, in turn, causing texture and rhytid improvement. Initial work on the feasibility of this concept was reported by Lask et al. (21) and Nelson et al. (22) in 1997. Early animal studies showed that this device can cause significant epidermal damage in pursuit of the desired dermal injury. Therefore, to protect the epidermis, a dynamic cooling system developed at the University of California, Irvine was incorporated into the device. With this system, a cryogen spray was delivered to the epidermis just prior to the pulsed laser exposure by tens of milliseconds. Studies have shown that short cryogen bursts do not offer enough epidermal protection at higher fluences, and longer spray times lead to a cryogen burn on the skin. Optimal cryogen spray times have been determined to avoid epidermal disruption while allowing dermal heating with the production of procollagen I. A thermal sensor was also implemented, which aids the user to adjust the fluence, to maintain ideal therapeutic temperatures for thermal injury to the dermis, and protection of the epidermis. The ideal epidermal temperature has been determined to be between 40°C and 46°C, which corresponds to heating at a temperature approximately 25°C higher in the dermis. To achieve this target, this device is generally used at fluences ranging from 20 to 36 J/cm^2 using a 3 to 5 mm spot, and by virtue of its wavelength, allows penetration of 100 to 500 μm into dermal tissue. The 1320 nm Nd:YAG laser has tissue water as its primary chromophore, and also notable is its significant horizontal scattering (23).

Kelly et al. (24) investigated the use of the 1320 nm Nd:YAG laser for the improvement of periorbital rhytides in 1999. Thirty-five patients were enrolled at three centers, and each received three bilateral treatments at two-week intervals. All patients received EMLA which was applied one hour prior to the procedure. Pre- and post-treatment photographs were evaluated. The authors reported the following results: no improvement in patients with mild rhytides, mild improvement in those with moderate rhytides, and significant improvement in those with severe rhytides. Patients developed transient post-treatment erythema. Four sites developed blisters, with two sites resulting in pinpoint scars. The etiology of blistering is unclear; however, the authors suggest that the failure of cryogen spray release to provide sufficient epidermal cooling could have led to this adverse effect.

A study by Menaker et al. (25) studied ten patients with facial rhytides, and showed improvement in only four patients. Three patients experienced postinflammatory hyperpigmentation, and three had pinpoint scarring at three months after treatment. In three patients, skin biopsies showed an increase in the amount and degree of homogenization of dermal collagen. In one patient, there was a slight decrease in the amount of collagen. In contrast to other studies, these authors concluded that the 1320 nm Nd:YAG system was not an effective treatment for facial rhytides. The thermal feedback system was not used in this study. This could explain the adverse effects in some patients as well as the minimal improvement seen in other patients.

A number of smaller studies followed in 1999 and 2000 using the 1320 nm Nd:YAG for collagen remodeling. Goldberg treated class I–II rhytides on 10 patients with four monthly sessions using the 1320 Nd:YAG laser (26). Laser pulsing was delivered 40 ms after a dynamic cryogen cooling was applied to the epidermis for 30 ms. Peak epidermal temperatures ranged from 40°C to 48°C. Eight of the ten patients showed improvement. There were no blisters. At six months, no erythema, scarring, or pigmentary alterations were noted, and histologic evidence of new dermal collagen formation was observed in all 10 subjects. Sriprachya-anunt et al., investigated the effectiveness of the 1320 nm Nd:YAG laser in inducing collagen tightening and neocollagenesis (27). They treated three to four areas on the inner arm or buttock of ten subjects. There was no epidermal disruption seen clinically and microscopically. Immediately after the laser treatment, no detectable collagen shrinkage was noted.

Histopathologically, plump fibroblasts and a zone of collagen damage were seen. The authors suggest that the presence of activated fibroblasts may have led to neocollagenesis. In another study, Alster (28) treated patients with mild rhytides with the 1320 Nd:YAG laser and found progressive, slow improvement over a 26-week period. Side effects were limited to transient erythema. Histologic studies showed a slight increase in collagen content at the end of the study. Ruiz-Esparza (29) evaluated the 1320 nm Nd:YAG laser for full-face rejuvenation. The author treated twenty-four patients using fluences below the threshold of pain. The patients received an average of 28 twice-weekly treatments for three consecutive months. The author reported modest improvements compared to traditional ablative resurfacing. Seventeen patients displayed increased skin turgor and fourteen patients showed improvement of rhytides. Skin biopsies were performed in five patients before treatment and at six months after the last treatment. Post-treatment biopsies showed more homogenous and eosinophilic collagen, and increased dermal thickness. This study demonstrated the use of the 1320 nm Nd:YAG laser for full-face rejuvenation without the need for anesthesia or convalescence. The number and frequency of treatments may be a disadvantages to this protocol, but this may be balanced by the absence of pain and morbidity experienced by the patients.

After the above mentioned studies, further full-fledged studies were published, which were not as promising. Trelles et al. (30) used the 1320 nm Nd:YAG laser on ten patients, each of whom received twice-weekly treatments at 30 to 35 J/cm^2 for four weeks, and were seen at two and six weeks posttreatment. While the authors noted histologic improvement in all cases, only two of the ten patients expressed satisfaction with the results at six weeks. The authors were disappointed with the results, but added that further refinement of treatment techniques along with better preparation and care of the epidermis in the form of superficial peels or exfoliants may be helpful. They suggested careful patient selection and realistic expectations, which is a view also held by Romero and Alster (31). Of note in this study was the lack of long-term follow-up. The most notable clinical improvements in earlier studies were seen at four to six months posttreatment. Although initially disappointed with the results, Trelles (32) later reported in 2001 that the long-term follow-up of the patients in the above study showed "clear clinical improvement" in patients who originally had little to no improvement at a few weeks of follow-up. This reconciliation of their studies with earlier data served to establish this laser as a safe and effective treatment for facial rhytides.

1064 NM Q-SWITCHED ND:YAG LASER

The 1064 nm Q-switched neodymium:yttrium–aluminum–garnet (QS Nd:YAG) laser was used in one of the earliest clinical investigations of nonablative rejuvenation. This laser has been used widely in cosmetic dermatology for several years for the removal of tattoos and other unwanted pigmented lesions. The 1064 nm wavelength allows penetration to the desired depth for collagen remodeling. The main targets in the skin for this radiation are reported to be melanin, hemoglobin, and water (33). In addition, its short pulse duration limits tissue destruction from heat diffusion.

After initial reports of improvement of facial rhytides and acne scars using the QS Nd:YAG laser with ablative parameters (34), Goldberg and Metzler followed in early 1999 with a study using a Q-switched Nd:YAG laser in a nonablative mode. They used a low fluence Q-switched Nd:YAG laser assisted by the use of a topical carbon suspension (35). Two hundred and forty-two sites on 61 patients were each treated three times with the following parameters: fluence of 2.5 J/cm^2, pulse duration of 6 to 20 ns, and a spot size of 7 mm. These sites were evaluated at 4, 8, 14, 20, and 32 weeks for skin texture, skin elasticity, and rhytid reduction. Skin casts were taken at baseline and at 32 weeks and compared with a digital imaging system. Side effects were limited to mild and transient erythema. The authors reported improvement in all clinical parameters at eight months. This early study suggested that the QS Nd:YAG laser may be a safe and effective system for nonablative skin rejuvenation.

Newman et al. (36) also used a topical carbon suspension in their study of the QS Nd:YAG laser in 2000. Twelve patients from each of the six skin types were treated with three passes of 2.5 J/cm^2, 10 Hz–pulsed laser light with a 6.7 mm spot size. The treated areas also received a glycolic acid–based lotion post-treatment. Four treatments at 7- to 10-day intervals were given. The authors noted improvement on an average of 25% in rhytides and 20% to 35% improvement in pigmentation, as judged by blinded observers. The rhytid improvement was slightly better in lighter skin and the pigmentary improvement was slightly better in darker skin. Adverse effects included erythema, mild stinging (worse in darker skin), and folliculitis. The folliculitis was thought to be due to the oil-based carbon solution; and, the authors also noted that the glycolic acid lotion used for aftercare in hopes of reducing the folliculitis may have contributed to the clinical improvement seen.

Goldberg and Samady (37) treated 15 patients (skin types II–III) three to five times with the QS Nd:YAG laser in 2001 as part of a comparitive study between this laser and the intense pulsed light (IPL) device, which is discussed later in this chapter. Both the patient and investigator evaluations showed "mild to moderate improvement" in most patients, irrespective of the device used. The authors noted fewer adverse effects with the QS Nd:YAG laser compared to the early IPL device used in this study.

In an attempt to objectively quantify laser-induced skin changes, Friedman et al. (38) used an in vivo digital imaging device in conjunction with the QS Nd:YAG laser treatment of facial rhytides and acne scars in 2002. The single rhytid patient was treated with five treatments at two to three week intervals with 3.0 to 3.5 J/cm^2 and 6 mm spot QS Nd:YAG laser light, and exhibited an 11% improvement in skin roughness after three treatments, which increased to 26% at six months. The authors stated that the digital system produced results that correlated with clinical impression, and speculate that the system may be of great utility in comparing various laser modalities in the future.

PULSED DYE LASER

Pulsed dye lasers (PDLs) emit yellow light at wavelengths between 577 and 600 nm that are well absorbed by hemoglobin. PDL systems having a pulse duration of 450 μs to 1.5 ms have been used for several years to treat vascular lesions by providing sufficient energy with a short pulse duration to specifically target blood vessels with minimal damage to the epidermis and surrounding tissue. At 577 nm, light penetrates to a depth of 0.5 mm, increasing the wavelength to 585 and 595 nm allowing greater depth of penetration. PDLs have a low incidence of scarring; however, depending on the parameters used, the PDL can produce cosmetically unacceptable purpura. Newer PDL systems have been developed with longer pulse durations that may decrease or eliminate the incidence of post-treatment purpura. Potential benefits of the PDL for skin rejuvenation stemmed from reports of dermal collagen remodeling after treatment of striae, hypertrophic scars, and keloids (39–41).

Following reports of improvement of acne scars (42) and mild rhytides (43) with the PDL, Zelickson et al. (44) treated facial rhytides on 20 patients with this laser in a study published in 1999. The devices used in this study had a wavelength of 585 nm, pulse duration of 450 μs, spot size of either 7 or 10 mm, and an energy ranging from 3.0 to 6.5 J/cm^2. Side effects, including purpura and edema that lasted for one to two weeks were universal; two patients had postinflammatory hyperpigmentation. A total of twenty-six treated sites were available for follow-up at 12 to 14 months. Of the sites, 6/26 (23%) maintained $\geq$50% improvement, another 4/26 (15%) maintained $\geq$25%, and 7/26 (27%) were below baseline. Histopathological examination of treated areas showed a band of well-organized elastin and collagen fibers in the superficial dermis as well as increased cellularity and mucin deposition. It should be noted that the 20 patients in this study actually comprise two 10-patient populations in two different centers; different treatment devices were used, as well as different systems for pre- and posttreatment gradation of the patients' rhytides. The authors state that this may account for the discrepancy seen in the results. Patients in whom all six sites (in six patients) reported to have greater than 50% improvement were from the same center and had mild to moderately wrinkled skin, and they also represented 100% of the population available for follow-up. The observers also knew which photographs represented pre- and posttreatment. The other center represented the other 20 sites available in seven patients. None of these moderate to severely wrinkled sites reached 50% improvement, and 35% of them were actually worse at 12 months. These observers were blinded as to which photographs were pre- and posttreatment.

Zelickson and Kist (45) further investigated into the concept of collagen remodeling after PDL treatments in 2000. Seven patients each received one PDL treatment to an area of photodamage and biopsies were performed at six weeks. They demonstrated increases in the dermal procollagen, collagen I, collagen III, collagenase, and elastin in 70% to 80% of samples, as well as hyaluronate receptor in over 50%. These results suggest a process of dermal remodeling that translates into the clinical improvement of rhytides seen after PDL treatment.

Bjerring et al. (46) studied the use of another PDL (N-Lite, SLS Ltd, Llanelli, Wales, UK) for nonablative skin rejuvenation. Thirty subjects with periorbital rhytides received one laser session with the following parameters: wavelength of 585 nm, pulse duration of 350 μs, fluence of 2.4 J/cm^2, and spot size of 5 mm. Patients had minimal intraoperative discomfort. There was no postoperative pain, purpura, or pigmentary change. The authors reported clinical improvement in all patients. In addition, in ten other subjects, forearm areas were treated using the above parameters: one area received one pass, another received two passes, and a third served as the control. Suction blisters were raised seventy-two hours after laser treatment. The fluid was analyzed to determine the concentration of aminoterminal propeptide of type III procollagen (PIIINP). A significant increase in PIIINP at the sites with single pass treatment was seen; however, no significant difference was seen between the control and double-treated sites. The authors suggest that the lower increase in procollagen production at the doubly treated sites indicates that the additional energy dosage has a negative effect. They further postulate that this may be the reason why cosmetic improvement of rhytides has not been reported with PDL treatments of vascular lesions. These lesions are usually treated at higher fluences compared with that used in this trial. In addition, the authors hypothesize that interaction with the vasculature, not just direct thermal injury to dermal collagen, contributes to the mechanism of dermal remodeling. They suggest that PDL light is absorbed in the blood vessels without the intensity to cause vessel rupture, but sufficient enough to induce the release of inflammatory mediators by endothelial cells. These mediators would in turn stimulate fibroblast activity to promote dermal remodeling.

It was later realized that delivering the PDL's fluence over a longer pulse duration with the addition of a coolant spray, much like that used with the 1320 nm laser, could eliminate the post-treatment purpura seen with the older PDL devices. Rostan et al. (47) used this device (V-Beam, Candela, Inc., Wayland, Massachusetts, U.S.) in a double-blind controlled trial published in 2001 on 15 patients. Rhytides on one side of the patient's face were treated with the 595 nm PDL at 6 J/cm^2, of 6 ms pulse duration, and coolant spray, while the other side was treated with coolant spray alone as a control. The authors noted improvement in 73% of patients compared to 20% with coolant spray alone, which was statistically significant. It should be noted, however, that the overall improvement in all patients' laser-treated rhytides was 12% (which increased to 18% in the "improved" patients).

Hohenleutner et al. (48) represent the dissenting opinion, as 12 patients received a single treatment with a 585 nm PDL (2.5 J/cm^2), and at six months' follow-up, only 1 of the 12 patients reported "very" mild improvement, and the other 11 no improvement at all. It should be noted that these ratings were performed by a questionnaire, and that the physicians' opinions were not included in the results.

INTENSE PULSED LIGHT

IPL system is a nonlaser light source that has been previously reported to be of use in the removal of pigmented and vascular lesions as well as unwanted hair (49,50). It emits noncollimated, noncoherent light at wavelengths between 500 and 1200 nm. Various filters are employed to selectively block therapeutically undesirable wavelengths. In addition, it can deliver various pulse patterns, usually single, double, or triple "micropulses" with variable delay times. IPL has also been reported to improve diffuse facial erythema seen with rosacea and systemic lupus erythematosus, poikiloderma of Civatte, as well as pigment irregularities resulting from photodamage (51–53). The shorter wavelengths with this device have been shown to improve vascular and epidermal pigmented lesions. The longer wavelengths are postulated to be effective for skin rejuvenation. IPL has been investigated for nonablative treatment of isolated cosmetic units as well as for full-face rejuvenation.

Bitter and Goldman (54) reported the use of IPL in improving the cutaneous changes associated with photoaging in 2000. Thirty patients received five full-face IPL treatments at three-week intervals. The investigators sought to use subpurpuric parameters as follows: 550 nm filter, fluences of 30 to 36 J/cm^2, and double 2.4 to 4.0 ms pulses. Transient erythema lasting a few hours was seen. Less than 2% of patients were reported to have purpura or swelling, requiring a one- to three-day recovery period; no scarring was reported. Clinical results from the patient's questionnaire revealed some subjective improvement: 49% of patients reported a 75% or greater overall improvement in the appearance of their skin, 73% reported a 25% or greater improvement of fine wrinkles, and 36% reported a 50% or greater improvement of fine wrinkles. In addition, patients noted an improvement in skin smoothness, pore size, and erythema. This early observation demonstrates the potential use of IPL for nonablative rejuvenation with minimal to no patient downtime. The authors followed this with a larger study of 49 patients, each of whom received four or more treatments at three-week intervals (55). Treatment parameters were as follows: 550–570 nm filler, fluences of 30 to 50 J/cm^2, double or triple pulses of 2.4 to 4.7 ms with delays of 10 to 60 ms. The investigators generally increased the fluence by 1 to 2 J/cm^2 at each subsequent treatment as tolerated. Again, the evaluation of results was by the subjects themselves. Overall, 88% of the subjects reported being satisfied with the results of the treatments. Most notably, 46% of subjects reported > 50% improvement of fine wrinkles, around 70% reported > 50% improvement in skin smoothness, and approximately 75% of subjects reported > 50% overall improvement.

In another study, Goldberg and Cutler (56) reported mild to moderate improvement of some rhytides without epidermal ablation using the IPL system. The investigators treated 30 subjects with skin types I and II and class I–II facial rhytides. One to four treatments were performed at two-week intervals over a 10-week period. Parameters included a cutoff filter of 645 nm, and fluences of 40 to 50 J/cm^2 delivered over triple pulses of 7 ms with a 50 ms interpulse delay. At six months, 9 of 25 patients showed substantial improvement of their rhytides; another 16 showed some improvement, and five showed no improvement. All patients experienced transient post-treatment erythema; however, no erythema, pigmentary changes, or scarring was seen at six months after treatment. It should also be noted that this study used independent observers rather than the subjects as the group performing the evaluation of the results.

Goldberg (57) followed this investigation with another study to evaluate the histological changes seen after multiple IPL treatments. Facial rhytides of five patients with skin types I and II were treated over a 10-week period using a filter of 645 nm and energies between 40 and 50 J/cm^2 with triple 7 ms pulses and a 50 ms delay. Pretreatment skin biopsies showed solar elastosis. Skin biopsies performed six months after the last treatment demonstrated some degree of superficial papillary dermal fibrosis with increased number of fibroblasts scattered in the dermis. The author concluded that the IPL is the first nonlaser light source to display clinical and histological evidence of new collagen formation.

Zelickson and Kist, in the same study, examining the effects of PDL on dermal remodeling, investigated the effects of IPL on various dermal proteins (14). Periorbital sun-damaged sites on two patients were treated with a single session of IPL. Skin biopsies at six weeks displayed increased amounts of collagen type I and III, elastin, procollagen, and hyaluronate receptor. One of the two specimens also showed an increase in collagenase. This study suggests a process of dermal repair and production of extracellular matrix proteins underlying the clinical reduction of rhytides seen after IPL treatments.

Negishi et al. (58) published a study of IPL use on Asian skin in 2001. Ninety-seven patients received three to six treatments at two-to-three-week intervals. Parameters were: cutoff filter of 550–570 nm, fluences of 28 to 32 J/cm^2 and double pulse (width 2.5–5.0 ms, delay 20–40 ms). This study took into account evaluations of both the treating physician and subject, and combining their opinions, approximately 88.8% of patients reported $> 55\%$ improvement in pigmented lesions (48.4% reported $> 75\%$), along with 83.3% reaching the same threshold for telangiectasias (33.3% $> 75\%$), and 66% for skin texture (13.4% $> 75\%$). The authors report that while earlier technologies have been avoided for the most part in type IV–V Asian skin owing to the risk of postinflammatory hyperpigmentation, IPL is safe and effective in these patients.

Kawada et al. (59) contributed a 60-patient study on the IPL treatment of solar lentigines and ephilides in 2002. They found that with a 500 nm filter and a fluence of 20 to 24 J/cm^2 for three to five treatments, 28% of patients' lesions were $> 50\%$ improved, and another 20% were $> 75\%$ improved. "Microcrusts" clearing within two weeks without hyperpigmentation in 57% of patients was the primary adverse event. On histological analysis (60), the clinical appearance of the "microcrusts" corresponded with effective improvement of lesions.

More recently, Hernandez-Perez and Ibiett (61) treated five Hispanic patients with five full-face IPL sessions, one every two weeks. The authors reported subjective improvement in the severity of wrinkles, thick skin, oily skin, and dilated pores from baseline, and graded the final appearance as "good" in all five patients. Microscopic analysis showed improvement with IPL treatment in both the dermal (elastosis, edema, telangectasias, and inflammation) and epidermal (atrophy, horny plugs, loss of polarity, and basal cell liquefaction) components of photodamage.

Prieto et al. (62) studied the histological effects of IPL treatment in five patients, and, interestingly, while they did not note an increase in new collagen, they did note a decrease in Demodex organisms in perifollicular skin, to which they attribute an esthetic improvement.

RADIOFREQUENCY DEVICES

Radiofrequency (RF) devices are the most recent development in the nonablative skin rejuvenation arena. Working on the principle of using electrical energy to generate heat in a resistor (in this case the skin) in conjunction with cryogen epidermal cooling, a new RF device (ThermaCool, Thermage, Inc., Hayward, California, U.S.) has been reported to cause selective dermal heating, which can result in skin tightening (63,64). This device is designed to cause a "volumetric heating", which is unaffected by the scatter and other dispersive phenomena that plague laser light. At the time of this writing, the first studies using this device were just published by Ruiz-Esparza and Gomez (65,66): one studying the effects of this device in nonablative skin rejuvenation, and another in acne vulgaris (66). The rejuvenation study was a report on 15 patients. Patient photographs were evaluated by four independent physicians for improvement in nasolabial folds, mandibular lines, cheek contour, and marionette lines. The degree of response was variable, but the authors state that 14 of the 15 patients showed clinical improvement with a single treatment of 52 J/cm^2, with an onset of improvement ranging from one week to three to four months. Of note in this study, the patients were treated with low energy pulses, and only in the preauricular area, which the authors view as an "anchor point" through which the improvement was effected. Treating the specific locations of lines or the entire face did not result in similar improvements, and increasing the energy pulses were equally ineffective. Early results are promising, and further studies are underway.

Also in preliminary studies is a combined RF/IPL device (Aurora, Syneron, Inc., Ontario, Canada), which is reported to use the pulsed light to increase the temperature of the target tissue over that of the surroundings, which in turn lowers its impedance to RF energy, thereby achieving selective thermolysis in the treatment area. This device also incorporates a precooling mechanism as well as safety monitors for both skin temperature and impedance. It has been suggested that in combination, the two modalities present in this device may create a favorable safety and effectiveness profile (67). For both this and the above device, more work is needed before definitive conclusions can be drawn.

CONCLUSION

Soft tissue fillers are an excellent media for targeting individual areas for improvement, but when treating the entire face, adjunctive treatments can be of great utility. In light of this, nonablative dermal remodeling techniques have been developed, which are reported to induce dermal damage without epidermal disruption. This can be achieved when the following requirements are met; first, the laser wavelength and radiant exposure must be sufficient to create selective dermal wounding or induce the production of inflammatory mediators that in turn, promote collagen remodeling. Second, the epidermis must be protected from thermal damage. The studies described previously have established the effectiveness of certain systems, and studies have recently been published, which have sought to determine the optimal cooling methods and parameters for their use (68–71).

In addition, while the mechanisms underlying the clinical improvement observed after nonablative laser rejuvenation have been investigated, they require further study. This aside, nonablative skin rejuvenation has been shown to be effective with a variety of different devices, and serves as a good complement to treatment with soft tissue fillers as well as botulinum toxin.

REFERENCES

1. Waldorf WA, Kauvar ANB, Geronemus RG. Skin resurfacing of fine to deep rhytides using a char-free carbon dioxide laser in 47 patients. Dermatol Surg 1995; 21:940–946.
2. Lowe NJ, Lask G, Griffin ME. Laser skin resurfacing: Pre- and post treatment guidelines. Dermatol Surg 1995; 21:1017–1019.
3. Lask G, Keller G, Lowe N, Gormley D. Laser skin resurfacing with the Silk Touch flashscanner for facial rhytides. Dermatol Surg 1995; 21:1021–1024.
4. Lowe NJ, Lask G, Griffin ME, Mawell A, Lowe P, Quilada F. Skin resurfacing with the Ultrapulse carbon dioxide laser: Observation on 100 patients. Dermatol Surg 1995; 21:1025–1029.
5. Ho C, Nguyen Q, Lowe NJ, Griffin ME, Lask, G. Laser resurfacing in pigmented skin. Dermatol Surg 1995; 21:1035–1037.
6. Hruza GJ. Laser skin resurfacing. Arch Dermatol 1996; 132:451–455.
7. Fitzpatrick RE, Goldman MP, Satur NM, Tope WD. Pulsed carbon dioxide laser resurfacing of photodamaged facial skin. Arch Dermatol 1996; 132:395–402.
8. Fitzpatrick RE. Laser resurfacing of rhytides (review). Dermatol Clin 1997; 15:431–447.
9. Nanni CA, Alster TS. Complications of carbon dioxide laser resurfacing: An evaluation of 500 patients. Dermatol Surg 1998; 24:315–320.
10. Bernstein EF, Chen YQ, Tamai K, Shepley KJ, Resnik KS, Zhang H, Tuan R, Mauvial A, Vitto J. Enhanced elastin and fibrillin gene expression in chronically photodamaged skin. J Invest Dermatol 1994; 103:182–186.
11. Bernstein EF, Chen YQ, Kopp JB, Fisher L, Brown DB, Hahn PJ, Robey FA, Lahhakorpi J, Vitto J. Long-term sun exposure alters the collagen of the papillary dermis. Comparison of sun-protected and photoaged skin by Northern analysis, immunohistochemical staining, and confocal laser scanning microscopy. J Am Acad Dermatol 1996; 34:209–218.
12. Fisher GJ, Wang ZQ, Datta SC, Varani J, Kang S, Voorhees JJ. Pathophysiology of premature skin aging induced by ultraviolet light. N Engl J Med 1997; 337(20):1419–1428.
13. Griffiths CEM, Russman AN, Majmudar G, Singer RS, Hamilton TA, Voorhees JJ. Restoration of collagen formation in photoaged human skin by tretinoin (retinoic acid). New Eng J Med 1993; 329:530–535.
14. Ditre CM, Griffin TD, Murphy GF, Sueki H, Telegan B, Johnson WC, Ru RJ, Van Scott EJ. Effects of alpha-hydroxy acids on photoaged skin: A pilot clinical, histologic, and ultrastructural study. J Am Acad Dermatol 1996; 34:187–195.
15. Nelson BR, Metz RD, Majmudar G, Hamilton TA, Gilard MO, Railan D, Griffiths C, Johnson TM. A comparison of wire brush and diamond fraise superficial dermabrasion for photoaged skin: A clinical, immunology, and biochemical study. J Am Acad Dermatol 1996; 34:235–243.
16. Nelson BR, Fader DJ, Gillard M, Marmudar G, Johnson TM. Pilot histologic and ultrastructural study of the effects of medium-depth chemical facial peels on dermal collagen in patients with actinically damaged skin. J Am Acad Dermatol 1996; 32:472–478.
17. Fitzpatrick RE, Tope WD, Goldman MP, Satur NM. Pulsed carbon dioxide laser, trichloroacetic acid, Baker-Gordon phenol, and dermabrasion: A comparative clinical and histologic study of cutaneous resurfacing in a porcine model. Arch Dermatol 1996; 132:468–471.
18. Cotton J, Hood AF, Gonin RM, Beeson WH, Hanke W. Histologic evaluation of preauricular and postauricular human skin after high energy, short-pulse dioxide laser. Arch Dermatol 1996; 132:425–428.
19. Ross EV, Naseef G, Skrobal M, Grevelink J, Anderson R. In vivo dermal collagen shrinkage and remodeling following CO_2 laser resurfacing. Lasers Surg Med 1996; 18:38.
20. Ross EV, Yashar SS, Naseef GS, Barnette DJ, Skrobal M, Grevelink J, Anderson RR. A pilot study of in vivo immediate tissue contraction with CO_2 skin laser resurfacing in a live farm pig. Dermatol Surg 1999; 25:852–856.

21. Lask G, Lee P, Seyfzadeh M, Nelson JS, Milner TE, Anvari B, Dave D, Geronemus RG, Bernstein LJ, Mittelman H, et al. Nonablative laser treatment of facial rhytides. SPIE Proc 1997; 2970:338–349.
22. Nelson JS, Milner TE, Dave D. Clinical study of nonablative laser treatment of facial rhytides. Lasers Surg Med 1997; 95:32–33.
23. Goldberg DJ. Full-face nonablative dermal remodeling with a 1320 nm Nd:YAG laser. Dermatol Surg 2000; 26:915–918.
24. Kelly KM, Nelson JS, Lask GP, Geronemus RG, Bernstein LJ. Cryogen spray cooling in combination with nonablative laser treatment of facial rhytides. Arch Dermatol 1999; 135:691–694.
25. Menaker GM, Wrone DA, Williams RM, Moy RL. Treatment of facial rhytides with a nonablative laser: A clinical and histologic study. Dermatol Surg 1999; 25:440–444.
26. Goldberg DJ. Nonablative subsurface remodeling: clinical and histologic evaluation of a 1320 nm Nd:YAG laser. J Cutan Laser Ther 1999; 1:153–157.
27. Sriprachya-anunt S, Fitzpatrick RE, Goldman MP. The effect of 1320 nm Nd:YAG laser with dynamic cooling on human skin [abstract]. Lasers Surg Med 1999; 11(suppl):25.
28. Alster TS. Nonablative cutaneous laser resurfacing: clinical and histologic analysis. Lasers Surg Med 1999; 11(suppl):25.
29. Ruiz-Esparza J. Painless nonablative treatment of photoaging with the 1320 nm Nd:YAG laser. Lasers Surg Med 2000; 11(suppl):25.
30. Trelles MA, Allones I, Luna R. Facial rejuvenation with a nonablative 1320 nm Nd:YAG laser: A preliminary clinical and histologic evaluation. Dermatol Surg 2001; 27:111–116.
31. Romero P, Alster TS. Skin rejuvenation with Cool Touch 1320 nm Nd:YAG laser: The nurse's role. Dermatol Nurs 2001; 13:122, 125–127.
32. Trelles MA. Short and long-term follow-up of nonablative 1320 nm Nd:YAG laser facial rejuvenation [letter]. Dermatol Surg 2001; 27:781–782.
33. Jacques S. Skin optics summary. http://www.omlc.ogi.edu/news/jan98/skinoptics.html.
34. Cisneros JL, Rio R, Palou J. The Q-switched Nd:YAG laser with quadruple frequency. Clinical histological evaluation of facial resurfacing using different wavelengths. Dermatol Surg 1998; 24:345–350.
35. Goldberg D, Metzler C. Skin resurfacing utilizing a low-fluence Nd:YAG laser. J Cutan Laser Ther 1999; 1:23–27.
36. Newman J, Lord J, McDaniel DH. Nonablative laser therapy in skin types I-VI: Clinical evaluation of facial treatment using QS 1064 nm Nd:YAG laser combined with carbon suspension solution [abstract]. Lasers Surg Med 2000; 12(suppl):17.
37. Goldberg DJ, Samady JA. Intense pulsed light and Nd:YAG laser nonablative treatment of facial rhytids. Lasers Surg Med 2001; 28:141–144.
38. Friedman PM, Skover GR, Payonk G, Kauvar ANB, Geronemus RG. 3D in-vivo optical skin imaging for topographical quantitative assessment of nonablative laser technology. Dermatol Surg 2002; 28:199–204.
39. McDaniel DH, Ash K, Zukowski M. Treatment of stretch marks with the 585 nm flashlamp-pumped pulsed dye laser. Dermatol Surg 1994; 32:332–337.
40. Alster TS. Treatment of keloid sternotomy scars with 585 nm flashlamp-pumped pulsed dye laser. Lancet 1995; 345:1198–1200.
41. Alster TS. Improvement of erythematous and hypertrophic scars by the 585 nm flashlamp-pulsed dye laser. Ann Plast Surg 1994; 32:186–190.
42. Alster TS. Improvement of facial acne scars by the 585 nm flashlamp-pumped pulsed dye laser. J Am Acad Dermatol 1996; 3579–3581.
43. Kilmer SL, Chotzen VA. Pulsed dye laser treatment of rhytids. Lasers Surg Med 1997; 9(suppl):44.
44. Zelickson BD, Kilmer Sl, Bernstein E, Chotzen VA, Dock J, Mehregan D, Coles C. Pulsed dye laser therapy for sun damaged skin. Laser Surg Med 1999; 25:229–236.

45. Zelickson BD, Kist D. Effect of pulsed dye laser and intense pulsed light source on the dermal extracellular matrix remodeling. Lasers Surg Med 2000; 12(suppl):17.
46. Bjerring P, Clement M, Heickendorff, Egevist H, Kiernan M. Selective nonablative wrinkle reduction by laser. J Cutan Laser Ther 2000; 2:9–15.
47. Rostan E, Bowes LE, Iyer S, Fitzpatrick RE. A double-blind, side-by-side comparison study of low fluence long pulse dye laser to coolant treatment for wrinkling of the skin. J Cosmet Laser Ther 2001; 3:129–136.
48. Hohenleutner S, Hohenleutner U, Landthaler M. Nonablative wrinkle reduction: Treatment results with a 585-nm laser. Arch Dermatol 2002; 138:1380–1381.
49. Raulin C, Werner S, Hartschuh W, Schonermark MP. Effective treatment of hypertrichosis with pulsed light: a report of two cases. Ann Plast Surg 1997; 39:169–173.
50. Raulin C, Goldman MP, Weiss MA, Weiss RA. Treatment of adult port-wine stains using intense pulsed light therapy (PhotoDerm CL): Brief initial clinical report. Dermatol Surg 1997; 23:594–597.
51. Bitter PJ. Noninvasive rejuvenation of photoaged skin using serial, full-face intense pulsed light treatments. Dermatol Surg 2000; 26:835–843.
52. Levy JL. Intense pulsed light treatment for chronic facial erythema of systemic lupus erythematosus: A case report. J Cutan Laser Ther 2000; 2:195–198.
53. Raulin C, Greve B, Grema H. IPL technology: A review. Lasers Surg Med 2003; 32:78–87.
54. Bitter P, Goldman M. Nonablative skin rejuvenation using intense pulsed light. Lasers Surg Med 2000; 12(suppl):16.
55. Bitter PH. Noninvasive rejuvenation of photodamaged skin using serial, full-face intense pulsed light treatments. Dermatol Surg 2000; 26:835–843.
56. Goldberg DJ, Cutler KB. Nonablative treatment of rhytides with intense pulsed light. Lasers Surg Med 2000; 26:196–2000.
57. Goldberg DJ. New collagen formation after dermal remodeling with an intense pulsed light source. J Cutan Laser Ther 2000; 2:59–61.
58. Negishi K, Tezuka Y, Kushikata N, Wakamatsu S. Photorejuvenation of Asian skin by intense pulsed light. Dermatol Surg 2001; 27:627–632.
59. Kawada A, Shiraishi H, Asai M, Kameyama H, Sangen Y, Aragane Y, Tezuka T. Clinical improvement of solar lentigines and ephelides with an intense pulsed light source. Dermatol Surg 2002; 28:504–508.
60. Kawada A, Asai M, Kamayama H, Sangen Y, Aragane Y, Tezuka T, Iwakiri K. Video-microscopic and histopathological investigation of intense pulsed light therapy for solar lentigines. J Dermatol Sci 2002; 29:91–96.
61. Hernandez-Perez E, Ibiett EV. Gross and microscopic findings in patients submitted to nonablative full-face resurfacing using intense pulsed light: a preliminary study. Dermatol Surg 2002; 28:651–655.
62. Prieto VG, Sadick NS, Lloreta J, Nicholson J, Shea CR. Effects of intense pulsed light on sun-damaged human skin: routine and ultrastructural analysis. Lasers Surg Med 2002; 30:82–85.
63. Hardaway CA, Ross EV. Nonablative laser skin remodeling. Dermatol Clin 2002; 20:97–111.
64. Sadick NS. Update on nonablative light therapy for rejuvenation: a review. Lasers Surg Med 2003; 32:120–128.
65. Ruiz-Esparza J, Gomez JB. The medical face lift: a noninvasive, nonsurgical approach to tissue tightening in facial skin using nonablative radiofrequency. Dermatol Surg 2003; 29:325–332.
66. Ruiz-Esparza J, Gomez JB. Nonablative radiofrequency for active acne vulgaris: The use of deep dermal heat in the treatment of moderate to severe active acne vulgaris (thermotherapy): a report of 22 patients. Dermatol Surg 2003; 29:333–339.
67. Kreindel M, Waldman A. Unpublished data.

68. Chang CWD, Reinisch, Biesman BS. Analysis of epidermal protection using cold air versus chilled sapphire window with water or gel during 810 nm diode laser application. Lasers Surg Med 2003; 32:129–136.

69. Svaasand LO, Randeberg LL, Aguilar G, Majaron B, Kimel S, Lavernia EJ, Nelson JS. Cooling efficiency of cryogen spray during laser therapy of skin. Lasers Surg Med 2003; 32:137–142.

70. Edris A, Choi B, Aguilar G, Nelson JS. Measurements of laser light attenuation following cryogen spray cooling spurt termination. Lasers Surg Med 2003; 32:143–147.

71. Aguilar G, Wang GX, Nelson JS. Dynamic behavior of cryogen spray cooling: Effects of spurt duration and spray distance. Lasers Surg Med 2003; 32:152–159.

12

ArteFill® Augmentation of Wrinkles and Acne Scars

Gottfried Lemperle
Division of Plastic Surgery, University of California, San Diego, California, U.S.A.

INTRODUCTION

Collagen was introduced in 1979 as the four dermal filler material and was extremely well received (1). This was the substance we were all waiting for. Although it is still one of the safest materials for injection into the dermis, early enthusiasm has quieted because of its short duration of action.

My experience for the last four decades with all kinds of autologous grafts, including dermis, fat, cartilage, bone, and tendon is that they disappear at sites where they do not maintain their native biological function. With most of these grafting materials there is little left behind after a few months, except scar tissue. In order to promote collagen deposition over a longer period of time, one has to stimulate the connective tissue constantly with a scaffold of nonresorbable foreign material (2). In an attempt to find a solution to this problem, we studied all types of powders from different synthetic materials already known to be successfully used in medicine (3). The material with least tissue reaction was the bone cement, which consists of various sizes of polymethyl-methacrylate (PMMA) microspheres and many attached impurities.

To further purify this powder and increase its biocompatibility, we isolated a certain fraction of microspheres, 30 to 42 μm in diameter (Fig. 1). This is the ideal size that is large enough to escape phagocytosis (4), but small enough to be pressed through a fine 27 G needle and be able to pass into the network of the collagen fibers of the deep dermal layer. The smaller the microspheres, the larger is the overall surface area and, therefore, the promotion of collagen deposition. Microspheres of a diameter of 100 μm promote only about 56% connective tissue; microspheres of a diameter of 40 μm promote about 78% connective tissue (2).

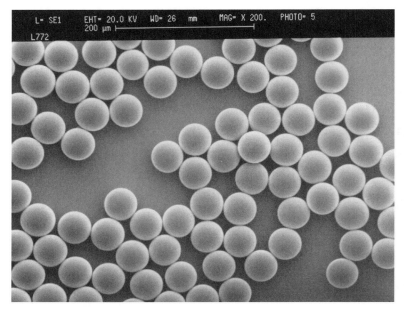

Figure 1
After sieving and multiple washing, the microspheres in Artecoll® have a
diameter of 32–40 μm and an absolute smooth surface (× 400).

MATERIAL

ArteFill® is a suspension of 20% PMMA microspheres of 30 to 42 μm
diameter in 80% collagen solution. For the reduction of pain during
implantation, 0.3% lidocaine is added. Its further purified success product
ArteFill is manufactured and distributed by Artes Medical Inc., 5870
Pacific Center Blvd., San Diego, CA 92121, U.S.A. ArteFill is supplied
in syringes of 0.9 and 0.5 mL content and designed for implantation into
the deep reticular dermis.

Artecoll received its certification, the CE mark as a medical
device for the European market as of September 1996, in Canada as of
September 1998, and in Mexico as of May 1999. Artecoll is distri-
buted and well accepted worldwide except in Japan and in the United
States. Clinical trials of ArteFill in United States (Artes Medical Inc.)
have been conducted at eight centers (5,6) and were completed in
September 2001. The results have been submitted to the U.S. Food and
Drug Administration (FDA) in March 2002. Final FDA approval of
ArteFill is expected in December 2005.

The advantages of ArteFill are:

1. modern "Aesthetic Tissue Engineering[TM]" technology,
2. absolute smooth surface of the microspheres,
3. indications similar to those of collagen and hyaluronic acid,

4. ease of injection despite higher viscosity than collagen,
5. permanent stimulation of connective tissue and collagen deposition,
6. long-lasting esthetic effect over many years, and
7. low rate of granuloma formation similar to collagen and hyaluronic acid injections.

BIOCOMPATIBILITY

Animal experiments have documented (2–4) that the key to ArteFill biocompatibility is the absolutely smooth surface of the microspheres. This accounts for its low incidence of granuloma formation. The effect of Artecoll is not only that of being a filler substance but also, a life-long stimulation of collagen deposition beneath the wrinkles. In comparison, some other longer lasting injectables contain particles with an irregular surface (2). Particulate materials such as polyurethane foam or silicone particles on the surface of textured breast implants are designed to cause a chronic granulomatous tissue reaction (2). Microscopically, the prevalent cells are foreign body giant cells or "frustrated macrophages" (13). ArteFill contains six million PMMA microspheres per ml. Therefore, there exist six million tiny capsules of connective tissue surrounding the microspheres like smooth walled breast implants. The microspheres provide merely a scaffold to promote connective tissue deposition. The carrier volume of 80% partly denatured collagen is replaced with the same percentage during the first month by the body's own fibroblasts and collagen fibers, and this process persists over the years (Fig. 2).

INDICATIONS

ArteFill is an excellent medium to achieve minimally invasive, lasting improvement of facial wrinkles and furrows.

There is a broad spectrum of well-defined medical and esthetic indications for the use of ArteFill outlined in Tables 1 and 2; most are similar to the indications of Zyplast® and Restylane®. The best candidates are patients with well-defined wrinkle lines and furrows and little excess skin. If a patient is unsure about the permanency of Artecoll or the achieved effect, an initial implantation of collagen or hyaluronic acid is recommended. Patients with sebaceous skin and big pore size, or extremely thin and loose skin are poor candidates for ArteFill as the implants might be palpable, shine through, or even be visible in such patients.

Allergy testing is required by the FDA to minimize the risk of hypersensitivity reactions, especially in patients who are treated with a collagen product for the first time. We recommend an intradermal test injection four weeks prior to the planned ArteFill implantation. Clinical

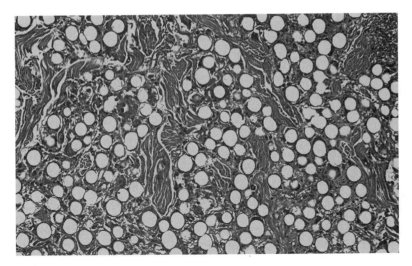

Figure 2
Histology ten years after an Artecoll® implantation shows still-active fibroblasts, micro-encapsulation of each single microsphere, capillary ingrowth, and little foreign body reaction (× 100).

trials (Rofil Medical International, B.V., Breda, The Netherlands) with the same collagen as contained in ArteFill, have revealed that the allergy rate to this special form of "denatured" bovine collagen is extremely low (0.1%).

Table 1 Aesthetic Indications for ArteFill® in the Face
Horizontal forehead lines
Glabellar frown lines
Shadowed lower lids
Single crow's feet
Oblique malar depressions
Malar bone augmentation
Irregularities of the nose
Augmentation of the tip of the nose
Nasolabial folds
Cheek lines
Preauricular lines
Lip augmentation
Philtrum augmentation
Unpleasant gummy smile
Perioral lip lines
Negative corners of the mouth
Marionette lines
Horizontal chin fold
Chin augmentation
Horizontal neck folds

> **Table 2**
> Medical Indications for ArteFill® with Demonstrated Successful Outcomes
>
> ---
>
> Depressed "rolling" acne scars
> Bony defects in the face and hand
> Small skull defects, drill holes
> Enophthalmos after blow out fracture
> Sunken eye prosthesis
> Tripod fracture of the malar bone
> Flat operated cleft lip, missing philtrum
> Depressed or asymmetric ala of the nose
> Uvula augmentation in snoring
> Alveolar ridge augmentation in toothless patients
> Scleroderma, mild Romberg's syndrome
> Facial wasting, facial lipodystrophy
> Visible borders of facial implants
> Vocal cord paralysis
> Inverted nipples, nipple augmentation
> Small funnel chest
> Gastro-esophageal reflux disease
> Urinary incontinence
> Fecal incontinence

TECHNIQUE

The method of implanting Artecoll is more technique-sensitive than injecting collagen or hyaluronic acid. It will take some practice and patience with a quick learning curve to develop a feel for the correct injection pressure. Therefore, it is best to start treatment on easier creases like the glabellar frown lines.

We recommend using the "tunneling technique," that is, moving the needle forth and back linearly just beneath the wrinkle (Fig. 3). Since the viscosity of ArteFill is three times higher than that of Zyplast (8), a higher and constant pressure must be applied throughout the injection procedure depending on the tissue and depth of placement. This simple addition to technique is easily and quickly mastered. ArteFill will give a long-lasting correction of facial folds if implanted correctly. It is important to place it in the right deep dermal plane and to not overcorrect, as this can be permanent.

Local anesthetic is suggested as there is slightly more pain on injection than with collagen. If there is no indication for a field block as in the lips, we suggest a topical anesthetic (EMLA®-cream) in very sensitive patients, applied 30 to 60 minutes before the procedure.

Generally, 27 or 26 G needles of 1/2 or 3/4 inch length should be used. Longer needles cause more resistance to thumb pressure, resulting in lower pressure within the tissue. The thickness of the needle is used to determine the thickness of the dermis much like a depth gauge. The outer diameter of a 30 G needle is 0.3 mm, of a 27 G needle is 0.4 mm (Fig. 4),

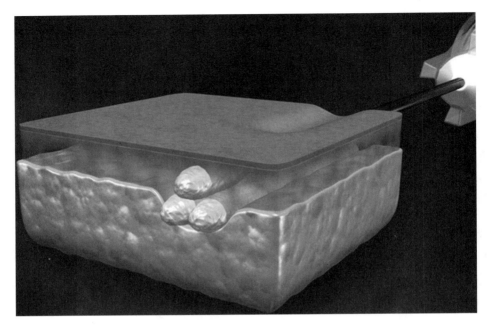

Figure 3
The "tunneling technique" is preferred over the microdroplet technique because
of even distribution of ArteFill®.

and of a 26 G needle is 0.45 mm. The thickness of facial skin varies
between 0.2 mm (lids), 0.4 mm (nasolabial folds), and 0.8 mm (frown
lines). The thickness of the skin in a deep crease is diminished to about
one-fourth of its normal thickness.

At the start of the procedure, make sure that the needle is not
blocked by gently squeezing one drop of ArteFill out of its tip. Now
insert the needle—while maintaining constant thumb pressure to the
syringe—into the skin beneath and along the line of the wrinkle and start
injecting, while withdrawing the needle. The dermis is much thinner than

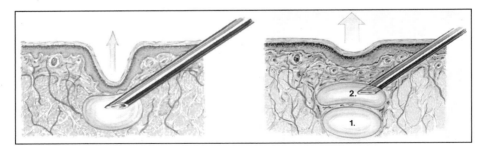

Figure 4
(*Left*) The first ArteFill® implant provides a "splint" to the wrinkle. (*Right*) A second
touch-up causes the diminished thickness of the dermis in a crease to recover to its
former thickness.

you think! *Artecoll should be implanted deep intradermally only, e.g., into the reticular dermis just above the junction between dermis and subcutaneous fat* (Fig. 4).

If the needle is in the right plane, resistance from the reticular dermis will be felt. If the needle is placed too deep, there will be only little resistance from the fatty tissue. If ArteFill is injected within the papillary dermis, a blanching effect will be seen. Should the needle be in the papillary dermis, stop injecting immediately and restart implantation one needle diameter (0.4 mm) deeper. You should always see the outline of the needle; however, the gray of the needle must never shine through the skin. ArteFill accidentally implanted within the papillary dermis will cause a blanch effect. To correct this easily, you should immediately distribute the injected material into the surrounding tissue with firm "scraping" motions of your fingernail.

At the end of each implantation, the implant is not massaged but palpated with the fingertip and slight pressure is applied to any detected lump only. Be aware that vigorous massage will spread the Artecoll deeper into the tissue, where it is lost. The theory and goal here is not only to augment the diminished thickness of the dermis but *to support the wrinkle* and thereby prevent it from further motion. If this is the case, the diminished thickness of the dermis recovers itself within three months! This fact is based on the observations of many patients, whose furrows disappeared only three months after implantation of ArteFill and has been documented on photographs during the clinical trial of ArteFill in the United States (6).

Interestingly, it has been observed in elderly patients with facial palsy or after a CVA, that in time, most furrows seem to disappear on the paralyzed side of the face. This serves to demonstrate that even in older patients, the dermis in a furrow is able to recover its previous thickness! The same mechanism may apply to facial creases after ArteFill implantation, as the creases are no longer wrinkled to the same extent as before.

Implant Volume

With the exception of the soft lips, overcorrection with ArteFill is not easy to create as there is usually a certain density in the reticular dermal tissue layer that will allow only a certain amount of this more viscous filler. Therefore, a second touch-up implantation of Artecoll on top of the first "splint" is often required at a later date for an optimal result [Fig. 4 (right)].

However, the amount of internal scar formation differs from patient to patient as has been learned from capsule formation around breast implants. As granulation tissue must invade the space between the microspheres (and will eventually make up to 80% of the implant) a few subsequent treatments are recommended rather than one "bulk" treatment.

For example, a first implantation of up to 0.8 cc ArteFill will be sufficient for the frontal furrows or both glabellar frowns, one nasolabial fold, either upper or lower lip, both corners of the mouth, both marionette lines, or two neck folds, respectively. A second treatment may become necessary after three to six weeks. In pedantic acne patients, up to 20 cc of ArteFill have been used over time; in facial bone augmentation up to 50 cc ArteFill.

Patient Instructions

ArteFill can be dislodged from the deep dermal site of implantation into deeper layers through pronounced facial muscle movement within the first three days, diminishing the expected result. Little nodules may form, especially in the lips and corners of the mouth. To prevent this, immobility is important within the first three days. As a reminder for the patient and to keep ArteFill evenly distributed, the implant site can be taped with Blenderm® or Transpore® (3M Company, Minneapolis, Minnesota, U.S.A.) for about three days. Patients are cautioned that there could be some swelling for the first 12 to 24 hours and areas of light pink coloration along the injection sites for two to five days that are easily covered with make-up.

Patients are told that the treated folds will improve over time. They must know that ArteFill can sometimes be felt as a rubber-like substance—or can be seen as a white substance eventually, when stretching the lips. A second implantation between the ArteFill "base" and the dermis of the wrinkles will give them a lasting effect.

ArteFill will receive FDA approval for the treatement of nasolabial folds only. However, in November 1997, a new provision was added to the Federal Food, Drug and Cosmetic Act, to allow any legally marketed, FDA-approved product to be administered for any condition within a doctor–patient relationship. This is called the "off-label use" of an FDA approved product.

SPECIFIC TREATMENT AREAS

Horizontal Forehead Lines

These respond well to treatment with ArteFill. The gray of the needle should not show through the wrinkle line. Superficial intradermal implantation may result in the formation of small granules like a string of pearls within the line. In deeper wrinkle lines, a second and third session is required.

Glabellar Frown Lines

Glabellar lines generally pose no problems as the dermis is thick and the connective tissue beneath provides a good support for the implant (Fig. 5). In case a slight overcorrection is necessary, care must be taken to not inject too far caudally—otherwise a lump produced by gravity may appear at the inner limit of the eyebrow. Deep lines and furrows require repeated treatments. Here, they can be placed intradermally because of the thickness of the skin.

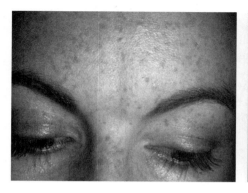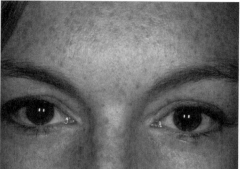

Figure 5
A median glabellar frown line augmented with 0.3 mL ArteFill®.

Shadowed Lower Lids

A dark ring along the nasal jugular groove or arcus marginalis is a good indication for ArteFill. The thin skin together with the orbicularis occuli muscle must be lifted from the infraorbital rim with a band of ArteFill of 2 to 3 cm in length. The implantation has to be strictly epiperiosteal, i.e., beneath the orbicularis occuli muscle and just in front of the insertion of the orbital septum. The bone can be felt with the tip of the needle. On retracting the needle slightly, ArteFill can be spread along the lower orbital rim. Care must be taken to withdrawing the needle without pressure, as implantation into the muscle will cause a nodule and bruising is easy in this area. In severe cases, the insertion of a small implant (9) may be more effective.

Single Crow's Feet

ArteFill is indicated only in single crow's feet in a patient with thick skin. However, multiple crow's feet in a patient with thin and flaccid skin are a contraindication, as the implant may be seen through and may appear as fine granules. A heavily wrinkled lid skin is better improved by laser resurfacing or botulinum toxin.

Facial Wasting and Cheek Depressions

Certain patients may develop a depression or hollowing of their cheeks in front of the canine fossa or in the submalar region. This circumscribed atrophy of the malar fat pad and adjacent subcutaneous fat is pronounced in patients with facial lipodystrophy who are on HIV medication (10). ArteFill implanted subdermally in mild cases, or epiperiosteally in severe cases, will be of great benefit. In severe cases, the atrophied Bichat's fat pad can be augmented by means of small silicone gel implants (11) or custom-made implants, which may be less expensive than a huge volume of ArteFill.

Irregularities of the Nose

Irregularities of the nose, especially after rhinoplasty or due to collapsed nostrils (12), can be improved easily through deep epiperiosteal or epichondreal placement of ArteFill. The patient should be instructed to mold the implant during the following three days, if necessary. In patients with an acute nasolabial angle, it may be helpful to implant a triangle of ArteFill subdermally at the columellar and nasal base.

Nasolabial Folds

Nasolabial creases are best supported by two to three bands of ArteFill implanted parallel and strictly medial to the fold (Fig. 6). During the first three days, Artecoll is still a paste and may be moved laterally by facial muscle movement. Therefore, it should be implanted directly beneath and about 1 to 2 mm medial to the crease. Care must be taken not to implant too superficially. In patients with very thin skin, the implant site may appear erythematous for several weeks and the implant may be visible in the form of little granules. A second implantation is often necessary, especially in the lower nasolabial crease adjacent to the corner of the mouth. Close to the nostrils, a fan-like injection technique is recommended.

Lip Augmentation

Lip augmentation is one of the most rewarding indications for ArteFill, if it is done correctly! There is a natural pocket between the white roll and the orbicularis oris muscle (13), which should be filled. We recommend the use of local anesthetic for the augmentation of the upper and lower lip. Our technique is to inject lidocaine 1 cc of a 2% solution beneath the mucosa of the upper and lower labiogingival fold to achieve a field block. After two minutes, one can direct the needle coming from lateral

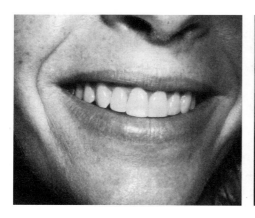 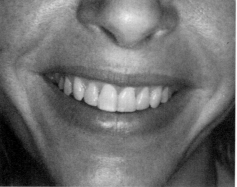

Figure 6
(*Left*) Nasolabial folds augmented with 1.7 ml ArteFill®. (*Right*) Eighteen months later.

into the correct plane. Usually, one half of the lip can be implanted by slowly withdrawing the needle while injecting. A volume of 0.5 to 1.0 cc of ArteFill is sufficient for each lip. A bigger volume may result in a dense mass and pain, so care is taken to augment the lips in stages. If ArteFill is well tolerated and the lips are soft after three months, more ArteFill can be added to the same pocket (Fig. 7) (14).

A flattened philtrum can be raised effectively by two vertical injections of ArteFill starting from below, e.g., from the two corners of Cupid's bow within the white roll. Only rarely does the implant dislodge into the surrounding tissue. In such a case, it becomes necessary to mold the implant between two fingers into the philtrum or the white roll. Injection should be by linear threading, and under no circumstances should the point injection technique be used in the outer lip.

However, microdroplets of ArteFill applied horizontally along the wet border increases the pouting effect (Fig. 8). ArteFill must never be implanted into the orbicularis oris muscle, since this may cause dislodging and nodule formation. ArteFill must not be superficially injected into the red vermilion of the lip as it will feel hard and may appear white when the lip is stretched. Be aware that submucosally implanted ArteFill may always be felt with the tongue or the teeth. Sensitivity to touch and kissing may last up to one year.

Avoid injecting ArteFill into an upper lip that has excessive vertical height, since this may further lengthen the lip and hide the front teeth even more. In this case, a prior or simultaneous lip lift through a subnasal excision is recommended.

ArteFill is not indicated in larger defects of the vermilion such as cleft lip whistle deformity because the implant may become hard. However, ArteFill implantation has resulted in an outstanding improvement of the missing white roll and philtrum after cleft lip surgery.

Gummy Smile

I am reminded of one of my patients who disliked her gummy smile so much that she kept a mass of chewing gum in her upper labiogingival sulcus. ArteFill 1 to 2 cc placed epiperiosteally in a horizontal direction in front of the roots of the upper incisors will remedy this. This works

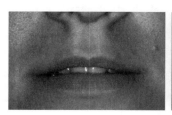 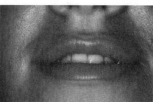 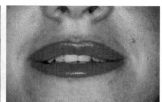

Figure 7
(*Left*) Small upper lip augmented with 1.8 mL Artecoll® in three sessions; (*center*) three years later; (*right*) ten years later. *Source*: From Ref. 12.

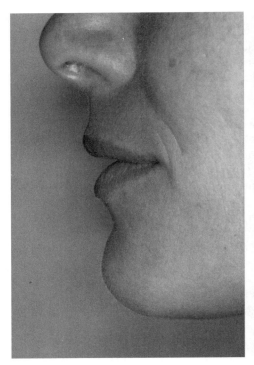 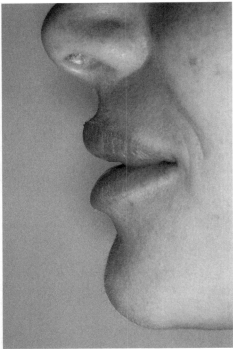

Figure 8
Microdroplets of ArteFill® implanted horizontally along the dry–wet border
increased the pouting effect of the upper lip.

even better if you elevate the muco-periosteum under local anesthesia,
inject the ArteFill, then close the incision. In severe cases, however, the
insertion of a small implant is preferable (16).

Perioral Lip Lines

Radial upper lip lines extend from tiny notches in the vermilion border,
both of which cause the lip to appear aged and lipstick to smudge. In a
younger patient with good projection of the white roll, these wrinkles
can be treated vertically from above. In patients with more than four
lines, the effect will be increased even by injecting transversely across
the entire white roll.

In the elderly patient, filling of the white roll and Cupid's bow prevents future development of radial lip lines (Fig. 9). Additional augmentation of the lost philtrum from below may give the lip a more youthful
look (15).

Negative Corners of the Mouth

They appear to be the most difficult but also a very rewarding site for
ArteFill treatment [Fig. 9 (right)]. First, the lower white roll is augmented

horizontally about 1 cm in length from the corner. Then, 5 to 10 vertical and horizontal threads of ArteFill should be placed using a criss-cross technique. This supports the area and slightly lifts the corner of the mouth. It may be helpful to extend some of the implant around the upper lip in a C-shaped fashion. Be aware that if the skin is relatively thin, implanting Artecoll too superficially may result in telangiectasias.

On the other hand, if the implant is placed into or close to muscle, nodule formation may result. Preferably, ArteFill should be implanted in many different tunnels and always in two sessions. If ArteFill is implanted into the orbicularis oris muscle, it will be formed into a pearl by the muscle movement and will be felt inside the cheek.

Marionette Lines

The vertical elongation of the dystopic corners of the mouth, as they extend to the mandibular border, can be greatly improved by linear threading and deep intradermal criss-cross implantation of ArteFill (Figs. 9 and 10).

Horizontal Chin Fold

The skin in the area of the mentolabial fold is relatively tight and this fold is difficult to fill with ArteFill (Fig. 10). Therefore, most patients will need a second or third implantation (Fig. 11). There is a danger of granule formation in the fold if ArteFill is implanted too superficially in the skin. If this happens, these can be removed easily by dermabrasion.

Horizontal Neck Folds

The dermis of the neck is extremely thin. Therefore, a test implantation of 2 cm in length is recommended to avoid subsequent overcorrection. Implantation results are favorable in the young patient, but often a second treatment is needed. An aged and flaccid neck is a contraindication

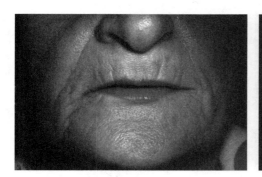 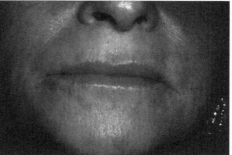

Figure 9
In elderly patients, filling of the white roll with 0.6 mL ArteFill® flattens radial lip lines up to 5 mm. Negative mouth corners must be filled very superficially and horizontally.

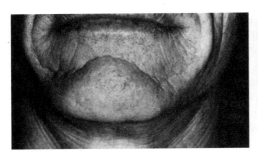
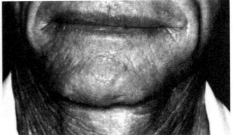

Figure 10
(*Left*) Deep horizontal chin fold augmented with 0.8 mL ArteFill® in one
session. (*Right*) Four years later.

for ArteFill. Patients with dark skin must know that underlying
hyperpigmentation in the folds could be more obvious after augmentation.

Nipple Augmentation

Flat nipples and inverted nipples grade 1 and 2, e.g., those, which can be
stimulated to protrude, and those with volume asymmetries can easily be

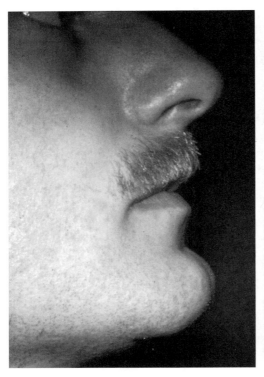
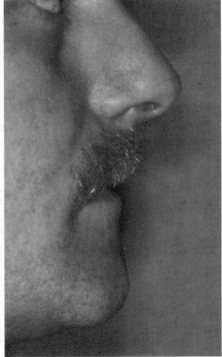

Figure 11
(*Left*) Young man who did not like his chin. (*Right*) Three years later after
augmentation of the horizontal chin fold with 2.4 ml ArteFill® in four sessions.

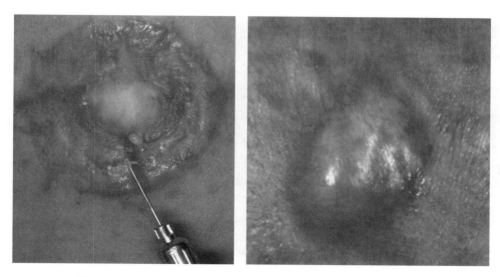

Figure 12
Nipple augmentation in a reconstructed breast. Artecoll® is especially suitable in equalizing asymmetries.

augmented with 0.25 to 0.5 cc of ArteFill (Fig. 12). Applying deep local anesthesia beneath the nipple, the amount of augmentation that the patient wants is estimated. After waiting for 10 minutes until the fluid has been resorbed, the nipple is lifted up and ArteFill is implanted from the side, moving the needle forth and back in order to avoid implantation into the ducts. If some material ends up in the ducts, this can easily be removed by massage. So far, there is no evidence that the ducts have been blocked by external implantation of ArteFill. The natural swelling during pregnancy will open these ducts anyway. If inverted nipples grade 3 and 4 are to be treated, ArteFill implantation without blind severance of all ducts would increase the crater! Therefore, the ducts are first cut as deep as possible and the ArteFill is implanted three to four days later.

Acne Scars

ArteFill is very effective for mature mildly depressed "rolling" (17,18) acne scars (Fig. 13). These can be filled either horizontally from a distance of 5 to 10 mm or in "boxcar scars" perpendicularly downwards directly into the center, continuously guiding the needle back and forth. Alternatively, a Microdroplet Delivery Device (MDD) can be used. Fresh scars should not be treated as they may not show improvement but may even worsen.

Ice-pick scars require pretreatment. They should be punched and sutured or subcised with a No. 11 blade or a double-beveled NoKor needle at a depth of about 1 mm (19). The fresh wound cavity can easily be

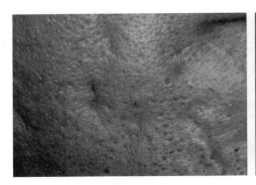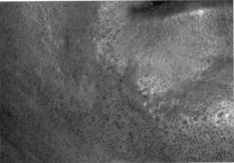

Figure 13
"Rolling" acne scars effectively leveled with 0.4 mL Artecoll®.

filled with ArteFill three to five days later, after the swelling has subsided and the incision wound has firmly closed.

COMBINED TREATMENTS

Laser Treatment

Laser treatment is no contraindication for ArteFill. It is a complimentary treatment, since both ArteFill and laser are effective in different layers of the skin. Laser peeling of the epidermis can be done either three to six months before or preferably immediately after ArteFill implantation. Swelling (edema) of the wrinkle lines and furrows enhances the laser effectiveness.

Dermabrasion and Chemical Peelings

Dermabrasion and chemical peelings are effective in the same superficial plane as laser resurfacing, e.g., in the epidermis and papillary dermis. Therefore, none of these three interfere with the implantation of ArteFill, which is deeper in the reticular dermis. ArteFill implantation can be performed weeks before or after the resurfacing procedure (Fig. 14).

Face-Lifts

Face-lifts in general do not affect sufficiently pronounced nasolabial folds and deep marionette lines. The treatment of choice for nasolabial folds should be a mid face–lift; however, this may cause scleral shows in certain patients (20). Therefore, deep nasolabial or labiomental creases can be augmented with ArteFill just prior to the surgical procedure in the same session (Fig. 15).

Botulinum Toxin

Since temporary paralysis of certain facial muscles does not permanently eliminate facial furrows or wrinkles, ArteFill is an excellent adjunct to

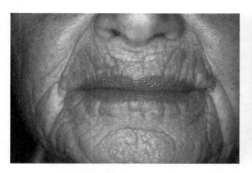 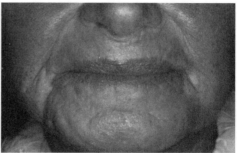

Figure 14
(*Left*) 75-year old patient, whose deep radial lip lines and right marionette line have been treated with 2.0 mL Artecoll® just before dermabrasion. (*Right*) Two years later.

BOTOX treatment. ArteFill can be implanted concomitantly or at a later time. In fact, the long-term augmentation effect resulting from ArteFill is enhanced by the paralyzing effect of BOTOX, which eliminates the motion in a particular wrinkle line and therefore enhances ArteFill's success as a collagen remodel.

POTENTIAL SIDE EFFECTS

Technical

Because of its long-lasting effect, ArteFill is not forgiving. Uneven distribution in the form of a string of pearls (Fig. 16) must be compensated by a second implantation of Artecoll into the created gaps. ArteFill implanted too deeply is ineffective and the procedure must be repeated. Implantation done too superficially can cause long-lasting itching and redness, which should be treated with corticosteroid cream or intradermal corticosteroid injections.

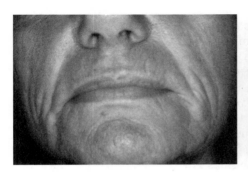 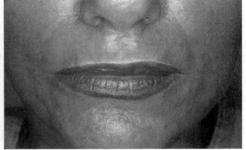

Figure 15
A 62-year-old patient with a face-lift after nasolabial folds, radial lip lines, and marionette lines had been augmented with 2.5 mL Artecoll®.

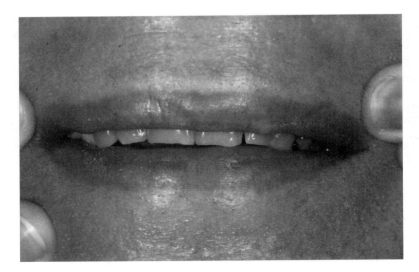

Figure 16
Pearl string of Artecoll® in upper lip after nonrecommended injection into vermilion. Symmetry was achieved by filling the white roll horizontally.

Intradermal granules may be removed by dermabrasion. Excision and suturing is rarely necessary. Dislodged nodules caused by intramuscular implantation should be softened through intralesional corticosteroid injections or, if caused by intraoral implantation, require excision. Excision of a nodule should always be thorough since any residual ArteFill may potentially cause secondary hypertrophic scarring.

Allergic Reactions

The PMMA microspheres are nonallergenic; however, as with all collagen preparations, allergic reactions to ArteFill are a possibility. There was only one patient with a systemic allergic reaction reported to the manufacturer of the same denatured collagen as in ArteFill (Resoderm®, Rofil Medical International) among 10,000 patients involved in a clinical trial. I have experienced only two acute allergic reactions among more than 3000 patients after Artecoll implantation: both patients had negative tests before treatment. Unfortunately, such an event cannot be prevented even by double testing.

One case of severe *anaphylactic shock* after the eighth treatment session with Artecoll occurred in Italy in 1997. The possibility of *sensitization to collagen* after multiple injections has been described and must be kept in mind for ArteFill as well. So far, the histology of excised granulomas or secondary allergy testing has not shown an allergic cause of nodule formation (21,22). Furthermore, all late allergy reactions of type IV described for collagen (23) must be expected after ArteFill implantation as well.

Telangiectasia

Telangectasia may occur at the implantation site in patients with very thin skin. It usually disappears within six months; however, it may require laser treatment.

Hypertrophic Scarring

Hypertrophic scarring has been reported and seen in our patients as well. ArteFill is supposed to evoke a tissue reaction with typical granulation tissue at the beginning, and later scar formation in the form of millions of microscopic capsules (Fig. 2). As known from smooth-walled breast implants, this capsule formation can be more or less pronounced in different individuals. After too superficial implantation of Artecoll, the treated fold may rarely convert into a hypertrophic scar (Fig. 17) but will react favorably to repeated intralesional Kenalog® injections.

Disappearance of the Implant

PMMA-microspheres are nonphagocytosable by macrophages or giant cells and nondissolvable by enzymes. Therefore, the microspheres will remain intact beneath the crease as long as the patient lives. However, if injected too deeply, it will remain in the subcutaneous fat without an effect on the crease. This often happens at the start of the learning curve.

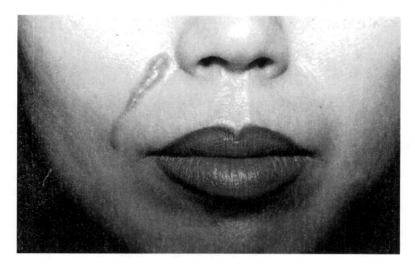

Figure 17
A single case of hypertrophic scarring in a Korean woman after Artecoll® was implanted too superficially. No reactions in the left nasolabial fold and in glabellar frown lines. One injection of Kenalog leveled the scar.

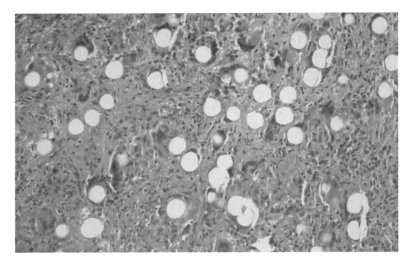

Figure 18
Histology of a rare case of a "true" Artecoll® granuloma. Multinucleate giant cells and epitheloid histiocytes increase the distance between the single beads three- to five-fold compared to a normal histological reaction. *Source*: From Ref. 22.

Another possibility is the implantation of the collagen carrier alone. Collagen melts at 40°C or under heavy pressure. If ArteFill is exposed to heat or sunlight, the gel may melt and the collagen fluid is pushed through the microspheres, which then remain in the syringe and block the needle.

On the other hand, facial muscle movement over several years will push the implant about one-tenth of a millimeter deeper and the crease may reappear after 5 to 10 years. Then, another ArteFill implant on top of the previous support [Fig. 4 (right)] is advisable.

Granuloma Formation

Today, true granuloma formation is a rare event in less than 0.02% of patients and may occur 6 to 18 months after Artecoll treatment (15). The pathologist will diagnose each normal granulation tissue surrounding the microspheres as a foreign body granuloma (21). Histologically, however, a growing Artecoll granuloma (22) shows a wide distance between the microspheres filled with macrophages, giant cells, fibroblasts, and broad bands of collagen fibers (Fig. 18). The cause is not understood as they appear to developed often after a second or third implantation of Artecoll. One half of the reported patients trace the onset of granuloma formation back to a severe infection (influenza) or facial injury. On the other hand, granuloma formation occurs in selected patients at a rate of 0.01% to 0.1% after treatment with all injectable tissue fillers like collagen (23), hyaluronic acid (24), and particulate injectables (21,22,25). Intralesional injection of corticosteroid crystals is the treatment of choice.

To be absolutely safe in certain patients, one can administer a test dose of ArteFill behind the ear and wait for a determined period of time prior to a more extensive ArteFill treatment.

TREATMENT OF COMPLICATIONS

Hypertrophic scarring, nodules, accidentally dislodged or too much ArteFill, as well as real granulomas, react well to intralesional long-term crystalline corticosteroids. Local steroids inhibit fibroblast activity and collagen deposition, macrophage activity and giant cell formation, and swelling, itching, or pain. A 1:1 mixture of lidocaine and triamcinolone (Kenalog® or Volon-A®) up to 20 mg or betamethasone (Diprosone®) up to 5 mg can be injected safely through a 1 ml syringe with Luer lock and a 30 G needle. It must be injected strictly into the nodule while guiding the needle back and forth, as corticosteroids injected into the surrounding tissue may cause temporary skin atrophy. In the case of skin atrophy, temporary filling with collagen or hyaluronic acid will level the indentation until natural recovery occurs within 3 to 12 months.

Since every patient reacts differently to corticosteroids, one has to increase the dose eventually. Two to five sittings in three-week intervals may be necessary. If this therapy is started early and aggressively, surgical excision will be of no issue. The danger of cortisone atrophy might be reduced by the injection of antimitotic agents (26). 5-Fluoro-uracil (mixed with 1/3 Diprosone and 1/3 Lidocaine), as well as Bleomycin, have been injected intralesionally (27) into keloids. Minocycline (2 × 100 mg daily) has been given systemically along with prednisone in diffuse silicone granulomas (28).

There is no longer-lasting result in plastic surgery than a bad result (James M. Stuzin). An early aggressive treatment of complications (29) or a simple touch-up may be preferred to a long-lasting untoward sequela.

CONCLUSION

During its ten years of clinical use, Artecoll has proved to be a reliable and predictable soft tissue filler substance. Having almost solved its initial problems of granuloma formation, ArteFill still requires a learning curve because of its higher viscosity and persistence. Technical mistakes in the form of uneven distribution, implantation into facial muscles, and injection into the subcutaneous fat are common at the beginning and have caused many physicians to stop implanting Artecoll. However, if the skills have improved, and the knowledge on the effect of crystalline corticosteroids has given self-confidence, the number of satisfied patients will increase.

There is a widening spectrum of rejuvenation procedures on the esthetic market (2), where each procedure may find its niche. Many of them are complementary to each other. Even the most sophisticated face-lifting procedure does not eliminate a deep nasolabial fold. Chemical peels or laser resurfacing of mouth, lids, and cheeks are effective ways to get rid of all superficial fine wrinkles but do not level the deeper radial lip lines, for instance. Botulinum toxin is a safe way of paralyzing the frontal and orbicularis oculi muscles for a short period; it may cause reversible but distressful muscle paralysis in the lower face. Implants for facial bone augmentation may not be of the right size or may not fit exactly. In all these cases, ArteFill can be used as a perfect adjunct at the same time or later.

The vast range of medical and esthetic indications of ArteFill (Tables 1 and 2) can be widened by new applications such as the implantation into shrunken gingival margins, as a stabilizer of a loose uvula in snoring, or as a bulking agent in cleft palate patients. The prospective use as a bulking agent in urinary and fecal incontinence, in gastro-esophageal reflux disease (GERD), or in vocal cord paralysis may be just a few of the many new indications.

SUMMARY

Most of the biological filler materials that increase the thickness of the corium in a wrinkle line are phagocytized within a certain time. Therefore, a lasting effect can be achieved consistently only with nonresorbable synthetic substances. ArteFill consists of 20 volume % microspheres of PMMA and 80 volume % collagen. Beneath the crease, the microspheres with their exceptional surface smoothness stimulate fibroblasts to encapsulate each one of the six million microspheres contained in 1 ml of Arte-Fill. Collagen is merely a carrier substance that prevents the microspheres from clumping during tissue ingrowth. The 20 volume % microspheres in ArteFill provide the scaffold for the 80 volume % of connective tissue deposition, a true replacement of the injected collagen. The filler material beneath a fold acts as a support and prevents the possibility of its further folding, thereby allowing the diminished thickness of the corium in the crease to recover. This recovery process is well known even in elderly patients with facial paralysis or following a stroke, whose facial wrinkles and furrows on the paralyzed side disappear over time.

Since 1994, its predecessor Artecoll has been used in more than 250,000 patients worldwide, except in the United States, with a low serious complication rate (29). Because of its higher viscosity and its persistence, technique-related side effects may occur at the beginning of its use. A steep learning curve on the physician's part and the knowledge of the effect of corticosteroids, however, prevents these solvable side effects. Patient satisfaction after ArteFill treatment is above 90%; they may experience an optimal result only after three months when the thickness of the dermis in a wrinkle or fold has recovered.

REFERENCES

1. Klein AW. Injectable bovine collagen. In: Klein AW, ed. Tissue Augmentation in Clinical Practice. Procedures and Techniques. New York: Marcel Dekker, 1998:125–144.
2. Lemperle G, Morhenn VB, Charrier U. Human histology and persistence of various injectable filler substances for soft tissue augmentation. Aesth Plast Surg 2003; 27:354–366.
3. Lemperle G, Ott H, Charrier U, Hecker J, Lemperle M. PMMA microspheres for intradermal implantation. Part I. Animal research. Ann Plast Surg 1991; 26:57–63.
4. Morhenn VB, Lemperle G, Gallo RL. Phagocytosis of different particulate dermal filler substances by human macrophages and skin cells. Dermal Surg 2002; 28:484–490.
5. Hamilton D. A pilot study of the first patients treated in United States with ArteFill implantation for the aging face. Cosmet Dermatol 2001(sept.):47–51.
6. Cohen SR, Holmes RE. Artecoll: A long-lasting injectable wrinkle filler material: report of a controlled, randomized, multicenter clinical trial of 251 subjects. Plast Reconstr Surg 2004; 114:964–976.
7. Eppley BL, Summerlin D-J, Prevel CD, Sadove AM. Effects of positively charged biomaterial for dermal and subcutaneous augmentation. Aesth Plast Surg 1994; 18:413–416.
8. McClelland M, Egbert B, Hanko V, Berg RA, DeLustro, F. Evaluation of ArteFill polymethylmethacrylate implant for soft-tissue augmentation: Biocompatibility and chemical characterization. Plast Reconstr Surg 1997; 100:1466–1474.
9. Yaremchuk MJ. Infraorbital rim augmentation. Plast Reconstr Surg 2001; 107:1585–1592.
10. Chastain MA, Chastain JB, Coleman III WP. HIV lipodystrophy: Review of a syndrome and report of a case treated with liposuction. Dermatol Surg 2001; 27:497–500.
11. Hasse FM, Lemperle G. Resection and augmentation of Bichat's fat pad in facial contouring. Eur J Plast Surg 1994; 17:239–242.
12. Lemperle G, Gauthier-Hazan N, Lemperle G. PMMA microspheres (ArteFill) for long-lasting correction of wrinkles: Refinements and statistical results. Aesth Plast Surg 1998; 22:356–365.
13. Feldman SG. ArteFill, Bioplastique, and beyond. In: Klein AW, ed. Tissue Augmentation in Clinical Practice. Procedures and Techniques. New York: Marcel Dekker, 1998:293–306.
14. Lemperle G, Hazan-Gauthier N, Lemperle M. PMMA microspheres (ArteFill) for skin and soft-tissue augmentation. Part II: Clinical investigations. Plast Reconstr Surg 1995; 96:331–334.
15. Lemperle G, Romano JJ, Busso M. Soft tissue augmentation with ArteFill: 10-year history, indications, technique and complications. Dermatol Surg 2003; 29:573–587.
16. Pessa JE, Peterson ML, Thompson JW, Cohran CS, Garza JR. Pyriforme augmentation as an ancillary procedure in facial rejuvenation surgery. Plast Reconstr Surg 1999; 103:683–686.
17. Jacob CI, Dover JS, Kaminer MS. Acne scarring: A classification system and review of treatment options. J Am Acad Dermatol 2001; 45:109–117.
18. Hirsch RJ, Lewis AB. Treatment of acne scarring. Semin Cutan Med Surg 2001; 20:190–198.
19. Lemperle G. Surgical methods of dermaplaning severely damaged acne skin. Plast Surg Products 2002; 12:21.
20. Lemperle G. Das Midface-Lifting. In: Lemperle G, ed. Aesthetische Chirurgie. Landsberg: Ecomed, 1998 (chapter IV-4).
21. Rudolph CM, Soyer HP, Schuller-Petrovic S, Kerl H. Foreign body granulomas due to injectable esthetic microimplants. Am J Surg Pathol 1999; 23:113–117.
22. Requena C, Izquierdo MJ, Navarro M, et al. Adverse reactions to injectable esthetic microimplants. Am J Dermatopath 2001; 23:197–202.

23. Hanke CW. Adverse reactions to bovine collagen. In: Klein AW, ed. Tissue Augmentation in Clinical Practice. Procedures and Techniques. New York: Marcel Dekker, 1998:145–154.

24. Shafir R, Amir A, Gur E. Long-term complications of facial injections with Restylane (injectable hyaluronic acid). Plast Reconstr Surg 2000; 106:1215–1212.

25. Bergeret-Galley C, Latouche X, Illouz Y-G. The value of new filler material in corrective and cosmetic surgery: DermaLive and DermaDeep. Aesth Plast Surg 2001; 25:249–255.

26. Fitzpatrick RE. Treatment of inflamed hypertrophic scar using intralesional 5-FU. Dermatol Surg 1999; 25:224–232.

27. Espana A, Solana T, Quintanilla E. Bleomycin in the treatment of keloids and hypertrophic scars by multiple needle punctures. Dermatol Surg 2001; 27:23–27.

28. Senet P, Bachelez H, Ollivaud L, Vignon-Pennamen D, Dubertret L. Minocycline for the treatment of cutaneous silicone granulomas (letter). Br J Dermatol 1999; 140:985.

29. Lemperle G, Gauthier-Hazan N, Wolters M, Eisemann-Klein M, Nievergelt H. Foreign body granuloma after all injectable dermal fillers: possible cause, and treatments. Plast Reconstr Surg 2006; 117(suppl): in press.

13

Restylane® and Perlane®

Fredric S. Brandt and Andres Boker
Department of Dermatology, University of Miami School of Medicine, Miami, Florida, U.S.A.

To many people, the coming of advancing age in the cycle of life and the numerous changes that accompany it is often bittersweet. Although there are scores of benefits that maturity and adulthood bring to human life, the passage of time certainly takes its toll. Because of modern society's constant preoccupation with beauty and youth, and the relentless pressure to preserve them, one great concern for many such adults is the esthetic evolution that goes along with their advancing age.

As a result, the continuously increasing demand for facial rejuvenation procedures and the equally broad array of available treatment options that emerge day to day, makes the optimal approach to facial renewal a task not to be taken lightly by the practicing dermatologist or plastic surgeon.

While plastic surgery remains an excellent option for long-term facial esthetic improvement, some patients may face monetary and time restraints as well as possible risk assessment uncertainty when considering this option for themselves. Surgery usually entails longer recuperation time, higher cost, and more risks, including the possibility of having a bad "job" done that will also last longer.

Other treatment options like facial resurfacing procedures, and the use of chemical peels and lasers, although satisfactory, usually yield subtle results, are not suited for all individuals and are sometimes considered to be aggressive or too invasive.

Injectable filler substances have long been used for the correction of wrinkles associated with aging and a wide selection of different materials have come and gone over the past 30 years. Until now, the gold standard of soft tissue augmentation was considered to be bovine collagen, which over the last 20 years has proved to be safe and durable and carries a high degree of patient satisfaction. However, the need for a material that lasted longer and was less immunogenic (e.g., required no skin testing), prompted the development of new products from both biologic and synthetic sources, which addressed these requirements. As a result of this came the development of hyaluronic acid (HA) and its derivatives, which since its initial isolation from the bovine vitreous in the 1930s, has been widely investigated and its chemical structure improved. Over the last decade, hylans have shown great clinical significance in a variety of medical conditions, including vesicoureteral reflux, urinary stress incontinence, osteoarthritis, and cellular therapy and encapsulation. Furthermore, its solid safety profile and increased longevity have prompted its use as an injectable substance for soft tissue augmentation. The most common sources of HA are rooster combs, umbilical cord, vitreous humor, tendons, skin, and bacterial cultures. In 1996, the Swedish company Q-Med launched the first commercial product of bacterial-derived HA for cosmetic use under the trade name Restylane®, and since then, approximately 500,000 patients have been treated successfully for wrinkle correction and/or lip enhancement worldwide (1). Two newer forms, Restylane Fine Lines and Perlane, were recently approved by the CE-mark in Europe and are now available. At present, with over six years of clinical experience in the cosmetic field worldwide, the Restylane family of products promises to establish themselves as the standard of treatment for soft tissue augmentation in the new millennium.

THE AGING HUMAN FACE

To better comprehend the appropriate use of injectable fillers for facial rejuvenation and soft tissue augmentation, it is of utmost importance to have a clear understanding of the underlying processes occurring in the aging face. Luckily, the skin represents an accessible and easily understandable model for the comprehensive study of factors that contribute to the complex phenomenon of aging. This subject has been the object of devoted research for decades, especially as one of its most advocated goals is the popular sought-after desire of facial wrinkle prevention.

The fundamental basis for facial esthetics is the existence of a harmonious relationship between the hard and soft tissues of the face (2). Various factors, including the force of gravity, muscular pull, and skeletal remodeling processes, affect this balance between the skeletal structure of the face and the soft tissue covering it. Therefore, with the progressive loss of soft tissues with the passage of time, the youthful appearance of a full face is lost, making the more evident bony structural elements a paramount sign of aging. Both inherent and environmental elements play an important role in this process and jointly contribute to the premature loss of facial structural balance.

Chronologic (intrinsic) aging affects the skin in a manner similar to that affecting other organs, in which a reduced collagen deposition resulting from diminished biosynthesis and reduced proliferative capacity of fibroblasts, results in an atrophy and apparent tissue volume loss in the dermal layer of the skin (3). Furthermore, the coexisting loss of elastin fibers, the oxidative stress imposed upon the lipid bilayer of cell membranes and dermal proteins, the nonenzymatic glycosylation of proteins, and the reduced repair capacity to re-synthesize both collagen and elastin fibers, contribute to and accelerate the degenerative changes occurring in the senescent skin (Fig. 1) (4,5).

Some authors explain this process as the result of a programmed change in gene expression in mitotic cells (keratinocytes and fibroblasts) and a cumulative damage in postmitotic cells, with a consequent disruption of tissue integrity and function due to loss of cellular components and accumulation of senescent cells and their byproducts (6).

Overall, this process can be regarded as an imbalance between the biosynthesis and degradation of dermal connective tissue proteins, with less regenerative capacity in face of ongoing degradation.

It is well known that collagen provides its tensile properties to the dermis and that it accounts for up to 80% of the dry weight of the skin, giving it its contour and providing underlying structures with a protective barrier against external trauma (3). Thus, substantial collagen and elastin depletion will ultimately result in a loss of skin fullness and a failure of proper tissue protection and support, making it look thin, with a paper-like appearance, while keeping a smooth wrinkle-free surface (Fig. 2) (7).

On histological examination, intrinsically aged skin shows general atrophy of the extracellular matrix with decreased elastin and disintegration of elastic fibers (7). Other features include the decline in epidermal turnover rates made evident by a decrease in epidermal thickness and a flattened dermoepidermal junction with effacement of dermal papillae (8).

These findings may collectively lead to an increased fragility of the skin and in conjunction with the previously discussed pathophysiological mechanisms, add to the decreased epidermal regenerative capacity that ensues with advancing age.

Superimposed on this inherent process is the injury resulting from environmental (extrinsic) factors, mainly sunlight ultraviolet–induced photodamage to the dermal connective tissue of the exposed skin. This may be the most important contributing factor responsible for the *premature* senescence of the skin and is, therefore, the main target of preventive measures in the maintenance of cutaneous health and preservation of youth.

The consequence of the combined effects of both intrinsic and extrinsic factors is a series of cellular changes and qualitative as well as quantitative alterations of dermal extracellular matrix proteins, resulting in a loss of recoil capacity and tensile strength of the skin, and ultimately leading to the formation of wrinkles (9,10).

Now, having understood the way by which the face loses its youthful and full appearance with advancing age, one can recognize that one of the cornerstones of facial rejuvenation is the replacement of lost volume using injectable filler substances. Thus, soft tissue augmentation aims to restore the natural facial biconvexity and accentuate individual features, as well as to fill in facial furrows and wrinkles to achieve an esthetically pleasing result.

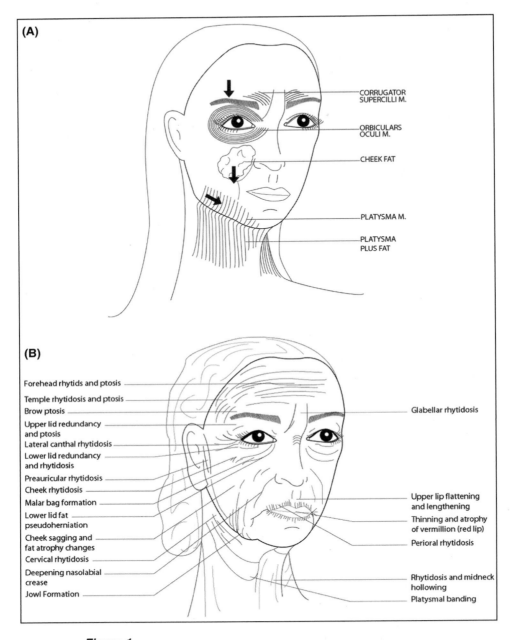

Figure 1
The effect of aging on the human face. (**A**) Gravitational and muscular pull on the facial structures. (**B**) Common topographic changes observed.

(A)

(B)

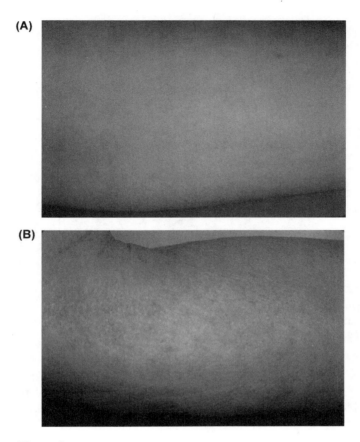

Figure 2
The effect of time on human skin. (**A**) Youthful skin. (**B**) Aged and photo-damaged skin.

OVERVIEW OF HA AND NASHA PRODUCTS

HA is a naturally occurring glycosaminoglycan biopolymer composed of linked alternating residues of the monosaccharides D-glucuronic acid and *N*-acetyl-D-glycosamine. It is an important structural element of the intercellular matrix in a variety of human tisses including the skin, subcutaneous and connective tissues, and synovial tissue and fluid. HA has an identical chemical and molecular form in all living organisms and is therefore, in its pure form, highly biocompatible and species nonspecific (11,12).

The importance of this viscoelastic substance in the extracellular space is reflected by its critical physiological activities, such as creating and maintaining tissue volume, providing structural support and cellular protection, and facilitating intercellular motility and communication (13). It has been noted that a direct correlation exists between the content of HA and the content of water in dermal tissue, and therefore, the

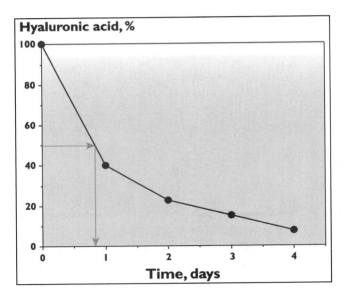

Figure 3
Disappearance rate of hyaluronic acid from the skin. *Source*: Q-Med AB, Uppsala, Sweden.

viscoelastic properties of the extracellular matrix. With advancing age, the concentration of HA acid in the skin decreases along with its ability to bind water, thus making the dermal matrix less voluminous and the overlying skin more prone to wrinkling (14).

In physiological circumstances, exogenous HA acid is degraded by the body's inflammatory processes at implantation sites almost immediately (Fig. 3) (15).

Consequently, it is evident that, to confer clinical usefulness to the material as an injectable filler, the chemical structure of natural HA must be modified to obtain a product with a reasonable in situ residence time. Various approaches have yielded different products, each with distinct chemical structures (16). As such, in the mid 1980s hylan B gel (Hylaform; McGhan Medical, Santa Barbara, California, U.S.A.) was developed using rooster combs as the source of HA. The cross-linking of the HA molecules was achieved through the addition of vinyl sulfone, which created an infinite molecular network based on bonds between the polysaccharide dimers. This method gave the product its viscous properties and water insolubility, and enhanced its resistance to degradation while preserving its extraordinary capacity to bind water (17,18). Nonanimal stabilized hyaluronic acid (NASHA) products (Restylane, Perlane and Restylane Fine Lines; Q-Med, Uppsala, Sweden) on the other hand, are produced with HA derived from bacterial cultures and are merely stabilized by a partial cross-linking method. The stabilization is a two-step process in which the addition of an epoxide results in a cross-link between a minor portion (< 1%) of the disaccharides in the

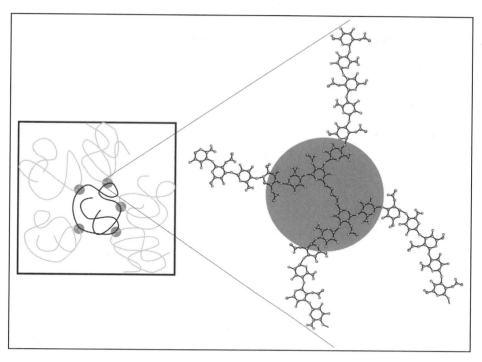

Figure 4
Stabilized NASHA molecule. *Source*: Q-Med AB, Uppsala, Sweden.

HA molecule. This allows the formation of a three-dimensional molecular network, which is stable and extremely elastic. NASHA products thus have a long duration with preserved biocompatibility (1,19; Fig. 4). Furthermore, neither chemical cross-linking nor stabilization changes the biological compatibility of the native polymer, hence preserving its inert nature and maintaining its vital functions in the extracellular matrix. It is also important to point out that the bioengineering process utilized for NASHA's production yields a highly pure form of HA, making it very unlikely for impurities or other contaminants to be present in the final product.

Although the gel particle size differs in the Q-Med products, the overall NASHA gel concentration is identical: 20 mg/mL of stabilized HA. This concentration has been selected to provide an optimal maintenance of volume for tissue augmentation and lifting, and is believed to increase residence time in the tissues. However, NASHA, like other biodegradable implants, is slowly broken down after injection. With conventional biodegradable implants, this has the disadvantage that the implant progressively shrinks and the esthetic benefit therefore quickly diminishes. In NASHA products, the slow biodegradation of the stabilized HA does not lead to gradual shrinkage, since the amount of HA in a NASHA gel bead is about five times greater than what is needed to maintain its volume. The surplus material supposedly makes the gel

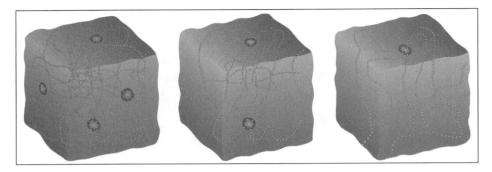

Figure 5
Isovolumetric degradation of NASHA products. *Source*: Q-Med AB, Uppsala,
Sweden.

last longer. This process is called isovolemic degradation and it allegedly
maintains the volume of correction until the stabilized gel is almost completely degraded (Fig. 5). When the gel is completely degraded, the
remaining HA fragments are metabolized along with the natural tissue
HA, and no trace of the original implant remains. Before degradation,
however, the size of the gel beads that remain in the tissue match the tissue matrix density at the level of injection (Fig. 6).

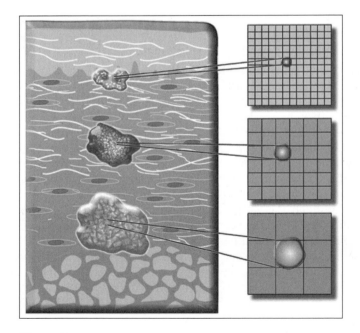

Figure 6
Injection level of Restylane® products. The mesh size in the illustration represents the density of extracellular structural elements—mainly collagenous and
elastic fibers—at varying levels. *Source*: Q-Med AB, Uppsala, Sweden.

The immunogenicity and allergic reactions elicited by NASHA products is a subject of ongoing debate. It is unclear whether some of these responses are due to protein components of the molecular complex or due to the HA acid itself. Some authors like Micheels suggest that the incidence of antibodies against HA directly is higher than in patients treated with ... although these findings remain to be corroborated and are inconclusive. Based on anecdotal surveillance data and preliminary data from recently completed clinical trials, however, the incidence of these allergic reactions and the frequency of antihyaluronic acid antibodies were extremely low. Nonetheless, if this new family of products promises to become the next generation for use in facial soft tissue augmentation, this issue clearly needs further investigation to draw more solid conclusions, and to reassure both physicians and patients about the safety and response of these materials.

Restylane®

Restylane (NASHA) has been approved in Canada, Australia, Europe, and South America as a medical device for the treatment of cutaneous contour deformities, and is widely used in the treatment of facial wrinkles and lip augmentation. It is currently undergoing clinical testing in the United States and the approval of the U.S. Food and Drug Administration (FDA) is being sought in the near future (Fig. 7).

As described earlier, Restylane is a stabilized form of HA acid moieties with highly elastic properties, which makes it an ideal material for soft tissue augmentation. It is extremely biocompatible and a number of pre-clinical animal studies have shown that Restylane does not induce dermal sensitization in guinea pigs and does not cause any significant reactions during rabbit muscle implantation tests. Additional testing has also revealed a lack of mutagenicity (Ames test), genotoxicity (mice

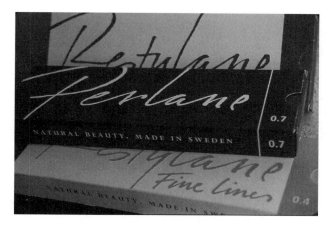

Figure 7
Product packages.

bone marrow micronucleus study and invitro chromosomal aberration study in mammalian cells), and cytotoxicity (20).

These findings were consistent with results obtained during the conduction of two clinical trials using Restylane for soft tissue augmentation therapy (21,22).

Olenius (22) conducted an open, nonrandomized multicenter trial for the assessment of the safety and efficacy of Restylane injections in the treatment of facial scars and wrinkles in a total of 112 patients (105 women and seven men) who received treatment (285 sites were treated) for depressed cutaneous scars and wrinkles. The most commonly treated areas were nasolabial folds (NLFs), glabellar lines, and lines at the corners of the mouth. Touch-up treatments were administered to 188 sites. Follow-up was performed at 1, 12, and 26 weeks following treatment. A week-52 evaluation was conducted on a subset of 20 patients selected at random. At each evaluation, the physician rated the site for degree of correction (VAS), feeling (firmness), texture (smoothness), color, and degree of improvement. Restylane effectively corrected the lesions, and the patient and physician evaluations were in close agreement. Based on the physician's evaluation, the average degree of correction was 79% at week 1 and 98% at week 2 (following the "touch-up" injections). The degree of correction declined slowly with time, from 82% at week 12 to 66% at week 52. Restylane was well tolerated and the most commonly observed side effects were erythema and swelling, which resolved in a few days. There were very few adverse experiences reported beyond the immediate procedure-related effects. These events included redness (six patients), acneiform changes (two patients), darkening of the treated area (two patients), tics (two patients), "bumps" at injection site (two patients), and telangiectasia (one patient).

Duranti et al. (22) conducted another open, nonrandomized trial for the assessment of the safety and efficacy of Restylane injections in the treatment of facial scars and wrinkles, and for lip augmentation or recontouring. A total of 158 patients (all female) received treatment (273 sites were treated). The most commonly treated areas were NLFs, glabellar lines, oral commissures, and the lips for augmentation. Touch-up treatments were administered after 8 to 10 days as required. Follow-up was performed at zero, one, two, four, and eight months following treatment. Unlike the VAS-based ratings used in the Olenius trial, this study utilized a five-point categorical rating: no improvement (0%), slight improvement (1–33%), moderate improvement (34–66%), marked improvement (67–100%), and overcorrection. Fifteen patients were excluded from the trial; 11 due to the requirement for "further implants," and four who were lost to follow-up. This left an effective sample size of 143 patients. At eight months 78.5% of patients had moderate or marked improvement based on the physician's assessment. The degree of improvement declined slowly with time, and appeared to be similar for most anatomic areas (although the degree of improvement for NLFs appeared to be somewhat higher than the others). The proportion of patients with "marked improvement" for lip augmentation was 88.5%, 79.5%, 64.1%, 43.6%, and 29.5% at zero, one, two, four, and eight months, respectively. The material was again well tolerated, and side effects ranged from mild erythema and swelling to bruising (three cases) and pain (one case). Typically, resolution was spontaneous within one to two days after injection into the skin and within a week after injection into the lips. Additionally, temporary palpable lumpiness has been noted after use in some patients.

Simultaneously, histological evaluations were conducted on a group of five subjects who received implants of both Zyplast® and Restylane on their arms. Four pairs of implants (0.05 mL) were placed intradermally (two pair on each arm) and were evaluated by visual inspection and blinded evaluation of biopsy specimens at 4, 12, 24, and 52 weeks. Biopsy samples were stained with hematoxylin, Pirco-Sirius (for Zyplast), and Toluidine blue (for Restylane). These histological methods resulted in a red staining of Zyplast (if present) and blue staining of Restylane (if present). The histological evaluation was performed by two pathologists who were unaware of the nature of the samples, and were asked to evaluate the tissue with respect to inflammation, foreign body reaction, and fibrosis. In addition, they were asked to describe the presence and the nature of the implant in the biopsy specimen.

The results revealed that Zyplast disappeared 12 to 24 weeks after implantation. In contrast, Restylane was qualitatively detected in all injection sites after 24 weeks and in 20% (4 of 20 implants) of injection sites after 52 weeks. Samples from both productions revealed a varying (grade 0–1) reaction as determined by histology. One subject had a slight histological reaction (grade 1–2) to Restylane.

In our experience, side effects have been similar to the ones reported and patient's response is generally very satisfactory. Furthermore, results are quite predictable and the material is easy to inject. Its composition is set to balance a normal tissue pressure; however, as the tissue pressure is sometimes disturbed to a higher value such as that during edema or to a lower value such as that during a low fluid intake, a small but significant change (swelling or shrinkage) of the material may occur. Restylane is injected into the mid-dermis through a 30 G needle.

Based on postmarket surveillance data, reactions thought to be of a hypersensitivity nature have been reported in about 1 in every 2000 treated patients. Other reports have indicated a higher incidence for antibodies to HA products in general (23). The reactions include swelling and induration at the implant site, sometimes with edema in the surrounding tissues. Erythema, tenderness, and rarely, acneiform papules may also occur. The reactions start either shortly after injection or after a delay of two to five weeks, and have been described as mild to moderate and self-limiting with an average duration of two weeks. In pronounced cases, a short course of oral steroids may prove effective. Patients who have experienced this type of reaction should not be re-treated with Restylane. These findings raise the question if skin testing is necessary for patients desiring the use of these products, and if it should be done regardless of the low incidence of allergic reactions (24).

There is a potential risk with the procedure that the material could be inadvertently injected into dermal blood vessels, which could lead to vascular occlusion and corresponding consequences. No such cases have been reported to date with Restylane.

Perlane®

Perlane is essentially the same material as Restylane, and is produced by the same method of stabilization of bacterial-derived HA molecules. The difference lies in the particle size of the gel beads. Thus, Perlane contains on average 8000 gel beads/mL in contrast to 100,000 gel beads/mL contained in Restylane. As mentioned, the concentration of NASHA remains constant (20 mg/mL). The thicker nature of Perlane also warrants the use of a larger 27 G needle to allow the easy passage of the material. Perlane is injected into the deeper layer of the dermis and is, therefore, intended for use in deeper cutaneous depressions and folds (Fig. 6).

Owing to the almost identical characteristics of both products, the results from pre-clinical studies with Restylane can also be applied to the pre-clinical assessment of Perlane.

Although there are no published data from studies on Perlane, a very similar array of side effects as those observed with Restylane injection can be expected in the clinical setting. Common injection-related reactions include erythema, swelling, pain, itching, and tenderness at the implant site. The injection of Perlane is usually reported to be more painful by patients, and sometimes warrants the use of an intraoral or infraorbital nerve block. Other side effects that are more frequent, but not unique, to Perlane are the formation of superficial bumps or blanching of the skin, when the injection is done too superficially.

Restylane® Fine Lines

Restylane Fine Lines is produced by the same manufacturing process as Perlane and consists of stabilized HA moieties. The difference lies only in the density of the gel and the particle size. It contains 200,000 gel beads/mL and the size of the beads is 150 μm. The concentration of NASHA is the same as with the other two products and is 20 mg/mL. Restylane Fine Lines is intended for the correction of thin, superficial lines like those surrounding the eyes and mouth. Its safety and side effect profile is very similar, if not identical, to Restylane and Perlane.

CLINICAL USE AND INJECTION TECHNIQUE

Augmentation of a cutaneous deformity essentially intends to fill a depression in the contour of the skin with an appropriate material. As such, it is not intended to alter the texture of the skin and would not correct any defects in pigmentation. An increase in the firmness of the underlying tissue, swelling, or discoloration would represent an adverse outcome. Initial correction of the contour deformity is an issue affected by the physician's injection technique, the volume administered, and the product's characteristics (e.g., viscosity and rapid or uneven volume loss). The desired result is one that is primarily esthetic; the patient seeks an improvement in the physical appearance of a contour deformity without causing any noticeable difference in the surrounding tissue. As the benefit of tissue augmentation is the correction of a visible defect, the clinical significance of any potential treatment can also be defined as a difference that can be detected visually.

UPPER FACE

Forehead Lines

The forehead region of the face is an area commonly used during facial expression, especially in patients who constantly elevate their eyebrows. In this part of the face, it is important to make a distinction between dynamic and nondynamic wrinkles, as they should have a different therapeutic approach. The more evident coarser horizontal lines are of muscular origin and are caused by the habitual use of the underlying frontalis muscle (25). Botulinum toxin is a valid and very effective treatment modality for this type of lines as paralyzing the muscle will prevent the overlying skin from wrinkling caused by repeated motion (26). However, finer lines resulting from chronic photodamage and chronologic aging of the skin, respond better to a filler agent as part of the fundamental mechanism is a loss of underlying dermal tissue and therefore, depletion of volume (Fig. 8).

Injection Technique

As forehead lines tend to be superficial, Restylane Fine Lines would be the treatment of choice for this area. It is injected into the superficial dermis with a 32 G needle, and no overcorrection is performed as this will result in visible papules that can last several months. When injecting the material, serial puncture technique is utilized (Fig. 9). Although injected superficially, the material should not be visible after injection.

Glabella—Worry Lines

Glabellar lines are bilateral and reasonably symmetrical, vertical wrinkles localized between the eyebrows. They arise as a result of prolonged muscular action and photodamage. The muscular group responsible for motion in this area is comprised of the corrugator supercilii, frontalis, and procerus muscles. Its function is brow adduction, moving the eyebrow and skin downward, and giving rise to the glabellar crease medially (27,28). The direction of these creases and wrinkles is usually

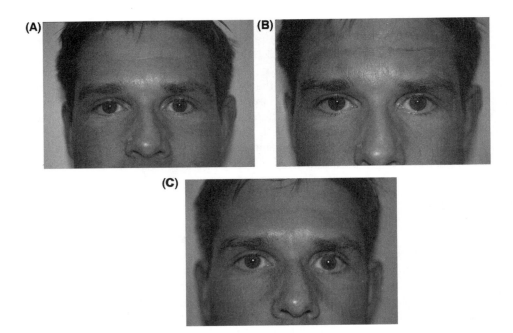

Figure 8
Patient with forehead lines (**A**) before, (**B**) immediately after, and (**C**) two weeks
after the injection of Restylane® Fine Lines.

perpendicular to the direction of the muscle fibers creating them. Once
again, the use of botulinum toxin injections in this area will help eliminate
deep furrows created by hyperactive muscular contraction (26). Nonetheless, filler agents can be used in the glabellar complex, but are not as effective as botulinum toxin injections (29,30). The ideal role for filler
materials in this area is to augment the result achieved with botulinum

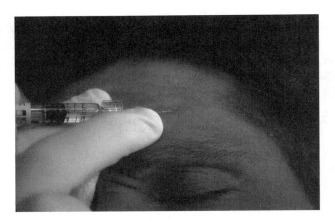

Figure 9
Injection technique of forehead lines.

(A)   **(B)**

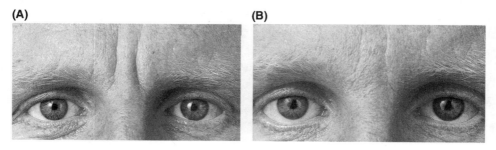

Figure 10
Patient with glabellar furrow (**A**) before, and (**B**) after the injection of
Restylane® Fine Lines. *Source*: Q-Med AB, Uppsala, Sweden.

toxin for lines that are extremely deep and cannot be eliminated by chemical denervation alone (31; Fig. 10).

Injection Technique

Although Restylane has been reported to be effective in the glabellar
complex, I prefer injecting the Fine Lines material in this area, as it
can be placed more superficially and thus minimize the risk of cutaneous
necrosis due to occlusion of a blood vessel. Again, this can be done prior
to the injection of BOTOX, but the ideal scenario would be to inject it
one week after complete chemical denervation has taken place. This will
allow to precisely identify the depth of the line remaining, and facilitate
the use of precise amounts of Restylane Fine Lines to fill in the volume
deficit. Again, Restylane is injected superficially with a 32 G needle to
100%; no overcorrection should be performed nor should the papules
be visible immediately after the injection. Serial puncture technique is utilized. Complications in this technique include bruising and cutaneous
necrosis if the material is placed too deeply.

Periorbital Wrinkles and Crow's Feet

Much of the wrinkling in the area around the eyes is the result of facial
chronologic aging and superimposed extrinsic photodamage. But a significant component can also be attributed to the hyperactivity of the
musculature underlying the skin around the eyes, resulting from repeated
smiling and grimacing over a long period of time.
     The wrinkles usually radiate outward and laterally from the lateral
ocular canthus and are perpendicular to the direction of the fibers of the
orbicularis oculi muscle. Weakening the muscles responsible for these
dynamic lines will impede their further contraction during common activities like squinting of the eyes, and as a result smooth out the overlying
skin (32). The use of filler materials to smooth out fine wrinkles around
the eyes is very effective, and should always be considered by itself or in

(A)   **(B)**

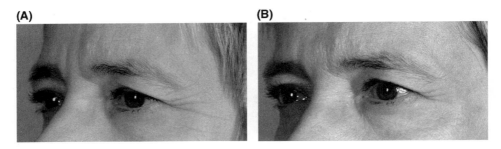

Figure 11
Patient with crow's feet (**A**) before and (**B**) after the injection of Restylane® Fine
Lines. *Source*: Q-Med AB, Uppsala, Sweden.

combination with botulinum toxin when attempting a rejuvenation of
this area of the face (Fig. 11).

Injection Technique

The ideal place for Restylane injection in this area are the periocular
rhytides that extend inferiorly into the upper cheek. These are difficult
to treat with chemodenervation as one can risk getting a lip ptosis from
inferior diffusion of the toxin into the levator labii superioris muscle
(33). Restylane Fine Lines should be injected utilizing the serial puncture technique with a 32 G needle and no overcorrection should be
performed.

Nonetheless, other periorbital rhytides, which may not be entirely
eliminated with chemodenervation, can also be treated with Restylane
Fine Lines. The most common complications are bruising and transient
pain, but persistent papules due to overcorrection can also be seen with
too superficial a placement of the material.

MID FACE

Nasolabial Fold

Owing to its multifactorial etiology and complex anatomic composition,
the NLF poses a challenge for the patient as well as the physician when
attempting a rejuvenation of the mid face. The fold is the result of diverse
factors that play a role in the development of the aging face, such as loss
of subcutaneous fat, gravitational ptosis and laxity of the skin, and over-
use of the muscles of facial expression (2). It is composed of subcutaneous fat and dense fibrous tissue, muscle fibers from the lip elevators
and their fascia, and excess skin hanging over the cutaneous attachment
of the zygomaticus major and minor, levator labii superioris, and levator
labii superioris alaeque nasi muscles (33).

(A)   **(B)**

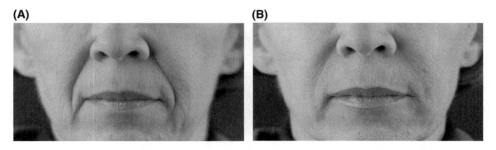

Figure 12
Patient with prominent nasolabial folds (**A**) before, and (**B**) after the injection of
Restylane®. *Source*: Q-Med AB, Uppsala, Sweden.

The NLFs are a common target for treatment with soft tissue augmentation, as they are fairly large, bilateral fissures that can be
augmented and measured with relative ease.

A variety of substances, including autologous fat (34), PMMA-
microspheres (35), Gore-Tex (36), bovine collagen (29,34,37), and other
substances (38) have been utilized to correct NLFs for a long period of
time. Implants intended to be permanent (e.g., Gore-Tex) are not usually
appropriate, as the outcome of an unwanted result is a long-lasting
adverse cosmetic effect that usually requires surgical correction.
Currently, only Zyplast has been approved by the FDA for correction
of contour deformities (including NLFs), and is therefore a defined standard for the safety and efficacy of any new biodegradable implant.
However, early clinical studies where Restylane was used to correct NLFs
show excellent duration and a very low frequency of side effects (30)
when compared to injectable bovine collagen (Fig. 12).

Injection Technique

The NLF can be treated with either Perlane or Restylane, or a combination of the two materials. Deep folds are best treated with Perlane alone
or a combination of Perlane and Restylane. Perlane is injected with a
27 G needle into the deep dermis either with serial puncture or linear
threading technique (Fig. 13). No overcorrection with this material is
necessary. If a deep NLF has a superficial component to it, Restylane
can be injected with a 30 G needle into the mid-dermis overlying the Perlane either with serial puncture or linear threading technique. If the NLF
is very shallow, Restylane alone should be injected with a 30 G needle
using the same technique. In all cases, the area should not be overcorrected and plaques should not be discernible in the dermis after material
placement. If injected too superficially, these visible papules can be
observed for at least six months following treatment. Bruising is the most
common side effect in this area and usually resolves within four to
seven days.

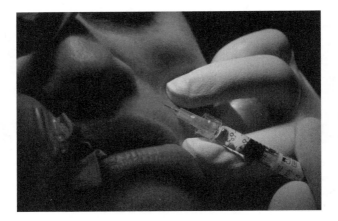

Figure 13
Injection technique of nasolabial folds.

Cheekbones

The youthful mid face is an even, convex surface outlined from the lower eyelid to the lower cheek. With advancing age, the effect of gravity pulls the underlying fat pad downwards, contributing to the formation of the NLF. This leaves behind a cheek depression, which is a very evident sign of aging (Fig. 2). Therefore, soft tissue fillers are the ideal treatment modality for this type of problem (Fig. 14).

Injection Technique

Facial contouring is an ideal use for Perlane. No other off-the-shelf biological material allows us to contour the face as well as this material.

The mid face, including the cheekbone area, can be augmented with Perlane. The material is injected with a 27 G needle into the lower dermis in the desired area and 100% correction is attempted. This can be used to

(A)   **(B)**

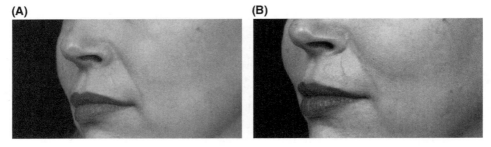

Figure 14
Patient with ptotic midface and cheekbones (**A**) before, and (**B**) after the injection of Perlane®. *Source*: Q-Med AB, Uppsala, Sweden.

(A)   **(B)**

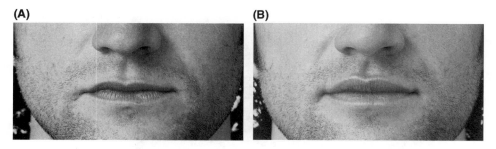

Figure 15
Patient with lip enhancement (**A**) before, and (**B**) after the injection of Perlane®.
Source: Q-Med AB, Uppsala, Sweden.

enhance the cheekbones, to fill in a hollow mid face, to fill in distensible deep scars, as well as to treat HIV lipodystrophy. The most common side effect is bruising, which usually resolves within a week. Overcorrection can persist for long periods yielding undesired cosmetic results and should therefore be avoided. Too superficial a placement of the material can lead to visible papules in the skin that can persist for several months. Serial puncture or linear threading, or a combination of the two can be used to eliminate contour defects of the face. These results should last for at least six months.

LOWER FACE

Lips

Full lips have long been considered the archetypal symbol of glamour and sensuality, especially in women. Over the course of years, however, the lips lose their fullness and change their shape, often becoming narrow and having drooping corners. These changes can readily result in a "sad face" appearance, and is therefore a common reason for patients to seek help for correcting it. Soft tissue fillers are ideal for this purpose as the replenishment of lost labial tissue will restore the pleasing esthetic look of a voluminous lip (Fig. 15).

Injection Technique

Lip enhancement should be performed with Perlane for results that last six months or longer (39). The material can be flowed into the upper and lower vermillion borders to create a more defined lip (Fig. 16). It can also be injected into the mucosa to enlarge the lips.

Perioral Region

In the perioral region, fine vertical lines extending above and below the vermillion border on the upper and lower lips are an evident sign of

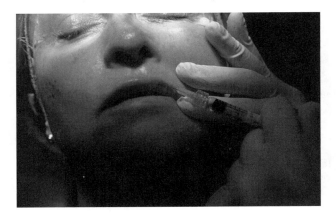

Figure 16
Injection technique of lips.

aging, particularly in women, and are therefore a common reason for patients to seek medical advice. They result from a combination of long-term use of the underlying musculature and actinic damage to the overlying skin. In addition, certain activities like smoking accentuate their depth and make them even more apparent.

Various treatment options, including botulinum toxin and abrasive resurfacing procedures, yield satisfactory results in most cases of fine rhytides surrounding the mouth. However, soft tissue augmentation has also been proven to effectively eliminate and smoothen out multiple, fine rhytides.

The corners of the mouth lose their structural support over time, and being subject to the forces of gravity, descend together with the rest of the facial soft tissues. As mentioned earlier, this signals sadness and old age, and is therefore another target for correction using soft tissue augmentation.

Injection technique

Upper lip lines should only be treated by the serial puncture technique with Restylane Fine Lines, without overcorrection, using a 32 G needle.

The oral commissures respond extremely well to the use of Perlane. The durability of this material provides an excellent longevity to this area. The corner of the mouth should be elevated prior to injecting Perlane into the upper and lower lateral oral commissures (Fig. 17). This will elevate the corner of the mouth and help efface the oral commissure (Fig. 18). The remaining defect extending from the lateral lip to the chin can then be filled in with Perlane.

Complications in this area include bruising, persistent beading when injected too superficially and not in a smooth line, and necrosis of the lip on injecting into a blood vessel.

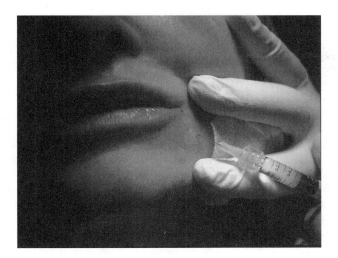

Figure 17
Injection technique to elevate the corners of the mouth.

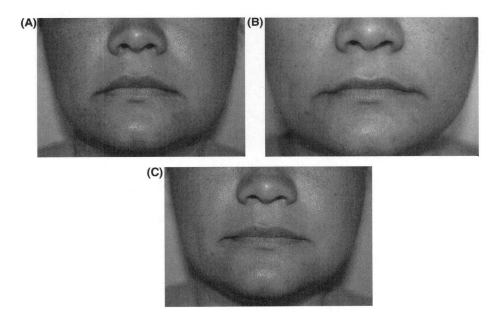

Figure 18
Patient with ptotic oral commissures (**A**) before, (**B**) immediately after, and (**C**) two weeks after the injection of Perlane®.

SCARS

Deep distensible scars can be corrected very well with Perlane. It should be injected into the deeper dermis directly underlying the scar.

FINAL CONSIDERATIONS

The usage of the Restylane family of products requires some form of anesthesia for most patients. Topical anesthesia in all areas except the perioral area seems to suffice. The use of topical betacaine or elamax before the procedure usually provides adequate pain relief for all areas except around the mouth. The treatment of the lip in most patients requires the use of a nerve block. This will also anesthetize the NLF region. Application of ice immediately after injection usually alleviates the postinjection burning that is associated with this material.

REFERENCES

1. Agerup B, Wik O. NASHA monograph, 2d ed. Uppsala, Sweden, 2001.
2. Zimbler MS, Kokoska MS, Thomas JR. Anatomy and pathophysiology of facial aging. Facial Plast Surg Clin North Am 2001; 9:179–187.
3. Uitto J. Connective tissue biochemistry of the aging dermis. Age-related alterations in collagen and elastin. Dermatol Clin 1986; 4:433–446.
4. Uitto J, Bernstein EF. Molecular mechanisms of cutaneous aging: connective tissue alterations in the dermis. J Invest Dermatol Symp Proc 1998; 3:41–44.
5. Goukassian D, Gad F, Yaar M, Eller MS, Nehal US, Gilchrest BA. Mechanisms and implications of the age-associated decrease in DNA repair capacity. FASEB J 2000; 14:1325–1334.
6. Campisi J. The role of cellular senescence in skin aging. J Invest Dermatol Symp Proc 1998; 3:1–5.
7. Braverman IM, Fonferko E. Studies in cutaneous aging: I. The elastic fiber network. J Invest Dermatol 1982; 78:434–443.
8. Hadshiew IM, Eller MS, Gilchrest BA. Skin aging and photoaging: The role of DNA damage and repair. Am J Contact Dermat 2000; 11:19–25.
9. Yaar M, Gilchrest BA. Skin aging: Postulated mechanisms and consequent changes in structure and function. Clin Geriatr Med 2001; 17:617–630.
10. Yaar M, Gilchrest BA. Aging versus photoaging: Postulated mechanisms and effectors. J Invest Dermatol Symp Proc 1998; 3:47–51.
11. Benedetti L, Cortivo R, Berti T, Berti A, Pea F, Mazzo M, Moras M, Abatangelo G. Biocompatibility and biodegradation of different hyaluronan derivatives (Hyaff) implanted in rats. Biomaterials 1993; 14:1154–1160.
12. Larsen NE, Pollak CT, Reiner K, Leshchiner E, Balazs EA. Biocompatibility and biodegradation of different hyaluronan derivatives (Hyaff) implanted in rats. Biomaterials 1993; 14:1154–1160.
13. Physiological function of connective tissue polysaccharides. Physiol Rev 1978; 58:255–315.
14. Ghersetich I, Lotti T, Campanile G, Grappone C, Dini G. Hyaluronic acid in cutaneous intrinsic aging. Int J Dermatol 1994; 33:119–122.
15. Reed RK, Laurent UB, Fraser JR, Laurent TC. Removal rate of [3H] hyaluronan injected subcutaneously in rabbits. Am J Physiol 1990; 259:H532–H535.
16. Manna F, Dentini M, Desideri P, De Pita O, Mortilla E, Maras B. Comparative chemical evaluation of two commercially available derivatives of hyaluronic acid (hylaform from rooster combs and restylane from streptococcus) used for soft tissue augmentation. J Eur Acad Dermatol Venereol 1999; 13:183–192.
17. Piacquadio D, Jarcho M, Goltz R. Evaluation of hylan b gel as a soft-tissue augmentation implant material. J Am Acad Dermatol 1997; 36:544–549.
18. Larsen NE, Pollak CT, Reiner K, Leshchiner E, Balazs EA. Hylan gel biomaterial: Dermal and immunologic compatibility. J Biomed Mater Res 1993; 27:1129–1134.
19. Duranti F, Salti G, Bovani B, Calandra M, Rosati ML. Injectable hyaluronic acid gel for soft tissue augmentation. A clinical and histological study. Dermatol Surg 1998; 24:1317–1325.
20. Investigator brochure, Restylane.
21. Olenius M. The first clinical study using a new biodegradable implant for the treatment of lips, wrinkles, and folds. Aesth Plast Surg 1998; 22:97–101.
22. Duranti F, Salti G, Bovani B, et al. Injectable hyaluronic acid gel for soft tissue augmentation. A clinical and histological study. Dermatol Surg 1998; 24:1317–1325.
23. Micheels P. Human anti-hyaluronic acid antibodies: Is it possible? Dermatol Surg 1998; 27:185–191.

24. Lowe NJ, Maxwell CA, Lowe P, Duick MG, Shah K. Hyaluronic acid skin fillers: Adverse reactions and skin testing. J Am Acad Dermatol 2001; 45:930–933.

25. Stennert E. Why does the frontalis muscle "never come back"? Functional organization of the mimic musculature. Eur Arch Otorhinolaryngol 1994; suppl:S91–S95.

26. Carruthers A, Carruthers J. Botulinum toxin in the treatment of glabellar frown lines and other facial wrinkles. In: Jankovic J, Hallet M, eds. Therapy with Botulinum Toxin. New York: Marcel Dekker, 1994.

27. Wieder JM, Moy RL. Understanding botulinum toxin: Surgical anatomy of the frown, forhead and periocular region. Dermatol Surg 1998; 24:1172–1174.

28. Macdonald MR, Spiegel JH, Raven RB, Kabaker SS, Maas CS. An anatomical approach to glabellar rhytids. Arch Otolaryngol Head Neck Surg 1998; 124:1315–1320.

29. Klein AW. Implantation technics for injectable collagen. Two and one-half years of personal clinical experience. J Am Acad Dermatol 1993; 9:224–228.

30. Olenius M. The first clinical study using a new biodegradable implant for the treatment of lips, wrinkles, and folds. Aesthetic Plast Surg 1998; 22:97–101.

31. Fagien S, Brandt FS. Primary and adjunctive use of botulinum toxin A (BOTOX®) in facial esthetic surgery. Clin Plast Surg 2001; 28:127–148.

32. Matarasso SL, Matarasso A. Treatment guidelines for botulinum toxin type A for the periocular region and a report on partial upper lip ptosis following injections to the lateral canthal rhytids. Plast Reconstr Surg 2001; 108:208–214.

33. Carruthers A, Carruthers J. Cosmetic uses of botulinum A exotoxin. Adv Dermatol 1997; 12:325–347.

34. Gormley DE, Eremia S. Quantitative assessment of augmentation therapy. J Dermatol Surg Oncol 1990; 16(12):1147–1151.

35. Lemperle G, Gauthier-Hazan N, Lemperle M. PMMA-microspheres (Artecoll) for long-lasting correction of wrinkles: refinements and statistical results. Aesth Plast Surg 1998; 22:h356–h365.

36. Cisneros JL, Singla R. Intradermal augmentation with expanded polytetrafluoroethylene (Gore-Tex) for facial lines and wrinkles. J Dermatol Surg Oncol 1993; 19:539–542.

37. Matti BA, Nicolle FV. Clinical use of Zyplast in correction of age- and disease-related contour deficiencies of the face. Aesth Plast Surg 1990; 14:227–234.

38. Pollack SV. Silicone, Fibrel, and collagen implantation for facial lines and wrinkles. J Dermatol Surg Oncol 1990; 16:957–961.

39. Bousquet MT, Agerup B. Restylane lip implantation: European experience. Operative Tech Oculo Orb Rec Surg 1999; 2:172–176.

14
AlloDerm® and Cymetra™

Justin J. Vujevich
Department of Dermatology and Cutaneous Surgery, University of Miami School of Medicine, Miami, Florida, U.S.A.

Leslie S. Baumann
Division of Cosmetic Dermatology, Department of Dermatology and Cutaneous Surgery, University of Miami School of Medicine, Miami, Florida, U.S.A.

INTRODUCTION

Physicians have various materials in their stockpile available for soft tissue augmentation. These materials can be divided into human- and nonhuman-derived tissues. Currently, the most popular substance used for soft tissue augmentation remains injectable bovine collagen. In fact, collagen injections have come to be regarded as the gold standard of filler materials with which other products are compared.

There are several drawbacks of bovine-derived collagen, however, including its temporary action and potential for allergic reaction. Therefore, new forms of human-derived materials for soft tissue augmentation are desired.

Human-derived materials are divided into autologous (self) and allogenic (human donor) tissues. Transplantation of intact allogenic human dermis is generally not performed for several reasons. First, tissue from another individual may contain mismatched epidermal, dendritic, and hematological cells. The recipient's immune system regards these cells as foreign, and would evoke an immunological response against the graft, which contains these foreign cells. Second, the process of preparing transplantation of intact autologous dermis may lead to an undesirable graft. When separating the epidermis from the dermis to process the autologous graft, cells may die or become damaged, releasing enzymes that may evoke an inflammatory response when transplanted into another site on the body. Thus, the immunological and inflammatory responses described above with allogenic grafts may lead to graft absorption and a poor clinical response.

Several human-derived human filler materials have been developed to address these issues with allogenic graft filler materials. Autologen

(Collagenesis Inc., Beverly, Massachusetts, U.S.) is composed of intact autologous collagen fibers extracted from skin procured from the patient during a previous elective surgery. Two square inches of donor skin are required to be extracted, frozen, and then mailed to the company, where the tissue is modified to remove all cellular elements of the dermis. The processed suspension of dermal protein fibers of the donor's skin is sent back to the practitioner for injection into the donor patient. Isolagen (Isolagen Technologies Inc., Paramus, New Jersey, U.S.) is a similar filler agent, which requires a 3-mm skin biopsy from the donor patient. The tissue is mailed to the company, where fibroblasts of the donor's skin sample are cultured. Several weeks later, a syringe is sent back to the practitioner for reinjection into the donor patient. Both Autologen and Isolagen do not cause an immune response because the collagen is human in origin. However, the long processing time and the necessity of undergoing a procedure to extract the tissue are drawbacks of the use these products.

Because of the problems of antigenicity and reabsorption and preharvesting hassles associated with allogenic filler materials, two products were developed: Alloderm® and Cymetra™ (LifeCell Corporation, The Woodlands, Texas, U.S.). These graft materials are the subject of this chapter.

BACKGROUND OF ALLODERM® AND CYMETRA™

AlloDerm and Cymetra are acellular, freeze-dried dermal graft materials processed from human cadaver dermis. AlloDerm is available in solid sheets, and Cymetra as an injectable. AlloDerm has been used for several years in United States for cosmetic and reconstructive soft tissue augmentation, as well as in the treatment of full-thickness burns. Cymetra became available as a micronized, injectable form of AlloDerm in 2000.

ALLODERM®

AlloDerm grafts are processed from human cadaver dermis. The process of graft preparation begins with the donor tissue undergoing several levels of testing and screening to assure its safety. Blood samples from each skin donor for AlloDerm are screened for Hepatitis B surface antigen (HBsAg), antibodies to hepatitis C, antibodies to the human immunodeficiency virus (HIV) types 1 and 2, antibodies to human T-lymphotropic virus (HTLV) type I and II, and syphilis (RPR or VDRL). In addition, the processing of AlloDerm includes a step in which donor skin is incubated in a solution containing a viral inactivation agent (VIA).

Next, a freeze-drying process removes all cells from the human tissue sample, yielding an acellular matrix of type IV and VII collagen, laminin, and elastin. Cell removal is achieved by uncoupling cell–matrix adhesion via low molecular weight–buffered detergents (1). In immunohistochemical staining, no class I or II histocompatibility antigens have been identified (Fig. 1). Once an acellular matrix is achieved,

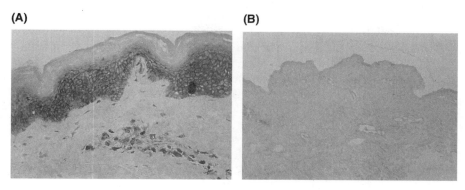

Figure 1
(**A**) Immunohistochemical staining of skin for major histocompatibility complex I (MHC-I) antigens, prior to processing into AlloDerm®. (**B**) Immunohistochemical staining of skin for MHC-I antigens, after processing of AlloDerm, demonstrating removal of all cells and transplantation antigens.

the dermal matrix is freeze-dried at a temperature that does not damage or distort the dermal framework (2).

AlloDerm has a two-year shelf life when unopened and refrigerated between 1°C and 10°C. After opening the packaging, the tissue is rehydrated for 10 to 20 minutes prior to use, in normal saline or lactated Ringer's solution (Fig. 2). Each pouch of AlloDerm contains one or two rectangular sheets of the acellular human dermis between pieces of an unattached, nonwoven backing (Fig. 2).

Alloderm is characterized by the capacity to integrate the surrounding tissue, allowing for rapid revascularization by the patient's blood

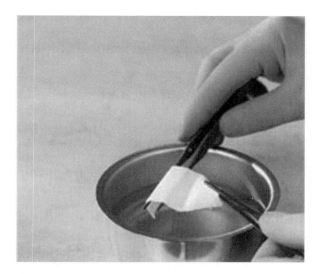

Figure 2
Hydrated AlloDerm® graft prior to implantation.

supply. Alloderm was originally developed as a surface skin graft for patients with burns. Livesey et al. (3) reported that skin grafts in pigs, which received processed acellular dermal matrix overlaid with a standard meshed split-thickness skin graft (STSG), showed a significant increase in dermal thickness at the graft site, when compared to STSG site alone at day 9 and day 60. Additional reports by Wainwright (4) and Wainwright et al. (5) revealed that the application of the graft between a debrided wound surface and a STSG resulted in decreased contracture and improved durability of the skin graft.

ALLODERM® PREPARATION

In cosmetic surgery, AlloDerm grafts are used for soft tissue augmentation of the lips, nasolabial folds, and depressed scars. Using sterile technique, the AlloDerm graft is transferred onto a lint-free sterile field, where the material can be shaped with scissors or scalpel, and rolled or folded to desired thickness. For implantation, the dermal side of the graft can be applied to open or closed surgical sites. If the surgical site is closed, a pocket or tunnel can be formed by blunt dissection down to the subdermal (or deeper) plane. After inserting an instrument (such as a tendon passer or alligator forceps) the graft is grasped and pulled into place. Insertion can be made easier by first moistening the tissue by dipping it in saline. It can then be anchored with absorbable sutures as the incision site is closed.

ALLODERM® APPLICATIONS

Lip Augmentation

AlloDerm grafts are ideal for rejuvenation of thin and ptotic lips since the grafted material is native to the surrounding tissue and gives a natural feel once implanted.

Anesthesia may be obtained locally with submucosally injected 2% Lidocaine with 1:100,000 epinephrine added for hemostasis. An intraorbital or metal nerve block may be added for postoperative anesthesia, or in case other procedures are performed that day. Generally, two rolled AlloDerm grafts are placed in the upper lip and one rolled graft is required for the lower lip. A 3.0×7.0-cm graft of 1 to 2 mm thickness is adequate. After hydrating the graft, it is trimmed to correspond to the amount of desired augmentation. After trimming, the graft is rolled and sutured circumferentially with a 5–0 plain gut suture.

The surgical area is prepped, and two small radial incisions are made just medial to the lateral commissure and at the peak of the cupid's bow on the upper lip. A blunt elevator is inserted through the incisions to create a tunnel. The grafts are inserted with an alligator forceps through the tunnel into place. This same procedure is then performed on the contralateral side of the upper lip.

In the lower lip, a similar technique is utilized with one graft. Radial incisions are made at the two lateral commissures and the midline lower lip. The graft is inserted in a similar manner described above.

All incisions are closed with 6–0 permanent sutures, and removed five to seven days later. Patients may be given oral cephalosporin for five days and a topical antibiotic ointment is applied at the incision sites. It is important to inform patients about subsequent swelling postgrafting and advise them to apply ice packs on the lips for 24 to 48 hours postprocedure. Swelling generally peaks three days postprocedure.

Nasolabial Folds

A 3×7-cm piece of AlloDerm is used and cut diagonally to divide the graft into two triangular segments. After hydration, the graft is folded along its long axis for insertion. Small incisions are made at the superior and inferior aspects of the nasolabial folds. Using a blunt-tip elevator, a tunnel is established at the dermal/subcutaneous junction. The hydrated AlloDerm graft is then pulled into place within the tunnel with alligator forceps. Once in place, the edges are trimmed with scissors and wound closure is accomplished using 6–0 permanent monofilament sutures.

Postprocedure ice compresses should be applied for the first 24 hours. Topical antibiotic ointment may be applied at the incision sites. A five-day course of an oral cephalosporin should be given postoperatively. Sutures should be removed five to seven days postprocedure.

Facial-Contour Defect Correction

AlloDerm grafts can also correct the depressed scars and contour defects. If the defect is small enough, then the AlloDerm graft can be inserted through a stab incision just lateral to the defect, with tunneling. If the skin defect is large enough, a longer incision may be necessary just lateral to the contour defect. After the incision is made, the grafting area should be undermined with scissors. Using forceps, the AlloDerm graft is inserted without folding over itself, through the incision site. If the defect is very deep, multiple grafts may be layered on top of one another. After implantation, the incision site is closed with 6–0 sutures.

Acne Scars

AlloDerm may also be used for augmentation of acne scars. In general, the graft is primarily used for softer, saucer-shaped defects, rather than for classic "ice pick" acne scars.

The prepped surgical area is anesthetized using 2% Lidocaine with 1:100,000 epinephrine added for hemostasis. A 1×2-cm or 1×4-cm AlloDerm graft is used. Depending on the needed contour, the grafts are cut into custom-fitted shapes using scissors or surgical blade. The pieces of graft are inserted just adjacent to the defect using an 18-gauge NoKor® needle. The bevel is angled to cut in a horizontal plane, parallel to the surface of the skin, and just underneath the scar. This creates a small pocket for the AlloDerm pieces. Adequate pieces of AlloDerm grafts are inserted with forceps to elevate and correct the skin defect. If necessary, the 18-gauge incisions may be sutured with dissolvable 6–0 chromic sutures.

CYMETRA™

Cymetra is an injectable, micronized form of Alloderm. Therefore, an incision is not required for soft tissue augmentation. Like Alloderm, Cymetra is processed from donated human tissue from U.S. tissue banks utilizing similar screening methods for AlloDerm. The allograft is processed into a particulate acellular dermal matrix, first by removing the epidermis and the dermal cells, then by converting the dermal matrix into micronized particles through a process called cryo-fracture. Finally, the micronized particles are dried, and placed in a 5-cc syringe for refrigeration. The collagen concentration is approximately 150 mg/mL with a median particle size of 123 μm (two-thirds of the particles measure between 59 and 593 μm) (6). However, twenty-seven percent of the particles measure 52 μm or less and are thus, subject to phagocytosis by host scavenger cells.

CYMETRA™ PREPARATION

Cymetra is stored refrigerated as a white pellet in a 5-cc syringe. A 3-cc syringe of 1% Lidocaine is mixed back and forth with the 5-cc Cymetra syringe until the pellet becomes a thickened, hydrated, creamy material. This process takes about 10 minutes and yields 1 cc of injectable Cymetra ready to be administered (Fig. 3).

CYMETRA™ APPLICATIONS

Nasolabial Folds

Cymetra may be used to improve the appearance of the nasolabial folds. After mixing the constituents and prepping the area, Cymetra is injected into each fold using a 26- or 27-gauge needle. While withdrawing the needle, the material is injected retrogradely into the subdermis of the wrinkle. After injecting the material, the practitioner massages the augmented area gently by pinching the cheek fold with the index finger and thumb. Additional Cymetra may be injected to fill in any unresolved areas. Alternatively, Cymetra can be injected subdermally using a serial puncture technique and repeating injections every few millimeters until the entire fold is corrected (Fig. 4).

Lip Augmentation

Cymetra may also be used to augment the appearance of the lips. For the vermilion border, a 22- or 23-gauge needle is inserted at the peak of the

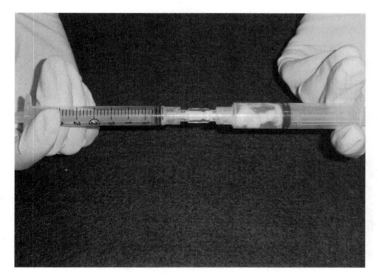

Figure 3
Preparation of Cymetra™ injection. Care should be taken to avoid clumping of the filler material within the syringe during mixing, as demonstrated in this photo.

cupid's bow, and threaded to the opposite commissure of the lip. While withdrawing and the bevel pointed up, the filler material is injected into the lip. This is repeated on the other side of the lip, with overlapping of the filler material on the middle third of the lip for proper augmentation of the lip. Depending on desired lip volume, approximately 0.5 to 0.6 ml will be injected per vermilion border (Fig. 5).

For vermilion area injections, a 23-gauge needle is inserted just anterior to the fascia of the orbicularis muscle one-third of the way across the lip. The needle is threaded across to the opposite side, and Cymetra is injected into the lip while withdrawing. Approximately 1 to 2 ml of Cymetra may be used per lip. After the procedure, patients should be told not to massage the injected area, nor to move the lips excessively for six hours or more.

Marionette Lines and Perioral Rhytids

Cymetra may be used for correction of the marionette lines and perioral rhytids. If further anesthesia is desired, the injection sites may be treated with topical or injectable Lidocaine prior to injecting Cymetra. After preparing the Cymetra, a 25-gauge needle is inserted distally into the inferior aspect of the wrinkle to be corrected. While tenting the skin and withdrawing the filler material bevel up, Cymetra is injected subdermally into the defect. After injection, the treated area should be gently massaged to distribute the filler material evenly along the wrinkle.

(A)

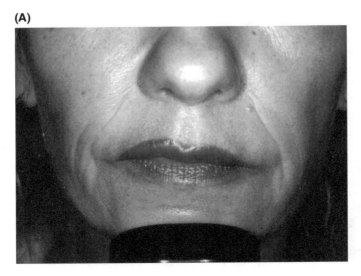

(B)

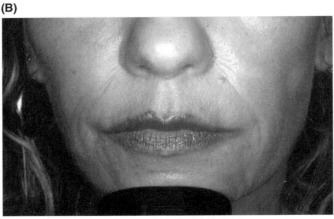

Figure 4
A 51-year-old female desiring nasolabial fold and perioral line correction. (**A**) Pre-operative view. (**B**) Twelve days postoperative view after injection with Cymetra™.

CLINICAL DATA ON ALLODERM® AND CYMETRA™

Clinical data on the two filler materials are scarce and primarily involve AlloDerm. One study by Sclafini et al. (7) evaluated the histological and clinical properties of subdermally implanted Alloderm versus Zyplast® (10 patients), and subdermally injected, micronized Alloderm versus Zyplast (15 patients). Host tissue incorporation with fibroblast ingrowth and collagen deposition was seen postAlloderm grafting and Cymetra injections. In addition, the mean percentage volume persistence of grafted Alloderm at one and three months (82.8% and 48.3%, respectively) was

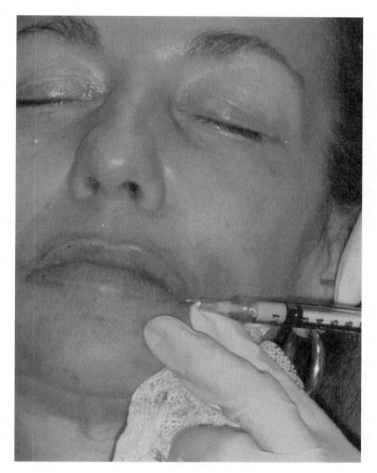

Figure 5
Cymetra™ injected with a 27 gauge needle into the vermilion border.

significantly greater than the volume persistence of injected Zyplast at one and three months (26.6% and 8.0%, respectively). The mean percentage volume persistence of the intradermally injected, micronized Alloderm at implantation and at four weeks (81.4%, 24.6%, respectively) was significantly greater than the volume persistence of injected Zyplast at implantation and at four weeks (56.6% and 12.6%, respectively).

A one-year follow-up study to this data by Sclafani et al. (8) reported that the AlloDerm volume persistence points at 1, 3, 6, and 12 months (82.8%, 48.3%, 21.9%, and 20.2%, respectively) was statistically greater than the volume persistence points at 1, 3, 6, and 12 months for Zyplast (26.6%, 8.0%, 1.1%, 0.9%, respectively). Furthermore, the 12-month biopsy specimens of the AlloDerm implants showed extensive host ingrowth with mature blood vessels and fibroblasts, while no evidence of Zyplast was identified in any of the specimens.

These results suggested that while at six months, approximately 20% of the implanted volume of implanted AlloDerm remained, further loss of this volume did not occur by one year. Therefore, overcorrection is necessary with AlloDerm, but "touch-up" procedures should be delayed until after six months postoriginal implant to allow for stabilization and equilibrium of the original implant material.

In terms of lip augmentation, Tobin et al. (9) reported 12 cases using the AlloDerm graft. From their clinical observation, the authors felt that the material had a 15% to 20% shrinkage rate, which stabilized after the first four to six weeks. Patients felt that the graft took a natural feel at approximately three months postimplantation. Their average follow-up was seven months, with the longest follow-up at one year.

In addition to the above studies, AlloDerm has been reported to improve acne scars, atrophic areas, and defects resulting from trauma or surgical resections. Cymetra is currently under investigation for its utility in treating acne scars, wrinkles, and AIDS-associated lipodystrophy.

COMPLICATIONS OF ALLODERM® AND CYMETRA™

In general, complications with Cymetra and Alloderm are uncommon. AlloDerm implantation may result in swelling, infection, and bleeding perioperatively, but this is technique-dependent. Furthermore, graft malpositioning and graft extrusion rarely occur. To date, there have been no reported cases of allergy to the graft material. Patients should be instructed to expect a postoperative "downtime" of their activities for approximately three to five days. For patients with history of herpes outbreaks, a five-day course of prophylactic acyclovir may be given.

Complications with Cymetra are also minimal. They include pain from injection, bleeding, and infection. To date, there have been no reported cases of allergy to the injected material.

SUMMARY OF ALLODERM® AND CYMETRA™

The advantages of AlloDerm and Cymetra are clear. Unlike with bovine collagen products, skin testing is not required with AlloDerm and Cymetra. Second, according to the literature, the longevity of correction with AlloDerm and Cymetra appears to be greater than that with bovine collagen. Finally, clinical testing on patients has not showed allergic or immunologic reactions to date. These characteristics have been found with bovine collagen products. There are disadvantages. AlloDerm requires time and skill to prepare (such as cutting, folding, and rolling) and implant the filler material (surgical procedure). Cymetra also requires a substantial time to mix the material with Lidocaine prior to injection. At present, these allogenic filler materials appear to be a promising modality for soft tissue augmentation.

REFERENCES

1. US Patent Office. Method for processing and preserving collagen-based tissues for transplantation. US Patent No. 5,336,616. Aug 9, 1994.
2. Livesey SA, del Campo AA, McDowall AW, et al. Cryofixation and ultra-low temperature freeze drying as a preparative technique for TEM. J Microsc 1991; 161:205–215.
3. Livesey SA, Herndon DN, Hollyoak MA, et al. Transplanted acellular allograft dermal matrix. Transplantation 1995; 60:1–9.
4. Wainwright DJ. Use of an acellular allograft dermal matrix (AlloDerm) in the management of full-thickness burns. Burns 1995; 21:243–248.
5. Wainwright DJ, Madden M, Lutterman A, et al. Clinical evaluation of an accelular allograft dermal matrix in full-thickness burns. J Burn Care Rehabil 1996; 17:124–136.
6. Ellis DA, Makdessian AS, Brown DJ. Survey of future injectables. Facial Plast Surg Clin North Am 2001; 9:405–411.
7. Sclafini AP, Romo T, Jacono AA, et al. Evaluation of acellular dermal graft in sheet (AlloDerm) and injectable (micronized AlloDerm) forms for soft tissue augmentation. Arch Facial Plast Surg 2000; 2:130–136.
8. Sclafani AP, Romo T III, Jacono AA, et al. Evaluation of accellular dermal graft (AlloDerm) sheet for soft tissue augmentation. Arch Facial Plat Surg 2001; 3:101–103.
9. Tobin HA, Karas ND. Lip augmentation using an Alloderm graft. J Oral Maxillofac Surg 1998; 56:722–727.

15

Other Temporary or Permanent Injectable Fillers

Arnold W. Klein
Department of Dermatology, David Geffen School of Medicine,
University of California, Los Angeles, California, U.S.A.

Frederick C. Beddingfield, III
Division of Dermatology, Department of Medicine, David Geffen School of Medicine,
University of California, Los Angeles, California, and Dermatology Research and
Development, Allergan, Inc., Irvine, California, U.S.A.

Besides the agents covered in other chapters, there are numerous products and techniques whose positions in the field of soft tissue augmentation have not yet been fully defined. The search for the perfect material to eradicate rhytides, smooth scars, and fill traumatic defects continues. New products appear, sometimes with great fanfare, but these sometimes fail to fulfill the promise of a better alternative to what we use. Fibrel, Autologen, Dermalogen, and Softform are no longer available. Isolagen was withdrawn from the market but is now undergoing clinical trials with the expectation that it will be reintroduced. Though no currently available implant fulfills the criteria for being the perfect material, many are adequate for a given task, satisfy patients, and offer excellent safety profiles; but efforts to develop the perfect soft tissue augmentation material continue. Permanent or temporary fillers lasting for many years are not necessarily ideal, however, because problems may persist indefinitely with such fillers. Additionally, the facial architecture with its delicate nuances changes over time and a filler placed in a certain location today may not be ideally placed years from now. Synthetic fillers are appearing in rapid succession, but thus far have failed to match the safety of hyaluronic acid fillers. Obviously, the techniques and substances used for soft tissue augmentation are increasing at an accelerated rate. The choice of implant material should be based on the location of the defect, potential for hypersensitivity reaction, desire for permanency, and the patient's feelings about the need for a "natural feel" of the implant. Choosing an appropriate injectable implant requires a thorough understanding of the materials available and the etiology of the wrinkle. Fine, superficial rhytides respond best to therapy at the intradermal level. Deeper, more substantial wrinkles typically have a subcutaneous component, with or without a facial-muscular element, and are best approached from the subcutaneous space. Often a wrinkle will have both a superficial and a deep component, such as the nasolabial fold, and both these components need to be addressed to obtain optimal results. Filler substances are essential tools to be used when treating the face either as stand-alone treatment or in conjunction with laser resurfacing, botulinum toxin, or chemical peels. The difficulty is in choosing the proper treatment techniques and in meeting patient expectations. As newer products develop, the methods of soft-tissue enhancement will continue to change, hopefully bringing improved results to patients. It is a fact that Europe is ahead of the United States in terms of filler availability. At the same time, the greater ease or approval for marketing of medical devices like fillers in Europe (the so-called CE mark), leaves a greater chance for unsafe fillers to be marketed there. While this means that Americans, to a degree, often have to wait for the latest fillers "to arrive" from Europe, this also means that we get the benefit of these products being tested overseas prior to their use here.

A better understanding has developed on the part of the cosmetically oriented physician that the three-dimensional aspects of the face must be preserved to achieve the best aesthetic result. Although one must be familiar with all the techniques, materials, and options, it is preferable to become proficient in only two or three different methods so that one can provide patients with the best results possible. Yet the patients can be provided with different options apart from those in which one is experienced.

It should be noted that autologous and allogenic products are not approved by the U.S. Food and Drug Administration (FDA). Because they are derived from human tissue, they are not required to undergo the FDA approval process.

Physicians should counsel patients about the risks and benefits of injectable substance therapy. Each physician should inform prospective patients about skin testing, the treatment procedure, and treatment expectations.

If one had looked at the list of filling substances ten years ago, there may have been five of them, but now there's a veritable encyclopedia of agents that are available to the practitioner for his/her use (Table 1). Injectable fat is the oldest of the materials used for tissue augmentation (1).

AcHyal is a non-animal derived 1% solution of the sodium salt of hyaluronic acid. It is provided in 2.5 cc prefilled syringes with 30-gauge needles. It can be stored at room temperature and has a shelf life of three years. Indications are for wrinkles, scars, lip and contour deformities. Adverse reactions are listed as reddening, inflammation, or bruising which dissipate in two to three days. There is no experience with the material in the United States and it is not FDA approved. It is manufactured by Tedec Meiji Farma, S.A. Ctra. M-300, KM 30,500 28802 – Alcalá de Henares, Madrid, Spain.

Aquamid® injectable is a hydrophilic polyacrylamide gel. It is 97.5% apyrogenic, and water bound to 2.5% cross-linked polyacrylamide. It has been CE marked since 2001. It is nonresorbable, nonallergenic, biocompatible, physically and chemically stable, immunologically inactive,

Table 1
Filler Substances

AcHyal[a]
Alloderm
Amazingel[a]
Aptos threads
Aquamid40[a]
Artecoll
Artefill[a]
Argiform[a]
Bio-Alcamid[a]
Biocell Ultravital[a]
Bioformacryl[a]
Bioplastique[a]
CosmoDerm NST and CosmoPlast NST
Cymetra
Dermal Grafting
Dermalive[a]/DermaDeep[a]
Dermaplant[a]
Dermicol[a]
Endoplast-50[a]
Esthelis
Evolence
Evolution[a]
Fascian
Fat
   Subcutaneous microlipoinjection
   Lipocytic dermal augmentation
Formacrill[a]
Goretex
Humallagen[a]
Hyacell[a]
Hyal-System[a]
Hylaform
Hylan Rofilan Gel[a]
Isolagen[a]
Juvederm[a]
Koken Atelocollagen
Kopolymer[a]
MacDeermol[a]
Macrolane
Meta-Crill[a]
Metrex[a]
New-Fill
Perlane[a]
Permacol[a]
Plasmagel
PMS 350
Procell[a]
*Pro*fill[a]

Continued

Table 1
Filler Substances (*Continued*)

Radiance/Radiesse
Resoplast[a]
Restylane
Restylane-Fine[a]
Reviderm Intra[a]
Rhegecoll[a]
Sculptra
Silicone[a]
Silicon1000
Surgisis
Teosyal[a]
Ultrsoft and Conform
Zyderm Collagen and Zyplast Collagen

[a]Not approved for use in the United States.

and migration resistant according to the manufacturer's claims. It is injected subcutaneously with a 27-gauge needle and is indicated for lips deformities, nasolabial folds, mentolabial folds, deep wrinkles, glabellar frowns, cheek augmentation, and aesthetic/reconstructive augmentation of the body, as well as other indications of facial and body contouring. In a European multi-center study, satisfaction exceeded 92% two years after treatment. It is not available in the United States but is available in Europe, Australia, Asia, Canada, and Mexico. It is manufactured by Contura International A/S, Sydmarken 23, 2860 Soeborg, Denmark. Tel: 45-3958-5960, website: http://www.aquamid.info/ and http://www.contura.com/.

Argiform[TM] *(a.k.a. Argyform)* is a hydrophilic polyacrylamide gel manufactured using a silver ion process to help repel bacteria. It has 0.03% residual unpolymerized acrylamide monomer. It is manufactured by Bioform Corp. (Krasnobogatyrskay Street, 42/1103, Moscow, Russia. Tel: 7 (095) 161-0524, e-mail: info@bioform.ru, website: http://bioform. ru). It is not available in the United States but is available in Europe.

Arteplast[TM], *Artecoll*[TM], *and Artefill*[TM] *(Non-FDA Approved)*: Arteplast is polymethylmethacrylate (PMMA) beads and Tween® 80. Arteplast is basically Plexiglas beads. It was part of the initial research before Artecoll (PMMA in a collagen suspension with lidocaine) was developed. It was removed from the market and is no longer in use; Artecoll has been used instead. Artecoll (a.k.a. Aretefill) has been associated with granulomas and nodules, especially when used in and around the lips and sometimes years after the procedure (2). Arteplast was manufactured and distributed by Rofil Medical International B.V., Breda, The Netherlands. Artefill, which is close to FDA approval by report, has been developed by Artes Medical, Corp., 4660 La Jolla Village Drive, Suite 825, San Diego, CA 92122.

Bio-Alcamid[TM] (BioAlcamid) is an injectable hydrophilic polyalkylamide gel. It is permanent and used for wasted areas of the face in HIV patients. It is manufactured by Progen, now Polymekon, Italy. It is approved in Europe and in Mexico. It is not available in the United States but is available in Mexico. Website: http://www.bioalcamid.com/.

Biocell Ultravital^TM is also called Biopolymere III. It is a biopolymer developed in Switzerland and contains Silicium (a derivative of silicon). According to the manufacturer, there is no need for allergy tests prior to treatment and results may be permanent. It is commonly used in South America. It is distributed by Biocell Laboratoires, CH 593 Vaduz, Lichtenstein. It is not approved by the FDA.

Bioplastique^TM is a suspension of textured composite silicone polymer of solid, vulcanized methylsiloxane rubber particles from 100 to 400 microns in size in a carrier vehicle (biocompatible plasdone hydrogel) (3). It is an investigational material for soft tissue augmentation with a controlled foreign body response. The size of the particles reportedly reduces migration. Several cases of granulomas requiring excision have been reported. It has a CE mark but owing to the controversy and resultant bad press surrounding the silicone gel implants, it is unlikely to be FDA approved and thus studies have been largely abandoned.

Dermalive^TM/*DermaDeep*^TM: Dermalive (for dermal injection) and Dermadeep (for subcutaneous injection) are composed of hyaluronic acid (60% volume) and acrylic hydrogel (40% volume) (HEMA) fragments. They are nonanimal in origin. The particle sizes are 45 to 65 microns. Collagen builds around the particles giving the fillers their volume. Skin tests are reportedly unnecessary. They come in preloaded syringes and are intended for use in the dermal and subdermal planes. Dermalive is used for augmenting lips and smoothing deep wrinkles. DermaDeep is very effective on nasolabial folds and for chin and cheek augmentation. It has a CE mark and has been available in Europe and South America for five years. They are produced by Dermatech, 28 Rue de Caumartin, 75009 Paris, France. Tel: 01-42-66-52-00, Fax: 01-42-66-52-24, website: http://www.dermadeep.com; http://www.dermalive.com.

DermiCol^TM is an uniquely formulated, injectable, cross-linked–collagen-based product. It has the ability to remain stable in the body for a significantly longer period of time than other collagen products. It is not available in the United States. Trials are underway for this product in Europe. It is manufactured by Colbar Life Sciences, Ltd., 9 Haminofim Street, PO Box 12206, Herzliya, Israel.

Endoplast-50^TM is a product of elastin-solubilized peptides with collagen (bovine, U.S.) for intradermal injection. Two skin tests are performed at 15-day intervals prior to treatment. Test syringes are available. It is provided in 0.5 ml or 1 ml syringes. A 30-gauge needle is used for injection. It is injected in a serial puncture technique in the reticular dermis and is then massaged. There is a rare possibility of hypersensitivity. After treatment, inflammation is expected for 24 to 48 hours. The material influences the proliferation of fibroblasts to produce collagen. Duration of correction is said to be 8 to 12 months. Distributed by Laboratories Filorga, 79 Rue de Miromesnil, 75008 Paris, France. Tel: 01-42-93-94-00, Fax: 01-42-93-79-65, E-mail: filorga@wanadoo.fr.

Esthelis^TM *(Non-FDA Approved)*: This product, which is CE marked and available in Europe, is a monophasic, non-animal hyaluronic acid filler manufactured by double cross-linking with BDDE, the hyaluronic acid into a "cohesive polydensified matrix" and was launched in March 2005 in Europe. As of this writing, it is not yet available in the United States or

Canada. The product comes in "Basic" or "Soft." The "Basic" product contains 25 mg/g sodium hyaluronate and is good for medium depth or deeper lines such as the nasolabial folds. The "Soft" product contains 20 mg/g sodium hyaluronate and is more suitable to finer lines with placement more superficially in the upper dermis. Both products are available in a 1-mL glass syringe and are very easy to inject with seemingly less pain than many hyaluronic acid fillers. Distribution agreements and additional regulatory approval in other countries are ongoing. The product is manufactured by Anteis S.A., 18 Chemin des Aulx, 1228 Plane-les-Ouates, Geneva, Switzerland.

Evolence™ *(Non-FDA Approved)*: This product is CE marked and available in Europe. It is a porcine-derived cross-linked collagen product. According to the manufacturer (no published data available at this writing), Evolence lasts for at least 12 months and was rated as having better wrinkle correction at 15 months compared to Zyplast® by blinded assessors, treating clinicians, and patients participating in a clinical trial. Evolence is produced in vitro by polymerization of monomeric porcine collagen followed by ribose glycation which, unlike many cross-linking technologies, does not require the use of potentially toxic chemicals that limit the degree of cross-linking achievable. The production process removes the most antigenic part of the collagen molecule—the telopeptides, which theoretically produces a treatment that is more immunologically compatible with human collagen. Evolence is manufactured by ColBar Lifescience Ltd, 9 Hamenofim St., PO Box 12206, Herzliya 46733, Israel: Tel +972-9-9718666, Fax +972-9-9718667.

Fascian® (Fascia Biomaterials, Beverly Hills, California, U.S.) is preserved, particulate fascia lata, derived from screened human cadavers. The material is freeze-dried and typically preirradiated. This injectable form of fascia lata can be injected when soft tissue augmentation is desired. Historically, preserved fascia grafts have proven efficacy and an excellent safety record over the past 73 years. In a clinical trial, Burres (4) followed-up 81 subjects for six to nine months after implantation without incidence of infection, allergic reaction, or acute rejection. Soft tissue augmentation was evident three to four months after grafting or longer in most cases. Injectable material is supplied in particle sizes of less than 0.25 mm, less than 0.5 mm or less than 2.0 mm. The Fascian particles are hydrated in 3 to 5 ccs of 0.3% lidocaine solution prior to injection. The injected area is preundermined with a 20-gauge needle and the material is injected into the preformed tunnel with a 16- to 25-gauge needle, depending on the size of the particles used.

Humallagen™ has poor rheology and cannot get through a 30-gauge needle.

Hyacell™ is composed of 40% hyaluronic acid and 20% embryonic tissue. It is not an actual filler but is used in facial and corporal mesotherapy. It stimulates collagen synthesis. Adverse reactions to Hyacell have recently made headlines in the New York area. It is not available in the United States but is undergoing clinical studies in Europe.

Hyal®-System is a higher concentration of hyaluronic acid. It has a molecular weight of 10^6 Daltons. It is available in preloaded syringes and is manufactured by Fidia S.P., Via ponte della Fabbria 3/A, 35031 Abano Terme (Padua), Italy.

Hylan Rofilan Gel is a hyaluronic acid, cross-linked with a natural acid instead of a chemical compound. The product is manufactured and distributed by Rofil Medical International B.V., Stationstaat 1B, 4815 NC Breda, The Netherlands. Tel: 31-76-531-5670, Fax: 31-76-531-5660, E-mail: RMI@rofil.nl.

Juvederm™, *Juvederm HV*™: These are not approved in the United States but are approved in the EU and Canada. Juvederm is nonallergenic hyaluronic acid derived from a nonanimal source. It comes in three versions: Juvederm 18 for fine lines and crow's feet; Juvederm 24 for forehead and cheek wrinkles; and Juvederm 30 to fill lips, sculpture cheeks, and fill deep nasolabial folds. Results can last for four to six months after treatment. Juvederm HV was developed to be more easily injectable than Juvederm itself. The Juvederm line has received good reviews from users in Europe and Canada. Inamed is seeking approval of Juvederm in the United States. It is available from Euromedical Systems Ltd., Connaught House, Moorbridge Road, Bingham, NG138GG, England. Tel: 44(0) 1949838111, E-mail: information@euromedicalsystems.co.uk.

Koken Atelocollagen implant is a 2% monomolecular solution of collagen of Japanese origin (5). It is supplied in cartridges and is to be injected using a dental syringe through a 30-gauge needle. The indications, contraindications, testing, and injection techniques are the same as those for Zyderm collagen implant. Unlike Zyderm, Koken Atelocollagen does not contain lidocaine. It is an aqueous solution of monomolecular collagen molecules, whereas Zyderm is a suspension containing molecules, fibers, and fibrils of collagen. It is manufactured by the Koken Co., Ltd of Japan but is not available in the United States. It is distributed by the Koken Co., LTD., 3-14-3 Mejiro, Toshima-KM, Tokyo 171, Japan. Tel: 81-3-3950-6600.

Macrolane™ is a nonanimal hyaluronic acid, manufactured by Q-Med. It is of greater density than Perlane and Restylane, possibly lasting longer than either. It is being studied for body contouring in Europe. It is available from Q-Med AB, Seminariegatan 21, 752 28 Uppsala, Sweden. Tel: 46 18 474 90 00, E-mail: info@q-med.com.

Metacrill™ is composed of microspheres (20–80 microns) of methacrylate in a colloidal suspension without protein. It is similar to Arteplast. It is distributed by Nutricel, Rua Sampaio Viana, 299-Rio Comprido, Rio de janeiro/RJ, Cep: 20,261-030, Brazil. Tel: 021-502-2314, 021-502-1481, Fax: 021-502-1527, E-mail: metacrill.com.br, website: www.metacrill.com.br.

New-Fill™, *Sculptra*™: New-Fill (or Sculptra in the United States, approved for HIV lipoatrophy) is a poly-lactic acid, not of animal origin. It is provided as freeze-dried material and can be stored at room temperature. After reconstitution with water, it is 4.45% poly-lactic acid and it is recommended that it be mixed 24 hours in advance to facilitate complete dissolution of the material in water, reducing the likelihood of the needles clogging. The material is biocompatible and biodegradable. The development of granulomas and/or nodules has been reported in some patients, especially shortly after the product was launched. Some prolific users of this product report that such complications can be avoided by newer injection techniques. It is injected into the dermis or subdermally using a

26-gauge needle. Indications are for nasolabial folds, lips, lipodystrophy of cheeks, acne scars, wrinkles, hands, and liposuction contour deformities. It is manufactured by Biotech Industry S.A., Siege social, 38 Ave du X Septembre, L2550 Luxembourg.

It was approved in Europe in 1999 to increase the volume of depressed areas, particularly for the correction of skin depression, including skin creases, wrinkles, folds, scars, and eye rings. In 2004, under the name Sculptra, the product was approved by the FDA specifically for the replacement of fat lost in the cheeks owing to the effect of antiretroviral therapy in HIV patients. The injections provide a gradual and significant increase in skin thickness, improving the appearance of folds and sunken areas. The correction using fibroplasia may last for months or longer. In a clinical trial of Sculptra in HIV patients, the treatment results lasted for two years after the first treatment session. Repeat injections may be necessary. Side effects of Sculptra may include the delayed appearance of small bumps or papules under the skin in the treated area. Generally these bumps are not visible and may only be noticed when pressing on the treated area. Other side effects may include injection-related events at the site of injection, such as bleeding, tenderness or discomfort, redness, bruising, or swelling. All patients have some edema and a experience significant proportion of pain during the injection procedure. Sculptra is available from Dermik Laboratories Inc., 1050 Westlakes Drive, Berwyn, Pennsylvania 19312. Tel: (484) 595-2700. Dermik Laboratories is a subsidiary of Aventis Pharmaceuticals, 300 Somerset Corporate, Boulevard, PO Box 6977, Bridgewater, New Jersey 08807.

Plasmagel is an autologous, blood-derived augmenting material. Ascorbic acid and lidocaine are added to blood plasma. The material is heated to form a gel, then injected. It is applicable for wrinkles, contour defects, acne scars, and lip augmentation (6).

Profill™ (or Profil) is provided as a translucent gel. It is a block copolymer of polyoxyethylene and polyoxypropylene with mineral salts, amino acids, and vitamins. The material contains no animal proteins. It is provided as a liquid which can be refrigerated until use. No skin test is required. The liquid material turns to gel upon implantation and can, therefore, be molded after implantation. It is provided in 1 mL syringes and injected with a 30-gauge needle in a serial puncture fashion. Several hours of redness are expected postimplantation. Correction reportedly lasts six to nine months. Profill has reportedly produced severe lipoatrophies of the face several months after injection (7). Profill is frequently used in concert with Endoplast-50. Similar to Endoplast-50, it is manufactured and distributed by Laboratories Filorga, 79 Rue de Miromesnil, 75008 Paris, France. Tel: 01-42-93-94-00, Fax: 01-42-93-79-65, E-mail: filorga@wanadoo.fr.

Radiance™/*Radiance FN*™/*Radiesse*™ is 40 micron spheres of calcium hydroxylapatite (CaHA) suspended in a patented pharmaceutical-grade aqueous polysaccharide gel carrier. Because calcium hydroxylapatite is a normal constituent of bone, it should not elicit a chronic inflammatory or immune response. Additionally, the gel carrier does not require allergy testing as is required with collagen. Radiance FN is the smaller particle and is the agent used for soft tissue augmentation in off-label manner. It is not yet approved by the FDA for esthetic uses but is approved for vocal fold insufficiency and Xray marking. It does not cause chronic inflammation, does not migrate, and requires no skin testing (8). Most patients have minimal to moderate pain and experience some bruising upon injection. There have been problems reported with the formation of submucosal nodules in the lip. Longevity is two to six years. The manufacturer is Bioform Inc., 4133 Courtney Road # 10, Franksville, Wisconsin, 51326, U.S.A. Tel: (262) 835-9800, website: www.bioforminc.com. There is an ongoing legal battle between Bioform and Artes over the ownership of this product.

Resoplast^{TM} (Rofil Medical International, Breda, The Netherlands) is bovine monomolecular collagen in solution. Concentrations of 3.5% and 6.5% are available. Indications and techniques of implantation are similar to Zyderm collagen. A skin test is provided.

Reviderm-intra^{TM} contains 40 to 60 micron dextran beads of the Sephadex type in hylan gel. It is of nonanimal origin. The material is non-immunogenic, biocompatible, and biodegradable. Intradermal injection is given with a 30-gauge needle. EMLA or a topical anesthetic can be used. No overcorrection is necessary. The material can be molded after injection to disperse the beads. Usually two injections are required, the second one coming six weeks after the first. Two hundred and seventy-four patients in a clinical study showed the material to be resistant to resorption and migration. Results usually last six to nine months. The product is manufactured and distributed by Rofil Medical International B.V., Stationstaat 1B, 4815 NC Breda, The Netherlands. Tel: 31-76-531-5670, Fax: 31-76-531-5660, E-mail: RMI@rofil.nl.

Sculptra^{TM}: See New-Fill.

Teosyal^{TM} *(Non-FDA Approved)*: This product is CE marked and available in Europe. It appears to be very similar to Juvederm and is a non-animal derived, monophasic, BDDE cross-linked, hyaluronic acid. It is available as "27g," "30g," and "Meso." The 27G product (27G stands for needle size) contains 25 mg/g of HA, is for the nasolabial lines and lips, and is placed in the deep dermis. The 30G product is injected through a 30G needle for perioral and finer lines and is placed in the mid-dermis. The meso product is injected through either a 30 or 32G needle and, per the company, is for "prevention of wrinkles, a deficit in elasticity and hydration involving the face, neck and low neck." This line of HA is manufactured by Teoxane, S.A., Les charmilles, Rue de Lyon, 105, CH 1203 Geneva. Tel: 41-22-3440-96-36, Fax: 41-22-340-29-33.

A variety of new fillers are available, most of them making their way to the United States after European and Canadian approval. The U.S. market may see a large number of fillers in the near future if many of the companies distributing these new filler products in Europe and Canada seek FDA approval. Caution is adivised when dealing with new fillers, especially permanent ones because they have as a class been associated with side effects, which do not resolve and may result in scarring. Improvements in cross-linking have been useful in improving upon both hyaluronic acid and collagen products, both or which have a long history of use and reasonable safety records.

REFERENCES

1. Neuhof H. The transplantation of tissues. New York: Appleton & Company, 1923.
2. Zuckerman D. Testimony on Artecoll; FDA Advisory Committee on General and Plastic Surgery Devices. February 28, 2003.
3. Ersek RA, Beisang AA. Bioplastique: a new textured copolymer microparticle promises permanence in soft-tissue augmentation. Plast Reconst Surg 1991; 87:693–702.
4. Burres S. Recollagenation of acne scars. Dermatol Surg 1996; 22:364–367.
5. Dierickx P, Derumeaux L. Comparative study of the clinical efficiency of a 2% collagen solution and a 3.5% collagen dispersion on 60 patients. 5th International Congress of Dermatology Surgery. Jerusalem, Israel, October 28–31, 1984.
6. Krajcik R, Orentreich DS, Orentreich N. Plasmagel: a novel injectable autologous material for soft tissue augmentation. J Aesthetic Derm and Cosmetic Surg 1999; 1:109–111.
7. Andre P. Facial lipoatrophy secondary to a new filler device (Profill) treated by lipofilling. J Cosm Dermatol 2002; 2:59–61.
8. Tzikas T. Collagen alternative for facial soft tissue augmentation offers good results. Cosm Surg Times, July 2003.

16

The Art and Architecture of Lips and Their Enhancement with Injectable Fillers

Arnold W. Klein
Department of Dermatology, David Geffen School of Medicine, University of California, Los Angeles, California, U.S.A.

In 1984, lip augmentation with injectable bovine collagen changed the goal of filling agents from eradicating lines to subtly increasing facial volume. Lip augmentation would soon become the number one use of agents for tissue augmentation. Soon it became apparent that the lips were the aesthetic focus of the lower face and a critical member of a small group of female facial landmarks that attracted the male species. These attractive female facial features were identical for males of all races and cultures. What were these facial sites that men were hot-wired to? More than simple sites, they were related to size and shape: a large upper face, smooth forehead, small nose, round eyes (bigger, wider apart with prominent eyelashes), a small lower face, and large lips with a plump yet sharp vermillion border (1). When we look at a person's face, the focus of the upper face is the eyes, and the focus of the lower face is the lips. For years and still to this day, models and actresses have attempted to enhance their lips and correct perioral radial rhytids by using lipsticks and covering agents. This is apparent in early screen stars who were able to create the illusion of any lip they desired through the use of make-up. From the work of Leonardo DaVinci (*Mona Lisa*) through the present day cinema (*First Wife's Club*), the importance of lips is continually emphasized. When full and well defined, lips impart a sense of youth, health, attractiveness, and sexuality to the bearer. Like many features of the face, as the lips age they become far less attractive. Losing volume, they become thin and flat. Also, owing to grinding and wear on the molars and age-related osteoporotic thinning of the mandible, the distance from the lips to the chin is greatly decreased. As dental height is lost, the face ages such that the ends of the lips hang down, contributing to the marionette lines [labio-mandibular grooves; (2)]; subtle enhancement would be the obvious goal. Some physicians felt compelled to define their personal esthetic for lip enhancement. They directed one to enlarge the cupid's bow, increase the relative length of the lower lip, and to augment the projection bulk of both the upper and lower lips. Additionally, it must be remembered that the Collagen Corporation itself attempted to market "The Paris Lip," which focused on vermilion injection with enhancement of the central portion of the lip and exaggeration of the philtral pillars. A study on lip augmentation was performed by the Collagen Corporation but never published owing to conflicts with the U.S. Food and Drug Administration (FDA) in that mucosal injection was an off-label use (3). The use of bovine collagen as a predictable injection agent allowed physicians to provide stable lip enhancement, which was very natural in appearance (4,5). As stated previously, lip augmentations heralded a movement toward the use of fillers for volumetric enhancement (4–11). Indeed, dermatologic and plastic surgical literature did not contain any information regarding the proper esthetic characteristics of lips. While women's magazines would present models with voluptuous lips and many celebrities were adored for their lips, no readily apparent guidelines existed to aid physicians in this area of enhancement (10). This resulted in esthetically improper lip enhancement by some physicians through unguided injection procedures. It was this author's opinion that injections should be performed in a subtle manner that would prevent the augmentation from being readily apparent. While enhancement of the vermilion border was an approved use of injectable bovine collagen, actual mucosal injection was again a frequent, albeit, off-label use of this agent. In 1984, I helped pioneer lip augmentation that began to focus on increasing volume and on an aesthetically pleasing appearance, rather than simply eradicating lines. My technique has evolved into an understanding of how lip enhancement must be done. Above all, it must never be detectable. Lips are about volume, but more importantly, shape and balance. Indeed, the areas of the cupid's bow and philtral pillars could only be slightly altered in that any distortions in these areas would draw attention to the lip enhancement, and possibly present an artificial appearance and detectable alteration.

Hyaluronic acid (HA) products are exciting new materials for soft tissue augmentation with great future potential. HA is a polysaccharide found naturally in the dermis. Its ability to bind water assists in hydration and provides skin turgor. Unlike collagen, it is identical across all species and is produced by many types of cells. In 2004, HAs were FDA-approved for use in tissue augmentation (12,13). They are biologically pure with low protein loads (14). Hylaform, Hylaform-Plus, Captique, and Restylane can all be used for this purpose. My preference is Restylane. It has four times the concentration (20 mg/cc of stabilized HA) as found in the other HA agents (5.5%). Even though there is a higher concentration of material, Restylane has a lower molecular weight, so a direct comparison of these agents based on published studies is impossible. Furthermore, whether the higher concentration is associated with a greater longevity of correction will only be determined by a direct head-to-head comparison. Restylane is a nonanimal stabilized HA gel (NASHA). As a concentrated HA gel, it is excellent for lip volume enhancement. This greater concentration alters the rheology, and, therefore, Restylane is more resistant to flow. It is provided in 1 cc and 4 cc preloaded syringes. Hylaform gel is processed from the cock's combs of domestic fowl. In clinical trials in wrinkles and scars, 80% reported moderate or greater satisfaction at 12 weeks with Hylaform. Hylaform and Restylane are widely used for facial augmentation throughout the world (Canada, England, Europe, Australia, etc.). They are especially popular for volume augmentation of the lips, which are the number one site for injection. Nevertheless, I have found Restylane suitable for almost any area. For fine areas, Restylane can be used with a 32 gauge needle rather than with a 30 gauge needle . Though this creates some shearing of the product and reduces the size of the beads, I have not found this to be problematic. This is excellent for fine lines above the lip, etc. There is reportedly no immunologic activity against Restylane. Indeed most of the reported reactions to Restylane are owing to injection technique although there have been some reports of redness as well as blue hues that persisted at the sites of implantation. Reported adverse reactions are less than two percent and include erythema, ecchymoses, and acne. However, there have been more serious adverse reactions reported with both Hylaform and Restylan (15–17). Furthermore, there remain many patients who prefer the subtlety of injectable collagen alone for lip augmentation.

It is this author's belief that permanent injectables (silicone, etc.) are a formula for disaster in the lips because, in addition to lumpiness, they frequently enlarge and distort the mouth over time. It is difficult to obtain a natural lasting result with a permanent filler. For example, the sharp edge of the upper lip (Glogau-Klien point) is destroyed, giving the upper lip an unnatural appearance with permanent fillers. Furthermore, problems can occur up to 15 years after injection; when reactions occur, surgery is the alternative to remove the agent. As for surgical procedures for lip enhancement as well as implantable materials such as Goretex, etc., they simply do not provide a natural result.

THE ARCHITECTURE OF THE LIP

Are there any rules we can establish for augmenting the perfect lip? In looking at the aging lip, there are two important factors to be considered. One is the shape of the lips themselves and other is the importance of the support provided to the lower third of the face by dentition and bone structure (18–21). These are all features dependent not only on injection of the lips themselves, but also on volumetric restoration of the lower third of the face. The lips should be full and well defined. They should be injected without blunting the edge of the vermilion border of the upper lip. A physician must also focus on the restoration of the ends of the lips, as well as the building of buttresses at these ends to restore height to the lower third of the face, correcting the labio-mandibular grooves/oral commissures. While dermatologic and esthetic journals deal with substances for implantation, these journals do not, in themselves, hold information regarding

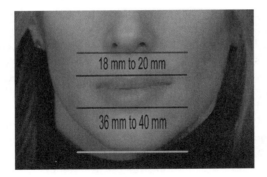

Figure 1
The upper lip should be 18 to 20 mm from the nose and the lower lip should be 36 to 40 mm from the chin.

the proper goal of lip enhancement. Instead, the answer is found in the dental literature where many articles have addressed the proper height, size, and location of the lips as produced by dental restoration (18–21).

With the patient in the postural head position (PHP), the lips should be parallel to a line drawn between the pupils of the eyes. With respect to spatial location, the upper lip should be 18 to 20 mm from the nose and the lower lip should be 36 to 40 mm from the chin (Fig. 1). Finally, in PHP, a line drawn from the mid-nares to the chin should just barely graze the upper and lower lip (Steiner's line) (Fig. 2). Lips must also maintain a natural profile. Unnatural fullness above the lip is to be avoided at all costs since it blunts the edge of the lip and gives

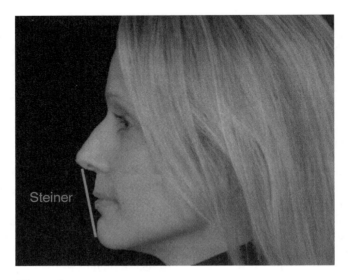

Figure 2
A line drawn from the mid-nares to the chin should just barely graze the upper and lower lip (Steiner's line).

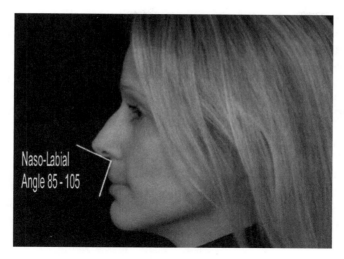

Figure 3
The nasolabial angle should be 85 to 105 degrees.

them a prognathic appearance. With respect to the facial profile, the nasolabial angle should be 85 to 105 degrees (Fig. 3). Finally, there is a slight elevation or ski-jump, which is a point of inflection as the lip turns from glabrous skin to mucosa. Since this site had not been formally noted before, it has been proposed to be called the G–K (Glogau–Klein) point (Fig. 4).

Prior to injection, suitable anesthesia should be administered. Dental blocks are very popular among many patients and physicians (22). However, at times, dental blocks can prevent normal motion of

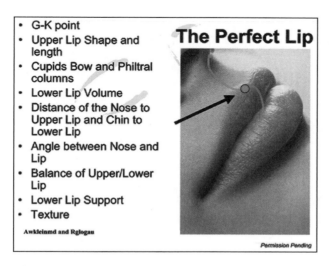

Figure 4
The perfect lip, showing the G–K point.

the lips during the injection session, and this could compromise the cosmetic result. Furthermore, blocks often allow the physician greater license for quick forceful injections with resultant lumpiness, severe bruising, and distortion of the injected site. Without a block, a very gentle injection technique is required. Topical anesthetic such as EMLA and Betacaine-LA (Canada) can be employed if desired. Betacaine-LA is also available in the United States. Additionally, even if HA products are to be used, injectable collagen can be used prior to the use of HA to create a flow track as well as deliver anesthesia to the site.

The patient should be seated upright in a chair with strong overhead lighting. Most authorities agree that aspirin, NSAIDs, and vitamin E should be avoided for a week prior to injection. Nevertheless, bruising and a certain degree of swelling with HAs are to be expected. The slower and more gentle the injection, the lesser pain and trauma. To the diminish swelling during injection, intermittent application of ice can be utilized postinjection. A prior history of herpes labial requires coverage with appropriate antivirals. Finally, an assistant can aid in the assurance of an excellent cosmetic result by being a separate pair of eyes to evaluate the degree of correction and asymmetry from a position in front of the patient while the physician is injecting from their side.

The patient is injected from right to center and then from left to center (Diagram 1). The preservation of the cupid's bow is critical because it is the defining aesthetic of the upper lip. Furthermore, the lower lip is to be injected not as a rounded wheel mass, but instead to produce central rollout or pout. When the lip is injected, the physician must stretch the lip to assure themselves that they are beginning at the end of the lip that is now part of the labio-mandibular groove (Diagram 2). Furthermore, with a firm surface to inject against, the stretched lip provides a better flow surface.

The tip of the needle should be dropped into the potential vermilion space at a 45 degree angle on the mucosal side. The needle is then redirected at a 20 degree angle from the lip. With the lip stretched, this will

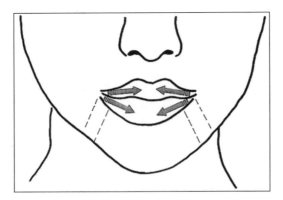

Diagram 1

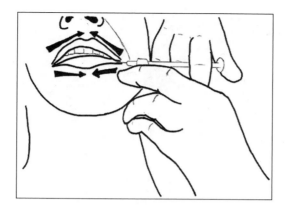

Diagram 2

allow the HA to flow along the potential space. Injection must be slow to ensure that the material stays uniform within this tubular potential. Again, adequate stretch of the lip is critical because a firm surface improves the volume uniformity of flow of the material, which can be hampered by the high viscosity of the agent. The finger can be kept at the G–K point to ensure flow within the channel.

Flow out of or flow above the channel can create an elevated lump, while flow below the channel is also to be avoided. As a point of resistance is met where the material will not flow, the continuation of the injection is moved to the next point. This technique, which I developed, was dubbed the "push-along" technique by Dr. Jean Carruthers. Once the material is injected past the midline of the lower lip, this section of the lip is complete. Next, the portion of the lip that connects the lower

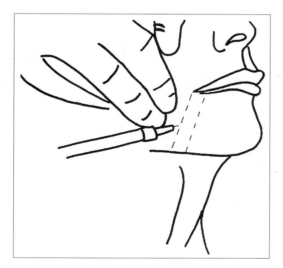

Diagram 3

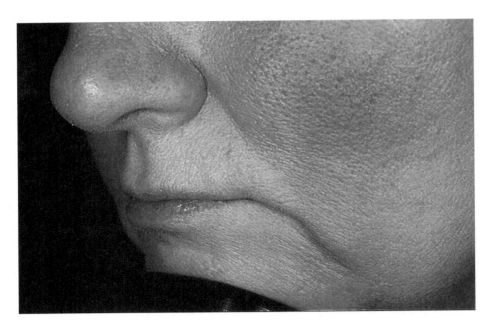

Figure 5
Before injection with Restylane®.

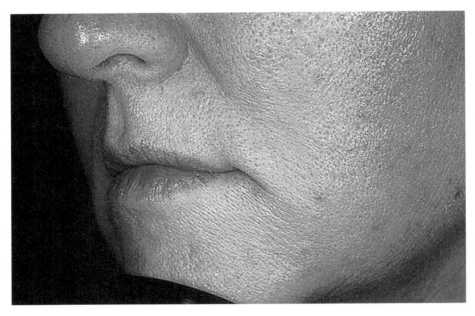

Figure 6
After injection with Restylane®.

lip to the upper lip along the side of the mouth is addressed (the Klein space). This will lift the lip and decrease the labio-mandibular groove. One may ask why this elevates the corner of the mouth. Theoretically, this is accomplished because the material flows around the modeolus as noted by Dr. Alastair Carruthers and securely elevates the corner of the upper and lower lip. The upper lip is injected in a similar manner paying particular attention to retaining the shape of the cupid's bow. Again, care must be taken to keep the material in the proper channel avoiding a lump above the lip. Once this is complete, buttresses from the jaw to the lip are injected in a sequential manner to support the lips and reestablish the vertical height, which has been lost due to bone resorption and any dental changes that may have occurred (Diagram 3). While there are other techniques for lip augmentation, hopefully, this framework will provide the basis for lip augmentation (Figs. 5 and 6). It is well described in a recent article by Carruthers et al. (23).

REFERENCES

1. Etcoff N. Survival of the Prettiest: The Science of Beauty. New York: Doubleday, 1999.
2. Robertson KM, Dyer WK, Dyer WK II. The use of fillers in the aging patient. Facial Plast Surg 1996; 12(3):293–301.
3. Brandt FD, Grekin DA, RA, Mittleman H. "Collagen Implants for Lip Augmentation," submitted then withdrawn to J Dermatol Surg Oncol 1990.
4. Klein AW. Injectable collagen: A tutorial. In: Dzubow LM, ed. Cosmetic Dermatologic Surgery. Philadelphia: Lippincott-Raven, 1998:19–34.
5. Klein AW. Injectable bovine collagen. In: Klein AW, ed. Tissue Augmentation in Clinical Practice. Marcel Dekker: New York, 1998:125–144.
6. Guerrissi JO. Surgical treatment of the senile upper lip. Plast Reconstr Surg 2000; 106(4):938–940.
7. Ergun SS, Cek DI, Baloglu H, Algun Z, Onay H. Why is lip augmentation with autologous fat injection less effective in the vermilion border? Aesth Plast Surg 2001; 25(5):350–352.
8. Castor SA, To WC, Papay FA. Lip augmentation with Allo Derma cellular allogenic dermal graft and fat auto graft: a comparison with autologous fat injection alone. Aesth Plast Surg 1999; 23(3):218–223.
9. Le Louarn C. [Botulinum toxin and facial wrinkles: a new injection procedure] Toxine botulique et rides facials: une nouvelle procedure d'injection. Ann Chir Plast Esthet 1998; 43(5):526–533.
10. Felman G. Direct upper-lip lifting: a safe procedure. Aesth Plast Surg 1993; 17(4):291–295.
11. Flageul G, Halimi L. Injectable collagen: an evaluation after 10 year's use as a complement of plastic surgery. Le collagene injectable: bilan après 10 ans d'utilisation en complement de la chirurgie esthetique. Ann Chir Plast Esthet 1994; 39(6):765–771.
12. Maloney BP. Cosmetic surgery of the lips. Facial Plast Surg 1996; 12(3):265–278.
13. Narins RS, Brandt F, Leyden J, Lorenc ZP, Rubin M, Smith S. A randomized, double-blind, multicenter comparison of the efficacy and tolerability of Restylane versus Zyplast for the correction of naso-labial folds. Dermatol Surg 2003; 29(6):588–595.
14. Friedman P, et al. Safety data of injectable nonanimal stabilized hyaluronic acid gel for soft tissue augmentation. Dermatol Surg 2002; 28:491–494.
15. Schanz S, et al. Arterial embolization caused by injection of hyaluronic acid (Restylane). Br J Dermatol 2002; 146(5):928–929.
16. Waddell DD. Acute reaction to intra-articular Hylan G-F. J Bone Joint Surg Am 2003; 85(8):1620.
17. Oswald A, Gachter A. Acute reaction to intra-articular Hylan G-F for treatment of gonarthrosis onset. Schweiz Rundsch Med Prax 2000; 89(46):1929–1931.
18. Rifkin R. Restoring vertical dimension to improve function, facial harmony, and dental esthetics. Contemp Esth Restor Prac 2004; 40–46.
19. McLaren EA, Rifkin R. Macroesthetics: Facial and dentofacial analysis. CDAJ 2002; 30(11):839–846.
20. Niamtu J. Cosmetic oral and maxillofacial surgery: the frame for cosmetic dentistry. Dent Today 2001; 20(4):88–91.
21. Cheng JT, Perkins SW, Hamilton MM. Perioral rejuvenation. Facial Plast Surg 2000; 8(2):223–233.
22. Elson ML. Anesthesia for lip augmentation. Dermatol Surg 1997; 23(5):405.
23. Carruthers J, Klein A, Carruthers A, Glogua R, Canfield D. Safety and efficacy of nonanimal stabilized byaluronic acid for improvement of mouth corners. Dermatol Surg 2005; 227.

17

HIV Facial Lipoatrophy: Etiology and Methods of Correction

Derek H. Jones
Department of Dermatology/Medicine, University of California,
Los Angeles, California, U.S.A.

HIV-associated lipodystrophy is an as yet undefined syndrome that may include hypertriglyceridemia, insulin resistance, diabetes, dorsocervical fat accumulation (buffalo hump), central visceral adiposity, and lipoatrophy, including thinning of the extremities, buttocks and face with sunken cheeks, and temporal wasting. It is unclear if a single disorder of lipid metabolism is responsible for the heterogeneity of findings. HIV *lipodystrophy* may represent a variety of different metabolic disorders, each with different pathophysiological mechanisms. This chapter will focus on the etiology and treatment of HIV-associated *lipoatrophy* as a distinct entity.

CLINICAL PRESENTATION AND EPIDEMIOLOGY

HIV-associated lipoatrophy manifests wasting of subcutaneous fat in the extremities and face. Lipoatrophy in the extremities often reveals underlying subcutaneous vessels, leading to a pseudo-athletic appearance. Loss of fat in the cheek, temporal, and periocular areas may create a gaunt and ill appearance. Individuals may feel very well, but look quite the opposite. Lipoatrophy may appear very rapidly over a few months, and often causes great distress among those affected. Whites have a greater risk of HIV lipoatrophy when compared to Blacks and Hispanics. Up to 50% of HIV-infected individuals may display lipoatrophy, with the incidence being on the rise (1). With over one million HIV-infected individuals in the United States alone, the numbers of individuals seeking treatment for facial lipoatrophy are staggering, particularly in major metropolitan areas.

ETIOLOGY

The etiology of HIV-associated lipoatrophy is unclear. Evidence points to a possible role of different antiretroviral medications, immune dysregulation, hormonal influences, and host factors including long-standing HIV infection.

The Role of Protease Inhibitors

The advent of protease inhibitors (PI) in the mid-1990s revolutionized the treatment of HIV. Combining PI with older nucleoside reverse transcriptase inhibitors (NRTI), referred to as HAART (Highly Active Anti-Retroviral Treatment), helped to rapidly suppress viral loads, raise CD4 counts, and reconstitute ravaged immune systems. HIV/AIDS changed from a once almost certain death sentence into a chronic, manageable disease. However, the syndrome of lipodystrophy shortly became evident [1]. The blame was initially placed squarely on PI therapy. Indeed, HIV protease, the target of PI, shares 60% homology with lipoprotein receptor–related protein and cytoplasmic retinoic acid–binding protein type 1 [2]. These proteins are involved in lipid and adipocyte metabolism. Inhibition of these proteins with PI therapy causes reduced differentiation and apoptosis of fat cells in peripheral areas [2,3]. In cultured fat cell models, PI causes decreased adipocyte differentiation, increased insulin resistance, and increased apoptosis [4,5]. Clinically, lipoatrophy is more prevalent with the use of PI, particularly indinavir, with the risk increasing with longer duration of its use [1]. However, although PI therapy may play a role in the pathogenesis of lipoatrophy, it is clear that it is not the sole cause.

The Role of NRTI Therapy

Clinically, lipoatrophy is associated with NRTI therapy, particularly stavudine [1]. It has been suggested that PI acts synergistically with NRTI [6]. One study shows that lipoatrophy is much less common in dual PI-treated patients if they did not receive NRTI therapy as well [7]. Etiologically, NRTI-related lipoatrophy may be secondary to NRTI-induced mitochondrial toxicity [8]. NRTIs may deplete mitochondrial DNA, resulting in fat cell apoptosis. More recently, thymidine-analog NRTIs have been proposed to be etiologically more significant. In one study, switching from a thymidine-analog NRTI (stavudine, zidovudine) to a nonthymidine NRTI (abacavir) actually increased peripheral limb fat at 24 weeks as measured by computed tomography (CT) and dual-energy X-ray absorptiometry (DEXA) scanning, although the effect was not clinically apparent [9].

The Role of Host Factors

Host factors are an especially relevant risk factor for HIV lipoatrophy. Among 1077 patients, lipoatrophy was more prevalent among patients with increasing age (> 40 years), Caucasian race, more severe HIV disease (i.e., AIDS), CD4 count < 100 or < 100 at nadir, longer duration of HIV infection, and body mass index loss (1). There were no dysmorphic changes if nondrug risk factors were absent. Therefore, lipoatrophy cannot be considered a simple adverse drug reaction. Lipodystrophy may be a consequence of prolonged survival in HIV (18).

The Role of Immune Dysregulation

There is an association of lipoatrophy with CD4 count at nadir, as well as CD4 increase during HAART, independent of specific antiretroviral drugs (1). HIV lipoatrophy may be secondary to the alteration of inflammatory cytokines in HIV. HAART-treated subjects have elevated numbers of CD8 lymphocytes containing tumor necrosis factor (TNF), and there is an association between lipoatrophy and serum concentrations of soluble TNF-receptors in HIV-infected patients (15,16). Release of TNF from subcutaneous adipocytes in vitro is higher among those with HIV lipodystrophy, regardless of antiretroviral use (17). TNF may mediate adipocyte differentiation and lipolysis. Therefore, adipocyte loss may be associated with TNF-related inflammation secondary to immune reconstitution or HIV itself.

The Role of Hormonal Influences

The occurrence of central obesity and buffalo hump in HIV lipodystrophy led to earlier speculation that the disorder may be secondary to Cushing's syndrome. However, no evidence of Cushing's syndrome has been demonstrated (10). Aggravation of lipodystrophy may be associated with low dehydroepiandrosterone (DHEA) levels, increased cortisol/DHEA ratios, and increased serum interferon levels (11,12). Furthermore, many patients with HIV are treated with anabolic steroids to prevent or treat HIV-related weight loss. A recent study has demonstrated that supplemental testosterone may decrease subcutaneous adipose tissue in HIV-infected men, which may be a complicating factor in HIV lipoatrophy. Moreover, lipodystrophy progresses despite the use of anabolic steroids (14).

PSYCHOLOGICAL EFFECTS OF LIPOATROPHY

Lipoatrophy is often devastating to those affected. In a study by Collins et al., it was demonstrated that individuals with lipoatrophy often had poor body image and low self-esteem, became depressed and socially isolated, and found that their sexual relationships were adversely affected. Furthermore, they often became noncompliant with HAART regimens, and felt that the doctor thought that their lipodystrophy was less of a concern than they did. There was also a negative economic impact of supplements and surgery undertaken to correct the problem (19). The scarlet letter of visible lipoatrophy frequently discloses these individuals as victims of a modern plague. Those affected are frequently desperate for treatments options, particularly options that have greater longevity than bioabsorbable fillers. Patients often seek more permanent forms of correction administered by unlicensed and untrained individuals in nonmedical settings. Such patients endanger themselves by undergoing correction with permanent filler substances not approved for use in the United States, and for which reliable toxicology data and human studies may not exist.

METHODS OF CORRECTION

Systemic Therapy

The thiazolidinediones (rosiglitazone, pioglitazone) are antidiabetic agents that improve insulin resistance in type 2 diabetes mellitus, and may also lead to fat gain in some patients. In vitro, they may rescue cultured fat cells from the harmful (apoptotic) effects of PI (4). Furthermore, they may increase fat mass in familial forms of lipodystrophy (20). Two studies have shown modest patient-perceived improvement in lipodystrophy after 24 weeks of rosiglitazone or pioglitazone, although effects on objective measurements, if any, are unclear (21,22). A more rigorous, prospective study comparing 8 mg q.i.d. rosiglitazone to placebo in 15 lipodystrophy patients showed no change in fat mass at 24 weeks, as measured by magnetic resonance imaging (MRI) (23). Therefore, it appears that a role for thiazolidinediones outside of clinical trials in the treatment of HIV lipoatrophy is not currently justified.

Switching HAART therapy away from drugs with more likelihood of causing lipoatrophy (PI, stavudine, zidovudine) has revealed that limited increases in leg-fat mass ($< 10\%$ of total limb fat mass, measured by DEXA and CT scanning) can be achieved after 24 weeks, but the change was not perceptible to the human eye (9,24). Furthermore, switching therapy in response to lipoatrophy incurs risks such as viral rebound and adverse drug events. Lastly, prolonged treatment interruption (> 6 months) does not yield a clinically evident improvement in lipoatrophy. In conclusion, systemic therapy, drug switching, or treatment interruption at this point does not appear to be an effective treatment for lipoatrophy.

Soft Tissue Augmentation

Soft tissue augmentation for HIV facial lipoatrophy may be grouped into two categories: (i) FDA-permissible versus FDA-prohibited and (ii) bioabsorbable versus permanent. FDA-permissible, bioabsorbable options include bovine collagen (Zyplast[TM]), human collagen (Cymetra[TM], Fascian[TM]), hyaluronic acid gel (Restylane[TM]), polylactic acid (Sculptra[TM]), fat transfer, and surgical Alloderm[TM] implants. FDA-permissible permanent options include ePTFE or custom-designed silastic implants, facelift, or microinjection silicone (off-label, investigational use only). FDA-prohibited,

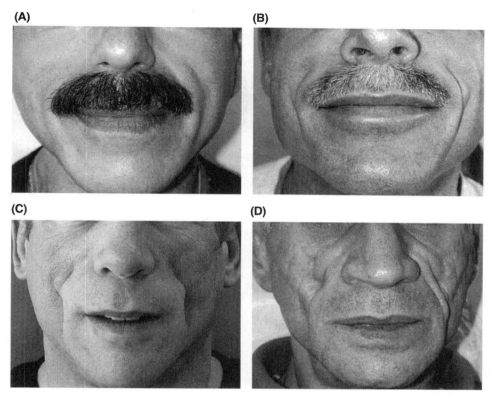

Figure 1
Lipoatrophy severity scale: stage 1 (**A**); stage 2 (**B**); stage 3 (**C**); stage 4 (**D**).

permanent options include polymethylmethacrylate (Artecoll^{TM}, Metacril^{TM}), mixtures of synthetic polymers (Kopolymer 4-E^{TM}, Metrex^{TM}), Biopolymere^{TM}, polyvinyl gel microspheres, and mixtures of synthetic polymers in water (BioAlacmid^{TM}, Aquamid^{TM}). A scale for rating the severity of facial lipoatrophy (Carruthers Lipoatrophy Severity Scale) has recently been proposed (25), and may be useful in the future for accurate inter-study comparison of different filler substances (Fig. 1).

FDA-PERMISSIBLE, BIOABSORBABLE OPTIONS

Zyplast^{TM} Collagen

The author performed a three-year retrospective analysis of more than 100 patients who underwent correction of HIV facial lipoatrophy with Zyplast, over 300 treatment visits. Zyplast was injected into the subdermal plane in aliquots of 0.1 cc to prevent lumpiness. Only cheek areas were treated. The average volume of collagen per treatment was 4 cc. Average time to follow-up for patient-initiated reinjection was 136 days (4.5 months), with 66% of patients returning for at least one reinjection. Adverse events occurred in 0.01% of treatments, and were limited to temporary palpable lumpiness in five patients and collagen necrosis leading to mild scar formation in one patient. Placing too much volume directly into the dermis may compress dermal vessels and create necrosis. Nodularity and necrosis may be limited by injecting into the subdermal plane, aspirating before injecting, limiting the volume to 0.1 cc per needle insertion, and placing injections 2 to 3 mm apart. Interestingly, no patient displayed collagen hypersensitivity, which may be related to a thy-2 shift–mediated decrease in delayed hypersensitivity seen in HIV. On average, there was a one-stage improvement on the Carruthers' lipoatrophy scale immediately postinjection. Forty percent of treated patients had only Stage 1 lipoatrophy (mild and localized), and it was these patients who seemed to get the best response and were most pleased with their Zyplast correction. Anecdotally, clinical persistence of correction in most patients was, at most, only 20% to 30% at six months. Most patients were very grateful for the correction achieved with Zyplast, but were uniformly disappointed when it became reabsorbed. Reasons for discontinuation of Zyplast treatments included short duration of correction, unnatural feel of collagen beneath the skin, and excessive cost related to repeat injections (Figs. 2 and 3).

Micronized AlloDerm® (Cymetra™)

Tsao evaluated 25 patients with HIV facial lipoatrophy treated with injectable micronized AlloDerm (40). AlloDerm was reconstituted with 3 cc of 1% lidocaine with 1:100,000 epinephrine to achieve a concentration of 330 mg/cc. Six to twelve cc of AlloDerm was injected into the mid-to-deep dermis of affected facial sites (medial cheeks and temples). Patients were evaluated at one and three months postinjection and retreated as needed. All patients experienced complete augmentation of their facial lipoatrophy. The results started to fade at one month and most patients

(A)   **(B)**

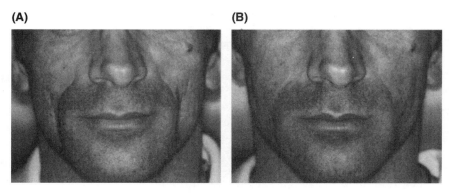

Figure 2
Pre- (**A**) and immediately post- (**B**) 7.5 cc of Zyplast™ collagen.

(A)   **(B)**

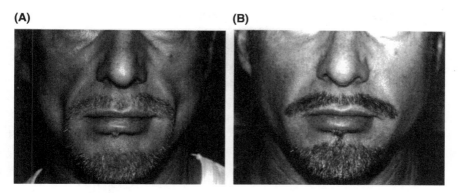

Figure 3
Pre- (**A**) and post- (**B**) 17-cc microinjection of Silikon 1000™, injected over 8 monthly visits (approximately 2 cc/visit).

had returned to their pretreatment lipoatrophy baseline within three months. Side effects were minimal and included expected post-injection erythema and edema lasting 24–48 hours. No infections, scarring, allergic reactions, or other adverse complications were seen. Injectable alloderm was considered a safe and effective treatment option. However, as with Zyplast collagen, excessive cost and necessity of frequent treatments with large volumes limit the utility of micronized AlloDerm for this indication.

Fascian™

Fascian is preserved human particulate fascia lata prepared for injection. Currently, there are no published studies on the use of Fascian for HIV lipoatrophy. It has been proposed that injection with Fascian typically generates new native collagen deposition in the treatment area (27). This hypothesis has stimulated some physicians to try Fascian for correction of HIV facial lipoatrophy. Physicians with significant experience of using Fascian for HIV lipoatrophy state that results are disappointing. Harold Brody, MD informally analyzed the results of 30 of his HIV facial lipoatrophy patients treated with Fascian. The substance reabsorbed very quickly, with less than 25% correction remaining on average at eight weeks posttreatment, when 240 to 320 mg of 1.0 mm particle size was used. (H. Brody, personal communication, 2002). With maintenance treatments performed every six to eight weeks with 160 to 240 mg of 1.0 mm particle size, most had persistence of less than 25% to 50% every time they came in at the six- to eight-week interval. Dr. Brody commented that "the results with Fascian, therefore, are not as sustaining as Zyplast and are disappointing." Many HIV lipoatrophy patients treated with Fascian confirm the rapid disappearance of Fascian postinjection. One physician has stated that after treating hundreds of HIV lipoatrophy patients, he has given up on any hope of its effectiveness for this condition (26). The idea that Fascian induces native collagen production apparently does not hold true for HIV lipoatrophy.

Fat Transfer

Since HIV lipoatrophy involves the loss of the patient's own subcutaneous fat, it seems logical that fat transfer would be the most appropriate augmentation option. Between 1997 and 1998, the author performed a series of fat transfers on 10 lipoatrophy patients. Donor fat was obtained from the abdomen or buttock. Excess fat, when available, was frozen and reinjected at three- to six-month intervals to help maintain correction. All did well, but the fat in almost all cases became reabsorbed over 6 to 12 months. Others have noted variable persistence of correction after fat transfer for HIV lipoatrophy (27). Factors initially stimulating fat loss may continue to promote the loss of donor fat after fat transfer. Indeed, HIV lipoatrophy patients often lose subcutaneous fat in the abdomen and buttocks, which are the usual donor sites (central abdominal lipoaccumulation in HIV usually occurs in the deep visceral fat, not the subcutaneous fat). Therefore, it makes sense that adipocytes from these donor areas would continue to dwindle. Currently, the biggest problem is that most affected with facial lipoatrophy have significant lipoatrophy of subcutaneous fat in the abdomen and buttock area, and therefore lack adequate fat reserves for transfer. An interesting potential donor site is fat from HIV-related dorsocervical lipoaccumulation. Liposuction is an excellent treatment option for dorsocervical lipoaccumulation (29,30). The author performed liposuction on a patient for this condition and transferred the aspirated fat to treat the patient's facial cheek lipoatrophy. The transferred fat has persisted over several intervening years, and the patient remains satisfied. Other physicians have noticed similar persistence of fat transferred from dorsocervical lipoaccumulation. (H. Brody, personal communication, 2002). This substantiates the idea that central (visceral) and dorsocervical adipocytes may be qualitatively and metabolically different from subcutaneous adipocytes elsewhere (31). In summary, in the few patients who have adequate donor fat, autologous fat transfer is a viable treatment option. However, incomplete persistence of correction with gradual reabsorption of fat over time, limits patient acceptance.

AlloDerm® Implants

A Los Angeles plastic surgeon has implanted AlloDerm (human cadaveric dermal tissue) sheets through a facelift incision to correct facial lipoatrophy in several patients. (Gregory Mueller, MD, personal communication, 2002). The initial correction is often quite satisfying to patients. However, implanted grafts often become reabsorbed over a two-year period. The great cost of this procedure and the possibility of graft absorption limit the utility of this procedure for HIV lipoatrophy.

NewFill™ (Polylactic Acid)

Polylactic acid (NewFill™, Medifill, London, W8 U.K., Biotech Industrie SA, Luxembourg; Sculptra®, Dermik Laboratories, Berwyn, PA) is an injectable bioabsorbable material for soft tissue augmentation. Poly-lactic acid is purported to be immunologically inert, and has been widely used as a vehicle for subcutaneously or intramuscularly injected drugs, or as a dissolvable bone implant or absorbable. Gradual reabsorption is typically expected over a two to three year period.

Polylactic acid has an interesting history within the U.S.'s HIV community. It has received significant press coverage worldwide in HIV patient-oriented periodicals and is often touted as a superior option for treating HIV facial wasting. During 2001 in the United States, prior to FDA approval of polylactic acid, Direct Access Alternative Information Resources (DAAIR) provided patients access to NewFill on their website www.daair.org. DAAIR stated that patients could legally obtain NewFill in the United States under FDA Personal Use Importation Regulations. Patients had to complete a Personal Use Importation Form downloaded from the website, obtain a prescription from a physician, and send it to DAAIR with payment for the substance. The substance was then shipped directly to the patient. U.S. physicians from Washington, D.C., New York, Florida, and California who were apparently trained for use of NewFill were listed on the website, and it was recommended that patients take the product to one of these physicians to have it injected. In October 2001, the FDA restricted the availability of NewFill through DAAIR, citing the following:

> NewFill is not approved for use in the United states. We have become aware that DAAIR, an AIDS buyer service, is attempting to bring in large quantities of NewFill under FDA's Compassionate Use/Personal Use Policy.
>
> I do not believe that NewFill qualifies for approval as a personal use item. A personal use item is one that is generally used at home, under the supervision of a licensed physician. In this case, the user is not actually using the device. One has to take it to his/her physician, who injects the substance in a three-stage process. If the Agency was to permit such an activity, it would open up a gigantic loophole for manufacturers of other devices like breast implants, heart valves, pacemakers, etc., to avoid the preapproval requirements of the Act, and simply have their patients order an unapproved device, and bring it to them so they could implant it.
>
> Another concern relates to the availability of legally marketed alternatives. According to FDA staffers, there are legal alternatives that have been cleared for use by the FDA. These devices have demonstrated their safety and effectiveness as they went through the approval process. DAAIR's website presents NewFill as safe and effective, but we are unaware of any such data.

The European VEGA study has followed patients treated with polylactic acid for 96 weeks (36). Fifty patients with severe facial lipoatrophy received four sets of injections at day zero and then every two weeks for six weeks. Patients were evaluated by clinical examination and facial ultrasonography and photography at screening and at weeks 6, 24, 48, 72, and 96. At entry, the median facial fat thickness was zero (range, 0.0–2.1 mm). The median total cutaneous thickness increased significantly from baseline: +5.1 mm at week 6, +6.4 mm at week 24, +7.2 mm at week 48, +7.2 mm at week 72, and +6.8 mm at week 96 ($p < 0.001$). No adverse events were observed. In 22 (44%) patients, palpable but nonvisible subcutaneous nodules were observed with a spontaneous resolution in six patients by week 96. Based on these data and data from other studies (37), on August 3rd 2004, the FDA granted conditional fast-track approval for polylactic acid to be marketed in the United States under the name Sculptra™, specifically for treatment of HIV-associated facial lipoatrophy. Conditions of approval include completion of a five-year registry study in the United States to further evaluate safety.

In the author's experience, patients achieving correction with polylactic acid generally state that the correction may dissipate after 6 to 12 months, and optimal corrections are difficult to achieve. In two patients treated with NewFill, the author has observed visible, small, firm, superficial red papules at the injection sites that have persisted over two years. Biopsy revealed a granulomatous foreign body reaction in the dermis. Therefore, injectable polylactic acid cannot be considered completely biologically inert (i.e., it is capable of triggering inflammatory reactions). It should be injected strictly into the subdermal plane, as more superficial injection may cause visible granulomatous papules. As with collagen, fat, and hyaluronic acid, the use of polylactic acid may be limited by high cost and the necessity over time of repeat treatments with large volumes.

Restylane™ (Non-animal Stabilized Hyaluronic Acid)

Hyaluronic acid is a polysaccharide component of soft tissue and is identical in all species and tissue types. Restylane (Medicis, Santa Barbara, California, U.S.A.) is an injectable form of hyaluronic acid, FDA-approved for soft tissue augmentation in December of 2003. Perlane™ (Q-Med Esthetics, Uppsala, Sweden) is composed of larger gel particles of hyaluronic acid and is intended for subdermal injection. Physicians in Canada have had success with Perlane (a larger gel-particle size of NASHA but not yet FDA approved) in treatment of HIV facial lipoatrophy, although large-scale studies have not been performed (50). The larger gel-particle size of Perlane may confer greater longevity of augmentation, perhaps up to 12 months or more (Kjell Rensfeldt, M.D., personal communication, 2002).

Calcium Hydroxylapatite (Radiance™, Radiesse™)

Radiance FN (recently renamed Radiesse) (BioForm, Franksville, Wisconsin, U.S.A.), consists of calcium hydroxylapatite (CaHA) microspheres suspended in an aqueous, polysaccharide gel. Apparently, it is long-lasting yet is ultimately bioabsorbable over months to years. It is FDA-approved as an augmenting agent for oral/maxillofacial defects, vocal cord insufficiency, and as a radiographic tissue marker. Some physicians in the United States are beginning to use it off-label for HIV facial lipoatrophy. The substance is radio-opaque. Formal studies evaluating the safety and efficacy of calcium hydroxylapatite for soft tissue augmentation are lacking. A recent report (49) describes the use of Radiance FN in three patients with HIV facial lipoatrophy. One patient required only one treatment, while two patients required a touch-up treatment at one month. The percentage of improvement following the initial treatment ranged from 75% to 90%. The authors report that although there has been some loss of improvement over time, there has been significant persistence for up to nine months. No complications were reported, and patient satisfaction was deemed high (49).

FDA-PERMISSIBLE, PERMANENT OPTIONS

Injectable Liquid Silicone

Among cosmetic dermatologists, off-label use of FDA-approved liquid injectable silicone is emerging as a safe, effective, and permanent treatment option for HIV facial lipoatrophy. Recently, Jones et al. (34) reported their experience with highly purified 1000 centistoke silicone oil for HIV facial lipoatrophy. Currently, over 1000 patients with HIV-associated facial lipoatrophy are being treated in an open pilot trial using a highly purified 1000 centistoke silicone oil injected by microdroplet serial puncture technique. Data on 77 subjects with a complete correction were analyzed to determine the number of treatments, amount of silicone, and time required to reach complete correction, relative to initial severity. The volume of silicone, number of treatments, and time required to reach a complete correction were directly related to initial severity of lipoatrophy ($p < 0.0001$). Supple, even facial contours were routinely restored, with all patients tolerating treatments well. No adverse events were noted. Currently, liquid injectable silicone appears to be the most cost effective treatment option in the United States. However, longer follow-up of treated patients is required to adequately assess the efficacy, durability and longer term safety of liquid injectable silicone for HIV facial lipoatrophy (34).

Silikon 1000 (Alcon Labs, Fort Worth, Texas, U.S.A.) is approved as an injectable intraocular fluid for treating retinal detachment. The background on the legality of silicone and descriptions of risks, benefits, and safe injection techniques were recently described (35). It is important for physicians wishing to perform this procedure to receive appropriate training in the microinjection technique. Physicians must also understand that use of injectable silicone for cosmetic purposes in the United States is currently not FDA approved, although physicians may legally use this product off-label. It is advisable to check with the State Licensing Boards and malpractice carriers prior to treating patients. Furthermore, physicians and patients must understand that the use of microinjection silicone for cosmetic purposes and for HIV facial lipoatrophy is investigational.

Pretreatment, patients must be medically stable with no evidence of active infection other than well-controlled HIV disease. Viral load and CD4 counts should be stable and there should have been no changes in the HIV treatment regimen for at least three months prior to injection. It is also important to use medical grade, FDA-approved silicone (Silikon 1000) and a strict microinjection technique (0.01 cc micro-aliquots through a 30-gauge needle injected at least 2 mm apart into the subdermal plane), and to keep the volume of injection to 1 cc or less per side. Larger volumes injected all at once may potentially increase the risk of complications, such as migration, granuloma, or abscess formation. Furthermore, injections must be performed at no less than one month intervals to allow for foreign body–induced collagen deposition, which will continue to augment the correction for up to three months postinjection. Doing so will ensure the buildup of a stable, smooth, and natural-feeling matrix of silicone microdroplets encased by the patient's own natural collagen. This requires great patience from both patient and physician, as noticeable corrections may take months to achieve, particularly with more severe lipoatrophy. With correctly performed injectable silicone, the cosmetic dermatologist can potentially achieve safe, cosmetically elegant, cost-effective, natural-feeling, and persistent correction of HIV facial lipoatrophy, with the potential to alleviate much suffering. The FDA has recently approved a phase I study to ascertain the safety and efficacy of a highly purified form of silicone, SilSkin[TM] (R-J Development Corporation, Peabody, Massachusetts, U.S.A.), for the treatment of facial wrinkles and HIV-associated facial lipoatrophy.

Expanded Polytetrafluoroethylene (ePTFE) Implants

Glougau has implanted SoftForm (ePTFE, in tube design) in a series of patients to correct HIV facial lipoatrophy (32). With ePTFE, permanent correction of HIV lipoatrophy is obtainable, but the correction is often incomplete. Although ePTFE implants fill the deep, triangular malar hollow, they do not address the more subtle facial contour distortions that may be seen in this condition. Often, palpable lumpiness may result. Carruthers has successfully addressed this problem by performing micro-injection silicone following ePTFE implantation (Alastair Carruthers, M.D., personal communication, 2002). It should be noted that implantation with ePTFE may carry the risk of extrusion, movement, infection and swelling (33).

Facelift

During consultations for HIV facial lipoatrophy correction, patients often manually pull up their redundant cheek skin at the preauricular area and ask, "Couldn't we just pull the excess skin to get rid of this problem?" Initial results with facelifts for lipoatrophy often reveal improvement, with attenuation of the malar hollows. However, in the author's experience, cheek hollows often return to baseline over a two-year period. The fundamental problem with HIV facial lipoatrophy is loss of subcutaneous fat. These patients are treated more effectively with fillers. To quote an adage of the cosmetic dermatologist, "lifts lift, and fillers fill." These patients most often do best with fillers.

Custom-Designed Midfacial and Submalar Implants

Binder et al. (47) recently reported on the use of custom-designed midfacial and submalar silastic implants for HIV facial lipoatrophy. The author has observed two patients whose lipoatrophy has progressed after implant placement, visibly revealing the edge of the implant. The unnatural feel of the rigid implant beneath the skin and the high cost of the procedure limit the attractiveness of this procedure.

Autologous Dermafat Grafts

Autologous grafts of de-epithelialized dermis with attached subdermal fat have been transferred from donor sites on HIV patients to the lipoatrophic facial area (48). Contour irregularities, high cost, and necessity of surgical risk and downtime limit the usefulness of this procedure.

FDA-PROHIBITED, PERMANENT OPTIONS

Polymethylmethacrylate (Artecoll™)

Polymethylmethacrylate (PMMA) is a nonbiodegradable synthetic polymer that may be used for soft tissue augmentation. Marcio Serra from Rio de Janiero, Brazil has recently reported results of 120 HIV facial lipoatrophy patients treated with injectable PMMA suspended in hydroxyethylcellulose and lidocaine. Minimum posttreatment follow-up was 12 months and maximum was 30 months. No infection, granuloma, or allergic reaction was observed, and the results were lasting with good esthetic results. Histopathology showed a diffuse granulomatous infiltrate in the subcutis, with extracellular vacuoles of different sizes but uniformly round shape. No change in CD4 count or viral load was attributable to the procedure. Some patients needed new injections after 12 to 18 months in previously untreated areas because of lipoatrophy progression. PMMA was deemed longer lasting and more cost-effective when compared with collagen or fat implants. The implants had a positive influence on the patient's psychological status, promoting improvement in self-esteem and quality of life (38).

Artecoll consists of homogenous PMMA microspheres suspended in bovine collagen, intended for soft tissue augmentation. FDA-approval studies for Artecoll are currently being conducted. As with all permanent injectable fillers, potential side effects of polymethylmethacrylate include development of granulomas, which may present as indurated nodules or plaques.

Polyvinyl Gel and Polyacramide Microspheres (Evolution™)

Vincento del Pino recently reported on the use of microspheres of polyvinyl gel and polyacrylamide (Evolution) for the treatment of HIV facial lipoatrophy. Thirty-five individuals were treated, and before and after photographs of half the group showed apparently convincing facial restoration. Of the 35 patients, 33 described the results as excellent or very good, one year after the first treatment, which usually consisted of two sets of injections. The treatments were well tolerated, with only mild facial swelling noted in two patients (39).

Kuhra Vital™ Implants (Rhegecoll™, Procell™, Metrex™, Kopolymer 4-E™)

Some HIV lipoatrophy patients in Los Angeles have received injection with the Kuhra Vital Implants (Dermabiol Institute, Lucerne, Switzerland), performed illegally by a non-physician practitioner. Apparently, Kopolymer 4-E and Metrex were the primary products used. For Kopolymer 4-E, the manufacturer-stated contents are polyoxiethylene-4 fatty acid ester, copolymers 4G, elastine spheres, and emulsifiers. For Metrex the stated composition is acrylate and methacrylate spheres, copolymers 4-G, polyethyleneglycol, cryptoxantine, ascorbic acid, and stabilizer (www.kuhravital.com). The manufacturer claims that the substances are biocompatible, nontoxic, and tolerated by 100% of patients. Unfortunately, there is no known legitimate clinical data supporting the composition, efficacy, or safety claims stated by the manufacturer. Furthermore, the products carry no CE mark for legal use in European (EEC) countries (equivalent to FDA-approval) and no U.S. FDA approval. Therefore, it cannot be medically justified to use these products for treatment of HIV lipoatrophy at present.

Polyacrylamide Gel and Other Synthetic Injectable Polymers

Del Pino has reported success injecting polyacrylamide gel (Aquamid™, Contura, Denmark), a non-FDA approved synthetic polymer, for the treatment of HIV facial lipoatrophy (41). The product reportedly contains 97.5% water with 2.5% polyacrylamide. The gel is injected subcutaneously in larger volumes. Apparently, a fibrous capsule ultimately forms around the periphery of the balloon-like implants and imparts a long-lasting correction. Advocates of polyacrylamide-in-water products claim that the substance can be easily removed through a small incision and drainage procedure, although formal studies supporting this are lacking. On Contura's website, claims of safety and efficacy of Aquamid are supported by descriptions of histologic studies and either retrospective or ongoing prospective human trials. None of the data, however, has been published in peer-reviewed medical journals. Recently, de Bree et al. (42) reported a case of severe granulomatous inflammatory response induced by injection of polyacrylamide gel into facial tissue. Another study analyzed the histologic and systemic effects of polyacrylamide gel injected subcutaneously in rats (43). The toxicity to the kidney was obvious. The local and histologic reaction was slight and a thin fibrous membrane formed around the implants, which gradually became stiff. The implants could not be withdrawn completely. The authors concluded that polyacrylamide gel has obvious cytotoxicity and is not a suitable material for soft tissue implantation. It should be noted that unpolymerized polymer is considered toxic to nerves and kidneys, and that different polyacrylamide gels may contain varying amounts of unpolymerized acrylic monomers.

Precursor products to Aquamid include the non FDA-approved Formacryl® and Bioformacryl®. These products anecdotally have been associated with cases of late-appearing infection, and impurities (unpolymerized acrylamide) may be toxic to nerves, kidneys and other organs. A new and molecularly very similar product, polyalkylamide (Bio-Alcamid™, Polymekon, Milan, Italy), is a non-reabsorbable acrylic acid-derived polymer with a reticulated structure characterized by alkylimide–amide groups. It is composed of 96% water and 4% synthetic polymer. Like the polyacrylamide products, advocates of Bio-Alcamid describe the product as biocompatible, nontoxic, nonallergenic, easily injectable and quickly removable. A recent study suggests that Bio-Alcamid does not interfere with morphological and functional characteristics of human skin fibroblasts (44). Another recent publication reports on the use of Bio-Alcamid in treating pectus excavatum, Poland syndrome, postoperative trauma, and facial aesthetic defects (45). Twelve of 2000 patients had postoperative *Staphyloccocus* infections. Aesthetic results were deemed excellent; tissues felt soft and the implants were uniformly distributed. No migration or dislocation of the implants, no granulomas, and no allergic responses were identified. It should be noted that long-term studies of safety and efficacy are lacking. Although Bio-Alcamid is not FDA-approved for any purpose, it has recently gained popularity among patients with HIV lipoatrophy, with large numbers of patients frequently traveling to Tijuana, Mexico where they often receive injections from a nonphysician, unlicensed practitioner who promotes the product to this population. A recent publication discusses the European experience with Bio-Alcamid for HIV-associated lipoatrophy. The report is descriptive but does not present formal objective data or long-term follow-up (46). Therefore, further well-designed, peer-reviewed studies are warranted.

REFERENCES

1. Lichentenstein KA, Ward DJ, Moorman AC, et al. Clinical assessment of HIV-associated lipodystrophy in an ambulatory population. AIDS 2001; 15:1389–1398.
2. Carr A, Samaras K, Chisholm DJ, Cooper DA. Pathogenesis of HIV-1 protease inhibitor-associated peripheral lipodystrophy, hyperlipidaemia, and insulin resistance. Lancet 1998; 351:1881–1883.
3. Zhang B, MacNaul K, Szalkowski D, Li Z, Berger J, Moller DE. Inhibition of adipocyte differentiation by HIV protease inhibitors. J Clin Endocrinol Metab 1999; 84:4274–4277.
4. Caron M, Auclair M, Kornprobst M, Capeau J. Differential in vitro effects of indinivir, nelfinavir and amprenavir on cell differentiation, insulin sensitivity and apoptosis in an adapted adipose cell model: Preventative impact of rosiglitazone [abstr]. Program and abstracts of the 3rd International Workshop on Adverse Drug Reactions and Lipodystrophy in HIV, Athens, Greece, Oct 23–26, 2001. Antiviral Therapy 2001; 6(suppl 4):14–15.
5. Caron M, Auclair M, Vigouroux C, Glorian M, Forest C, Capeau J. The HIV protease inhibitor indinavir impairs sterol regulatory element-binding protein-1 intranuclear localization, inhibits preadipocyte differentiation, and induces insulin resistance. Diabetes 2001; 50:1378–1388.
6. Mallal SA, John M, Moore CB, James IR, McKinnin EJ. Contribution of nucleoside analogue reverse transcriptase inhibitors to subcutaneous fat wasting in patients with HIV infection. AIDS 2000; 14:1309–1316.
7. Cohen C, Ryan J, Jiang P, et al. Effect of nucleoside (NRTI) intensification on prevalence of morphologic abnormalities (MOAS) at year 4 of ritonavir plus saquinavir therapy in an HIV-infected cohort [abstr]. Program and abstracts of The 1st IAS Conference on HIV Pathogenesis and Treatment, Buenos Aires, Argentina, July 8–11, 2001.
8. Brinkman K, Smeitank JA, Romijn JA, Reiss P. Mitochondrial toxicity induced by nucleoside-analog reverse-transcriptase inhibitors is a key factor in the pathogenesis of antiretroviral-therapy-related lipodystrophy. Lancet 1999; 354:1112–1115.
9. Carr A, Smith D, Workman C. Switching stavudine or zidovudine to abacavir for HIV lipoatrophy: A randomized, controlled, open-label, multicenter, 24-week study [abstr]. Program and abstracts of the 9th Conference on Retroviruses and Opportunistic Infections, Seattle, Washington, Feb 24–28, 2002.
10. Lo JC, Mulligan K, Tai VW, Algren H, Schambelan M. "Buffalo hump" in men with HIV-1 infection. Lancet 1998; 351:867–870.
11. Christeff N, Nunez EA, Gougeon ML. Changes in cortisol/DHEA ratio in HIV-infected men are related to immunological and metabolic perturbations leading to malnutrition and lipodystrophy. Ann NY Acad Sci 2000; 917:962–970.
12. Christeff N, de Truchis P, Melchior JC, Gougeon ML. Serum cortisol: DHEA is the best predictor of clinical evolution and lipid variations associated to lipodystrophy [abstr]. Program and abstracts of the 3rd International Workshop on Adverse Drug Reactions and Lipodystrophy in HIV, Athens, Greece, Oct 23–26, 2001. Antiviral Therapy 2001; 6(suppl 4):33–34.
13. Ford P, Tenzif S, Wobeser W, Ross R, Jenkins D. Dyslipidemia and body composition effects of testosterone cipionate in a group of people living in Ontario, Canada [abstr]. Program and abstracts of the 3rd International Workshop on Adverse Drug Reactions and Lipodystrophy in HIV, Athens, Greece, Oct 23–26, 2001. Antiviral Therapy 2001; 6(suppl 4):33–34.
14. O'Mahony C, Price LM, Nelson M. Lipodystrophy despite anabolic steroids. Int J STD AIDS 1998; 9:619.
15. Ledru E, Christeff N, Patey O, de Truchis P, Melchior JC, Gougeon ML. Alteration of tumor necrosis factor-alpha T-cell homeostasis following potent antiretroviral therapy:

Contribution to the development of human immunodeficiency virus-associated lipody-strophy syndrome. Blood 2000; 95:3191–3198.

16. Mynarcik DC, McNurlan MA, Steigbigel RT, Fuhrer J, Gelato MC. Association of severe insulin resistance with both loss of limb fat and elevated tumor necrosis factor receptor levels in HIV lipodystrophy. J Acquir Immune Defic Syndr 2000; 25:312–321.

17. Johnson JA, Ablu JB, He Q, Engelson ES, Kotler DP. Elevated in vitro tumor necrosis factor release from abdominal subcutaneous adipose tissue in HIV-infected subjects with lipodystrophy [abstr]. Program and abstracts of the 3rd International Workshop on Adverse Drug Reactions and Lipodystrophy in HIV, Athens, Greece, Oct 23–26, 2001. Antiviral Therapy 2001; 6(suppl 4):16–17.

18. Buss N, Duff F. Protease inhibitors in HIV infection. Lipodystrophy may be a conse-quence of prolonged survival. BMJ 1999; 318:122.

19. Collins E, Wagner C, Walmsley S. Psychosocial impact of the lipodystrophy syndrome in HIV infection. The AIDS Reader 2000; 10(9):546–551.

20. Arioglu E, Duncan-Morin J, Sebring N, et al. Efficacy and safety of troglitazone in the treatment of lipodystrophy syndromes. Ann Inter Med 2000; 133:263–274.

21. Calmy A, Hirschel B, Karsegaard L, et al. A pilot study for the use of pioglitazone in the treatment of highly active antiretroviral therapy lipodystrophy syndromes [abstr]. Pro-gram and abstracts of the 3rd International Workshop on Adverse Drug Reactions and Lipodystrophy in HIV, Athens, Greece, Oct 23–26, 2001. Antiviral Therapy 2001; 6(suppl 4):32.

22. Visnegarwala F, Maldonado MR. Use of PPAR-[gamma] modular rosiglitazone in nor-moglycemic patients with HIV lipodystrophy syndrome [abstr]. Program and abstracts of the 3rd International Workshop on Adverse Drug Reactions and Lipodystrophy in HIV, Athens, Greece, Oct 23–26, 2001. Antiviral Therapy 2001; 6(suppl 4):82.

23. Sutinen J, Hakkinen AM, Westerbacka J, et al. Rosiglitazone in the treatment of HAART associated lipodystrophy (HAL): A randomized, double-blind, placebo-con-trolled study [abstr]. Program and abstracts of the 9th Conference on Retroviruses and Opportunistic Infections, Seattle, Washington, Feb 24–28, 2002.

24. John M, James I, McKinnon E, et al. A randomized, controlled, open-label study of revi-sion of antiretroviral regimens containing stavudine (d4T) and/or a protease inhibitor (PI) to zidovudine (ZDV)/lamivudine (3TC)/abacavir(ABC) to prevent or reverse lipoa-trophy: 48-week data [abstr]. Program and abstracts of the 9th Conference on Retro-viruses and Opportunistic Infections, Seattle, Washington, Feb 24–28, 2002.

25. James J, Carruthers A, Carruthers J. HIV-associated Facial lipoatrophy. Dermatol Surg 2002; 28:979–986.

26. Abrams H. HIV Matters lipodystrophy update. Symposium sponsored by AIDS Project Los Angeles, Los Angeles Shanti, Being Alive, and the Los Angeles Gay and Lesbian Center, Los Angeles, CA, Mar 27, 2001.

27. Burres S. Preserved particulate fascia lata for injection: A new alternative. Dermatol Surg 1999; 25:790–794.

28. Hadley M, Brody H. Autologous fat grafting for lipoatrophy in the HIV patient. Annual Meeting of the American Society of Dermatologic Surgery, Dallas, TX, Oct 24–28, 2001.

29. Chastain MA, Chastain JB, Coleman WP. HIV lipodystrophy: Review of the syndrome and report of a case treated with liposuction. Dermatol Surg 2001; 27:497–500.

30. Jones D. Commentary on HIV lipodystrophy. Dermatol Surg 2001; 27:610.

31. Carr A. HIV Protease inhibitor-related lipodystrophy syndrome. Clin Infect Dis 2001; 30(suppl 2):S135–S142.

32. Glougau R. HIV associated lipodystrophy and e-PTFE implants. Annual Meeting of the American Society of Dermatologic Surgery, Denver, CO, Nov 2–5, 2000.

33. Brody H. Complications of expanded polytetrafluoroethylene (e-PTFE) facial implant. Dermatol Surg 2001; 27:792–794.

34. Jones DH, Carruthers A, Orentreich D, Brody H, Lai MY, Azen S, Van Dyke G. Highly purified 1000 centistoke oil for treatment of HIV-associated facial lipoatrophy. Dermtol Surg 2004; 30:1279–1286.

35. Orentreich D, Jones D. Liquid Injectable Silicone. In: Carruthers J, Carruthers A, ed. Soft Tissue Augmentation. New York:Elsevier, 2005:77–91.

36. Valantin MA, Aubron-Olivier C, Ghosn J, Pauchard M, Schoen H, Bousquet R, Katz P, Costagliola D, Katlama C. Polylactic acid implants (NewFill®)to correct facial lipoatrophy in HIV-infected patients: results of the open-label study VEGA. AIDS 2003; 17: 2471–2477.

37. Moyle GJ, Lysakova L, Brown S, Sibtain N, Healy J, Priest C, Mandalia S, Barton SE. A randomized open label study of immediate vs. delayed polylactic acid injections for the cosmetic management of facial lipoatrophy in persons with HIV infection. HIV Medicine 2004; (5)2:82–97.

38. Serra M. Facial implants with polymethylmethacrylate for lipodystrophy correction: 30 months follow-up. Program and abstracts of the 3rd International Workshop on Adverse Drug Reactions and Lipodystrophy in HIV, Athens, Greece, Oct 23–26, 2001. Antiviral Therapy 2001; 6(suppl 4):75.

39. Del Pino V. Successful surgical therapy with polyvinyl gel microspheres of severe facial lipoatrophy: Results after one year of follow up. Program and abstracts of the 3rd International Workshop on Adverse Drug Reactions and Lipodystrophy in HIV, Athens, Greece, Oct 23–26, 2001. Antiviral Therapy 2001; 6(suppl 4).

40. Tsao S. Injectable alloderm for augmentation of HIV-positive protease inhibitor-induced facial lipoatrophy. Presented at the ASDS-ACMMSCO Combined Annual Meeting, Chicago, IL, Oct 31–Nov 3, 2002.

41. Del Pino V. Surgical therapy with polyacrylamide gel of facial lipoatrophy. Presented at the 3rd European Workshop on Lipodystrophy and Metabolic Disorders, Marbella, Spain, April 25–27, 2002.

42. de Bree R, Middelweerd R, Van der Wall I. Severe Granulomatous inflammatory response induced by injection of polyacrylamide gel into the facial tissue. Arch Facial Plast Surg 2004; 6:204–206.

43. Huo M, Huang J, Qi K. Toxicities of polyacrylamide gel implants. Zhonghua Zheng Xing Wai Ke Za Zhi 2002; 18:79–80.

44. Pacini S, Ruggiero M, Morucci G, Cammarota N, Protopappa C, Gulisano M. Bio-alcamid, a novel prosthetic polymer, does not interfere with morphological and functional characteristics of human skin fibroblasts. Plast Reconstr Surg 2003; 111:489–491.

45. Pacini S, Ruggiero M, Morucci G, Cammarota N, Protopappa C, Gulisano M. Bio-alcamid: a novelty for reconstructive and cosmetic surgery. Ital J Anat Embryol 2002; 107:209–214.

46. Protopapa C, Giuseppe S, Caporale D, Cammarota N. Bio-Alcamid™ in drug-induced lipodystrophy. J Cosmet Laser Ther 2003; 5:226–230.

47. Binder W, Bloom DC. The use of custom-designed midfacial and submalar implants in the treatment of facial wasting syndrome. Arch Facial Plastic Surg 2004; 6:394–397.

48. Berish S, Baum T, Robbins N. Treatment of human immunodeficiency virus-associated lipodystrophy with dermafat graft transfer to the malar area. Plast Reconstr Surg 2004; 113:363–370.

49. Comite SL, Liu JF, Balasubramanian S, et al., Treatment of HIV-associated facial lipoatrophy with Radiance FN (Radiesse). Dermatol Online J (United States) 2004; 10(2):2.

50. Gooderham M, Solish N. Use of hyaluronic acid for soft tissue augmentation of HIV-associated lipoatrophy. Dermatol Surg 2005; 31(1):104–108.

18

Common Questions About Tissue Augmentation

David Charles Rish
Los Angeles Medical Center, University of California, Los Angeles, California, U.S.A.

There are several commonly asked questions regarding substances and techniques for soft tissue augmentation. In this chapter an attempt is made to anticipate these questions and to provide answers.

QUESTION 1. WHERE DO I GET THE SUBSTANCE?

Artecoll®
>   Arsis Medical BV
>   Ambachtsweg 38, NL-3606 AP Maarssen
>   The Netherlands
>   Approved in Europe, Canada, Mexico.
>   Submitted to FDA for approval, March 2002.

ArteFill®
>   Artes Medical Corp.
>   4660 La Jolla Drive, Suite 825
>   San Diego, California 92122

Bioplastique™
>   Susan Doherty
>   Corporate Office: Uroplasty, Inc.
>   2718 Summer St. NE
>   Minneapolis, MN 55413
>   Tel: 612-378-1180
>   Fax: 612-378-2027
>   International Headquarters: Uroplasty BV
>   6214 Maastricht
>   The Netherlands
>   Tel: 011-31-043-26-0700
>   Fax: 011-31-043-26-1133
>   Note: Bioplastique is not yet available in the United States.

BOTOX® and BOTOX® Cosmetic
   Allergan
   Irvine, California
   Tel: 714-246-4599
   www.allergan.com

Restylane™, Restylane Touch™, and Perlane
   Q-Med
   Seminariegatan 21
   SA 75228, Uppsala, Sweden
   Tel: 011-46-18-504-210
   Fax: 011-46-18-503-145
   E-mail: info@q-med.se
   Distribution in the United States:
   Corporate Headquarters
   Medicis Aesthetics, Inc.
   8125 North Hayden Road
   Scottsdale, Arizona 85258-2463

Alloderm®
   Life Cell Corporation
   3606 Research Forest Drive
   The Woodlands, Texas 77381
   Tel: 800-367-5737
   Fax: 713-363-3360
   Kathleen Dennis
      Marketing Representative
      Life Cell Corporation
      3849 Pacific Avenue
      Long Beach, CA 90807
      Tel: 800-819-5202

Resoplast™
   Rofil Medical International BV
   Chasseveld 3a
   4811 DH Bredia, The Netherlands
   Tel: 31-76-520-9537
   Fax: 31-76-520-9276

Koken Atelcollagen
   Koken Co., KTD
   3-14-3, EJIRO, TOSHIMA-KU
   Tokyo 171, Japan
   Tel: 81-3-3950-6600
   Fax: 81-3-3950-6602

Recollagenation
   Steven Burnes, MD
   100 UCLA Medical Plaza, Suite 522
   Los Angeles, California 90024

Zyderm®, Zyplast®, Zyderm® II
Inamed Aesthetics
71 South Carneros Road
Goleta, California 93117
Tel: (800) 624-4261
www.inamed.com

Myobloc™
Solstice Neurosciences, LLC

Hylaform®
Inamed Aesthetics
71 South Carneros Road
Goleta, California 93117
Tel: (800) 624-4261
www.inamed.com

Isolagen™
US Corporate Headquarters:
Belinda Long, Customer Relations
Isolagen, Inc.
2500 Wilcrest, 5th Floor
Houston, Texas 77042
Phone: 713-780-4754
Fax: 713-781-9396
E-mail: info@isolagen.com

Cosmoderm®, Cosmoplast®
Inamed Aesthetics
71 South Carneros Road
Goleta, California 93117
Tel: (800) 624-4261
www.inamed.com

QUESTION 2. WHERE DO I OBTAIN THE NECESSARY SURGICAL EQUIPMENT?

The surgical equipment used in these various procedures can be obtained from most medical/surgical equipment companies. There are many companies that rent, lease, and sell lasers equipment.

QUESTION 3. HOW DO I LEARN THE PROPER TECHNIQUES FOR USING THE SUBSTANCE?

Learning the proper techniques requires a combination of reviewing written information, spending time visiting and observing at trained physicians' offices, and taking courses and training sessions at meetings and at symposiums. The following approaches are suggested:

Artecoll: Visits with foreign physicians who utilize this substance.
Zyderm: Videos, and seminars, and in-office observation.
BOTOX: Workshop courses on filling substances and in-office observation.
Laser: Various laser companies offer training courses and laser meetings offer hands-on courses.
Subcision: Articles have been written describing this technique; in-office observation is recommended.
Restylane: Videos, seminars, and in-office observation.
Dermal grafting: Dr. Swinehart's video and visit to his office.
Artecoll: Visits with foreign physicians who utilize this substance.
Hylaform: Workshop courses on filling substances, in-office observation.

QUESTION 4. WHAT ARE THE BEST INDICATIONS ACCORDING TO AUTHORS?

See Table 1.

QUESTION 5. WHAT ARE THE COMPLICATIONS REPORTED BY AUTHORS?

See Table 2.

QUESTION 6. WHAT SERIOUS COMPLICATIONS HAVE BEEN SEEN?

Any invasive procedure may have serious complications. Fortunately these complications are rare. Injections used for soft tissue augmentation have, rarely, caused vascular occlusion leading to blindness. Scarring and abscess formation have rarely been reported. Resurfacing with lasers and peels has caused serious scarring and pigmentation problems. Hemorrhage and excess volume reduction with liposuction procedures have caused death. These serious complications are rare and usually avoided by proper training and good medical judgment.

QUESTION 7. HOW CAN ONE BEST AVOID COMPLICATIONS?

Most surgical complications can be avoided by good planning and good surgical techniques. Taking a complete medical and drug history is important.

Table 1
What to Use

	Lip Augmentation	Nasolabial Fold	Depressed Scar	Contour Defect	Revision Mentoplasm	Acne Scars	Glabella	Perioral	Corners of the Mouth/Marionette Lines	Crow's Feet	Forehead Lines	Necklines	Chin Lines	Superior Horizontal Nasal Furrows	Sun-Damaged Skin	Back of Hands	Liposuction Depression	Chicken pox scars	Lipoatrophy	Wrinkle Depression Lines
Alloderm	X	X	X	X	X															
Artecoll	X	X				X	X	X	X									X		
Autologen		X				X	X		X					X						
Bioplastique																				
Botox							X			X	X	X								
Cosmoderm	X	X																		
Derma Graft		X				X	X	X										X	X	
Fibrel			X			X		X												
Hylaform	X	X				X	X	X												
Koken																				
Laser						X		X		X					X					
Lipocytic Dermal Augmentation		X	X											X						
Microlipoinjection		X													X	X				
Perlane/Restylane	X	X				X	X	X	X	X	X	X								
Recollagenation						X														
Resoplast																				
Subcision						X											X		X	
Zyderm	X	X				X	X	X	X											

Table 2
Complications

	Persistent ecchymosis, bruising	Discoloration	Extrusion	Elevation	Redness	Swelling	Cyst formation	Pain and itching	Herpes outbreak	Palpable implant	Uneven distribution	Sensitive to pressure	Persistent redness	Visible implant	Overcorrection	Acne flare	Ptosis	Infection	Undercorrection	Contact Dermatitis	Hyperpigmentation	Hypopigmentation	Scar	Seroma	Hypertrophic scar	Acute allergy reaction	Blindness (very rare)	Cyst/abcess	Tissue necrosis	Hypersensivity response	Angioedema	Prolonged nodulation and induration
Alloderm						X		X	X				X				X															
Artecoll					X	X		X	X	X	X	X	X												X	X	X					
Autologen	X		X					X		X			X							X												
Botox	X							X							X																	
Cosmoderm	X																															
Derma Graft					X		X												X													
Fibrel	X				X			X						X														X	X			X
Hylaform	X				X	X		X					X	X	X	X																
Koken	X				X									X	X												X	X	X	X	X	
Laser					X														X	X	X	X	X									
Lipocytic Dermal Augmentation	X															X			X													
Microlipoinjection	X																															
Perlane / Restylane	X			X	X	X		X		X																				X		
Recollagenation	X	X	X	X																			X					X	X	X	X	
Resoplast	X				X																							X	X	X	X	
Subcision	X	X			X	X									X						X											
Zyderm	X				X								X	X														X	X	X	X	X

Most infections can be avoided with sterile technique and, when appropriate, systemic and/or topical antibiotics. Herpes simplex infections can be avoided by taking a history and using prophylactic Zovirax® (acyclovir), Famvir®, or Valtrex®.

Bleeding and bruising can be diminished by taking a good history and confirming that the patient has not taken anticoagulants, aspirin or other Nsaids, or other drugs that promote easy bruising. Pregnant patients may bruise more easily. Good techniques are helpful and posttreatment application of icepacks is beneficial in preventing bruising. Pressure after surgical procedures may help avoid bruising.

Scarring with lasers may be minimized with shorter pulse duration, use of less energy to minimize thermal damage, and fewer passes.

Vascular occlusion with injected augmentation substances may be avoided by more superficial techniques. Most allergic reactions to Zyderm can be avoided by double testing and retesting if more than a year has elapsed since the last injection.

Intramuscular glucocorticoids have been used with some augmentation and resurfacing procedures to help avoid postprocedure swelling.

Index

Ablative resurfacing, 253
Accessory cell, 210
AcHyal, 328
Acids, natural commonly used, 242
Actinic purpura, 244
AdatoSil 5000^{TM}, 153
Adhesion molecules, 187, 210
Adjuvants, 177, 205
Adulterants
  role of, 155, 163, 165, 178
Aesthetics facial, 292
Aging of the face
  expression, 240
  gravity factor, 240
  intrinsic aging, 240
  photoaging, 240, 247, 257
  sleep lines, 240
Allelic, gene alternative, 211
Alligator forceps, 57, 318
AlloDerm®, 56, 318, 364
AlloDerm® graft hydrated, 328
  acne scars, 319
  facial-contour defect correction, 319
  nasolabial folds, 319
  implants, 323, 354
  preparation, 318
  transplant, 315
Allogenic filler material, 315, 316, 324
  AlloDerm®, 316
  Cymetra^{TM}, 316, 320, 352
Allografts
  dura mater, 60
  human dermis, 56
  human fascia lata, 58, 59

[Allografts]
  human placental collagen, 59
  human-cultured skin derived from
    neonatal foreskin, 59
  recombinant human collagen, 60
Alpha hydroxy acids, 240, 242, 252
American Association of Tissue Bank
  (AATB), 56
Ames test, 299
Anchor point, 260
Anesthetics
  EMLA®-cream, 272
  ice–saline–xylocaine, 25
  tumescent solution, 10
Antigens, 166, 181, 211
Antigen-presenting cells (APC), 211
Antimitotic agents, 287
Aquamid®, 328
Argiform^{TM}, 330
Argyform^{TM}, 330
Artecoll®, 363
  advantages of, 268
  aesthetic indications, 270
  anaphylactic shock, 284
  biocompatibility of, 269
  boxcar scars, 281
  composition, 267
  granuloma, 286
  hypertrophic scarring, 285
  ice-pick scars, 22, 281, 319
  implantation, 270, 273
  side effects of, 283
  telangiectasia, 67, 285
ArteFill®, 267, 330